M000272828

Atlas of
INFECTIOUS DISEASES

Volume V

SEXUALLY TRANSMITTED DISEASES

Atlas of
INFECTIOUS DISEASES

Volume V

SEXUALLY TRANSMITTED DISEASES

Editor-in-Chief

Gerald L. Mandell, MD

Professor of Medicine
Owen R. Cheatham Professor of the Sciences
Chief, Division of Infectious Diseases
University of Virginia Health Sciences Center
Charlottesville, Virginia

Editor

Michael F. Rein, MD

Professor of Internal Medicine
Division of Infectious Diseases
University of Virginia Health Sciences Center
Charlottesville, Virginia

With 22 contributors

**Churchill
Livingstone**

DEVELOPED BY CURRENT MEDICINE, INC.
PHILADELPHIA

CURRENT MEDICINE
400 MARKET STREET, SUITE 700
PHILADELPHIA, PA 19106

Library of Congress Cataloging-in-Publication Data

Sexually transmitted diseases / editor-in-chief, Gerald L. Mandell; editor, Michael F. Rein ; developed by Current Medicine, Inc.
      p. cm. – (Atlas of infectious diseases ; v. 5)
  Includes bibliographical references and index.
  ISBN 0-443-07720-7 (hardcover)
  1. Sexually transmitted diseases–Atlases. I. Mandell, Gerald L.
II. Rein, Michael F. III. Current Medicine, Inc. IV. Series.
    [DNLM: 1. Sexually Transmitted Diseases–atlases. WC 17 S518
1996]
RC200.1.S477 1996
616.95' 1–dc20
DNLM/DLC
for Library of Congress   95-32207
                                                  CIP

Development Editors:	**Lee Tevebaugh and Michael Bokulich**
Editorial Assistant:	**Jabin White**
Art Director:	**Paul Fennessy**
Design and Layout:	**Patrick Whelan and Patrick Ward**
Illustration Director:	**Ann Saydlowski**
Illustrators:	**Elizabeth Carrozza, Sue Anne Fung-Ho, Beth Starkey, Lisa Weischedel, Wieslawa Langenfeld, and Gary Welch**
Production:	**David Myers and Lori Holland**
Typesetting Director:	**Colleen Ward**
Indexer:	**Elinor Lindheimer**
Managing Editor:	**Lori J. Bainbridge**

Printed in Hong Kong by Paramount Printing Group Limited.

10 9 8 7 6 5 4 3 2 1

PREFACE

The diagnosis and management of patients with infectious diseases are based in large part on visual clues. Skin and mucous membrane lesions, eye findings, imaging studies, Gram stains, culture plates, insect vectors, preparations of blood, urine, pus cerebrospinal fluid, and biopsy specimens are studied to establish the proper diagnosis and to choose the most effective therapy. The *Atlas of Infectious Diseases* will be a modern, complete collection of these images. Current Medicine, with its capability of superb color reproduction and its state-of-the-art computer imaging facilities, is the ideal publisher for the atlas.

Infectious diseases physicians, scientists, microbiologists, and pathologists frequently teach other health-care professionals, and this comprehensive atlas with available slides is an effective teaching tool.

Dr. Michael F. Rein has a long and distinguished career in the field of sexually transmitted diseases. This experience has enabled him to assemble an outstanding group of experts who have prepared superb chapters. The images are instructive and comprehensive. This volume will be a valuable resource for clinicians caring for patients and for teachers of the discipline of sexually transmitted diseases.

Gerald L. Mandell, MD
Professor of Medicine
Owen R. Cheatham Professor of the Sciences
Chief, Division of Infectious Diseases
University of Virginia Health Sciences Center
Charlottesville, Virginia

CONTRIBUTORS

Lawrence Corey, MD
Professor of Laboratory Medicine
Division of Virology
University of Washington School of Medicine
Seattle, Washington

Nicholas J. Fiumara, MD, MPH
Clinical Professor of Dermatology
Tufts University School of Medicine
Clinical Professor Emeritus
Boston University School of Medicine
Boston, Massachusetts

Laura T. Gutman, MD
Associate Professor
Departments of Pediatrics and Pharmacology
Duke University Medical Center
Durham, North Carolina

Gavin Hart, MD, MPH
Director, Sexually Transmitted Diseases Control Branch
South Australian Health Commission
Adelaide, South Australia

Sharon L. Hillier, PhD
Associate Professor of Obstetrics, Gynecology, and
  Reproductive Sciences
University of Pittsburgh School of Medicine
Director, Reproductive Infectious Disease Research
Magee-Womens Research Institute
Pittsburgh, Pennsylvania

Robert B. Jones, MD, PhD
Chief, Division of Infectious Diseases
Professor of Medicine, Microbiology, and Immunology
Indiana University School of Medicine
Indianapolis, Indiana

Franklyn N. Judson, MD
Director, Denver Public Health
Professor, Departments of Medicine and Preventive
  Medicine
University of Colorado Health Sciences Center
Denver, Colorado

John N. Krieger, MD
Professor of Urology
University of Washington School of Medicine
Seattle, Washington

Sandra A. Larsen, PhD
Chief, Treponemal Pathogenesis and Immunology Branch
Division of Sexually Transmitted Diseases Laboratory
  Research
Centers for Disease Control and Prevention
Atlanta, Georgia

Per-Anders Mårdh, MD, PhD
Professor of Medicine
University of Uppsala
Uppsala, Sweden

William M. McCormack, MD
Professor of Medicine and of Obstetrics and Gynecology
Chief, Infectious Diseases Division
State University of New York Health Sciences Center
Brooklyn, New York

Birger Möller, MD
Department of Obstetrics and Gynecology
University of Odense
Odense, Norway

Daniel M. Musher, MD
Chief, Infectious Diseases Section
Professor of Medicine
Veterans Administration Hospital
Houston, Texas

Jorma Paavonen, MD
Department of Obstetrics and Gynecology
University of Helsinki
Helsinki, Finland

Richard Reid, MD
Assistant Professor
Department of Obstetrics and Gynecology
Wayne State University School of Medicine
Detroit, Michigan
Director, Gynecologic Endoscopy
Crittenton Hospital
Rochester, Michigan

Michael F. Rein, MD
Professor of Internal Medicine
Division of Infectious Diseases
University of Virginia Health Sciences Center
Charlottesville, Virginia

Allan Ronald, MD, FRCPC, FACP
Professor of Medicine and Medical Microbiology
Associate Dean of Research
University of Manitoba
Winnipeg, Manitoba
Canada

Navjeet K. Sidhu-Malik, MD
Assistant Professor of Dermatology
University of Virginia Health Sciences Center
Charlottesville, Virginia

Jack D. Sobel, MD
Professor of Medicine
Chief, Division of Infectious Diseases
Wayne State University School of Medicine
Detroit Medical Center
Detroit, Michigan

Lars Weström, MD
Department of Obstetrics and Gynecology
University of Lund
Lund, Sweden

Barbara B. Wilson, MD
Associate Professor of Dermatology
University of Virginia Health Sciences Center
Charlottesville, Virginia

Jonathan M. Zenilman, MD
Associate Professor
Johns Hopkins University School of Medicine
Chief, Sexually Transmitted Diseases Services
Baltimore City Health Department
Baltimore, Maryland

CONTENTS

CHAPTER 1

Gonorrhea

Jonathan M. Zenilman

EPIDEMIOLOGY

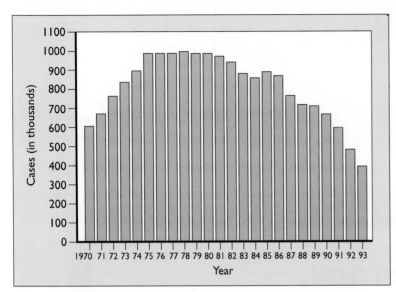

FIGURE 1-1 Reported cases of gonorrhea in the United States between 1970 and 1993. Gonorrhea is the most common reportable infectious disease in the United States, with over 500,000 cases reported annually and an estimated 1 to 1.5 million unreported cases. The overall incidence of gonorrhea has been declining since 1975, due to two major factors. First, as the baby boom generation aged, the number of individuals at highest risk for sexually transmitted diseases (ages 15 to 34) peaked in 1975. Also, the national gonorrhea screening program, instituted by the Centers for Disease Control and Prevention in 1972, contributed to this decline. (*Adapted from* Centers for Disease Control and Prevention: Surveillance for sexually transmitted diseases. *MMWR* 1993, 4(SS-3):1–13; with permission.)

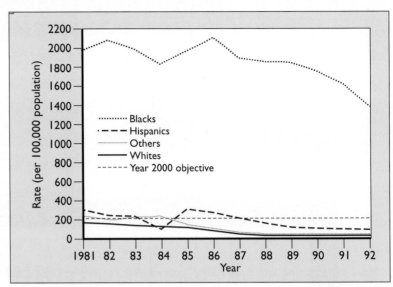

FIGURE 1-2 Incidence of gonorrhea by ethnic and racial group in the United States between 1981 and 1992. With the decline in overall incidence, gonorrhea increasingly has become a disease concentrated in minorities. However, some of the disparity may be explained by reporting bias. (*Adapted from* Centers for Disease Control and Prevention: Surveillance for sexually transmitted diseases. *MMWR* 1993, 42(SS-3):1–13.)

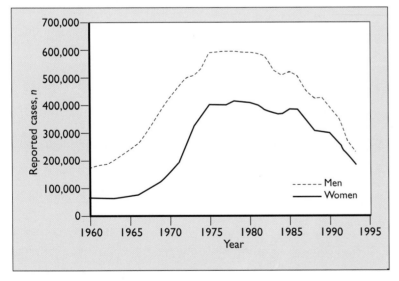

FIGURE 1-3 Incidence of gonorrhea by gender in the United States between 1960 and 1993. The incidence of gonorrhea peaked in the United States in the mid-1970s and has decreased to 430,000 cases (total) in 1993. The decrease has been attributed to increased screening and intervention. An alternative hypothesis is that due to demographic shifts in the US population as the generation of "baby boomers" aged, the number of "persons at risk" decreased. (*Adapted from* Centers for Disease Control and Prevention: Summary of notifiable diseases, 1993. *MMWR* 1993, 42(53):28; with permission.)

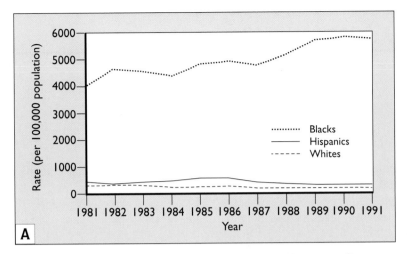

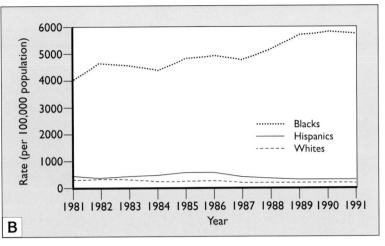

Figure 1-4 Incidence of gonorrhea among adolescents. Gonorrhea is a disease primarily of adolescent young adults, with over 90% of cases reported from individuals aged 15 to 34 years. Despite the overall decline in incidence of gonorrhea since 1975, the rate among US adolescents, and especially among minority adolescents, has not decreased over the same period. Gonorrhea disproportionately affects men and women within the reproductive age groups, with the highest rates seen among 15- to 19-year-olds. **A,** Rates of gonorrhea among 15- to 19-year-old men, by ethnic group, between 1981 and 1991. **B,** Rates of gonorrhea among 15- to 19-year-old women, by ethnic group, between 1981 and 1991. (*Adapted from* Webster LA, Berman SM, Greenspan JR: Surveillance for gonorrhea and primary and secondary syphilis among adolescents, United States, 1981–1991. *MMWR* 1993, 42(SS-3):1–13; with permission.)

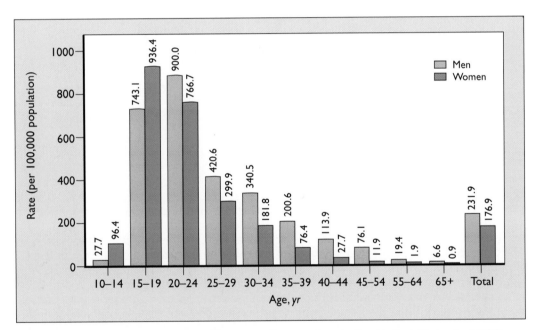

Figure 1-5 Age- and gender-specific rates of gonorrhea in the United States in 1992. The incidence of gonorrhea is highest in adolescents and young adults aged 15 to 34 years. Epidemiologists have suggested that incidence rates should be calculated using the number of persons aged 15 to 34 years as the denominator, which would encompass > 90% of gonorrhea cases.

PATHOGENESIS AND TRANSMISSION

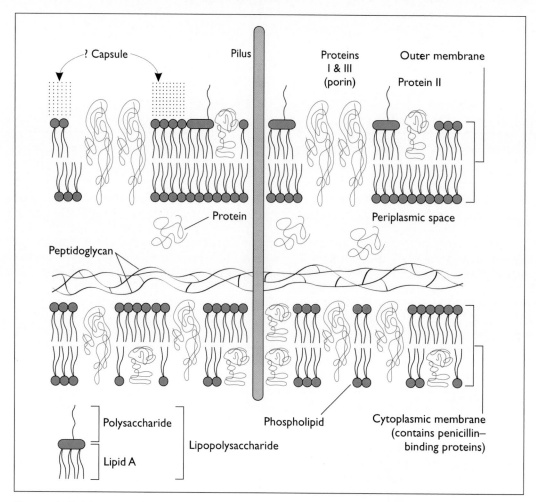

FIGURE 1-6 Diagram of cell wall of *Neisseria gonorrhoeae*. The cell wall of *N. gonorrhoeae* is a trilaminar structure consisting of the outer membrane, peptidoglycan, and inner cytoplasmic membrane. The pathogenicity of the organism is largely due to structures in the outer membrane. This membrane consists of a lipopolysaccharide capsule and various proteins and is similar to outer membrane structures seen in other gram-negative bacteria. The periplasmic space is immediately beneath the outer membrane and is adjacent to the peptidoglycan, which forms the major cell wall constituent. Inhibition of peptidoglycan synthesis is the mechanism of action for the penicillins and cephalosporins. There is an inner cytoplasmic membrane that contains penicillin-binding proteins. Traversing the entire membrane are pili, which are filamentous projections responsible for mucosal adhesion. In addition, the other outer membrane proteins of *N. gonorrhoeae* also function as porins, or hydrophilic channels, which in turn trigger host cell endocytosis of the organism, an important step in early inflammation. The outer membrane proteins have enormous genetic and antigenic variability. Therefore, repeated gonococcal infections are common, and efforts to prepare mucosal-based vaccines have been unsuccessful to date. (*Adapted from* Tramont EC, Boslego JW: *Neisseria gonorrhoeae. In* Gorbach SL, Bartlett JG, Blacklow NR (eds.): *Infectious Diseases*. Philadelphia: W.B. Saunders; 1992:1443–1445; with permission.)

Virulence factors of *Neisseria gonorrhoeae*

Pili
Lipo-oligosaccharide
Opacity proteins
Adhesions
Iron-repressible proteins
IgA protease
"Blocking" antibiotics

FIGURE 1-7 Virulence factors of *Neisseria gonorrhoeae*. In contrast to the commensal *Neisseria*, which are widely prevalent, gonococci have a number of virulence factors that make this organism pathogenic. These factors include adhesion mediators, mediations of inflammation, and mediators of mucosal invasiveness.

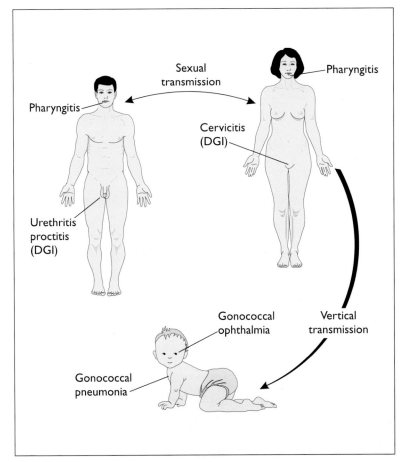

FIGURE 1-8 Common modes of gonorrhea transmission. Transmission of gonococcal disease occurs almost exclusively by sexual contact. Transmission via inanimate objects is extremely uncommon. The only major exception to sexual transmission is vertical (mother-to-infant) transmission during parturition. (DGI—disseminated gonococcal infection.)

Risk factors for gonococcal infection

Adolescence
Multiple sexual partners
Nonbarrier contraception
Low socioeconomic status
Concomitant use of intravenous drugs or crack cocaine
Previous history of gonorrhea

FIGURE 1-9 Risk factors for gonococcal infection. Epidemiologists have associated gonococcal infection with a number of behavioral and social risk factors. In large part, these factors are related to socioeconomic status and access to health care.

CLINICAL SYNDROMES

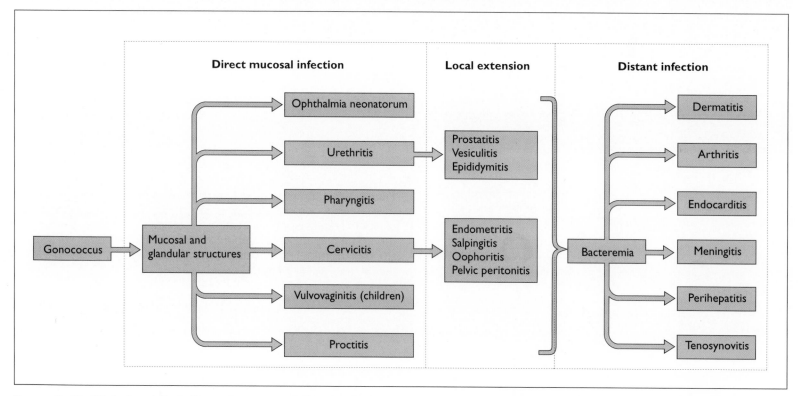

FIGURE 1-10 Clinical manifestations of gonococcal disease. Gonorrhea is usually manifest as a mucosal disease, although a minority of patients develop disseminated gonococcal infection. Mortality is extremely low, but the morbidity of and cost for treating gonococcal complications, especially pelvic inflammatory disease, are substantial. Additionally, gonococcal infections have been shown to facilitate transmission of HIV. (*Adapted from* Washington JA II: Medical bacteriology. *In* Henry JB (ed.): *Clinical Diagnosis and Management by Laboratory Methods*, 17th ed. Philadelphia: W.B. Saunders; 1984:1089; with permission.)

Clinical Manifestations in Men

Common signs and symptoms of gonorrhea in men		
	Symptoms	**Signs**
Urethritis	Dysuria	Discharge
	Discharge	Lymphadenopathy
	Testicular pain	
Proctitis	Tenesmus	Discharge
	Constipation	Friable mucosa
	Discharge	

FIGURE 1-11 Common signs and symptoms of gonorrhea in men. Gonococcal urethritis is the most common syndrome seen in men. Symptoms include urethral discharge and dysuria and typically begin 2 to 5 days after sexual exposure. On physical examination, a urethral discharge, which is usually purulent, is seen. Approximately 5% to 10% of men are asymptomatic. The complications of gonococcal urethritis include gonococcal tysonitis (inflammation of the periurethral glands) and gonococcal pyoderma. The major differential diagnosis of gonococcal urethritis is nongonococcal urethritis.

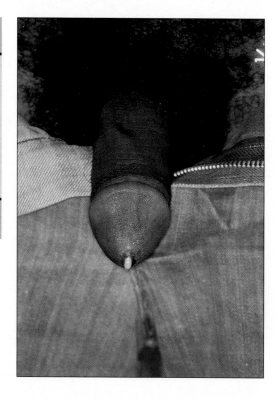

FIGURE 1-12 Gonococcal urethritis with urethral discharge. On physical examination, a urethral discharge, which is usually purulent, is seen in 90% to 95% of men. The purulent discharge may appear spontaneously at the urethra, without urethral manipulation (stripping). Such appearance of discharge prior to stripping is more common in gonococcal than in nongonococcal urethritis. (*Courtesy of* M.F. Rein, MD.)

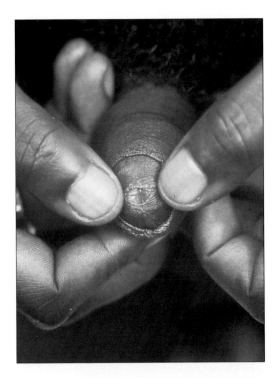

FIGURE 1-13 Inspection of urethra for discharge. Gonococcal urethritis manifests visible inflammation of the urethra proximal to the meatus. This observation may be particularly useful in patients who have recently urinated, thereby washing away discharge.

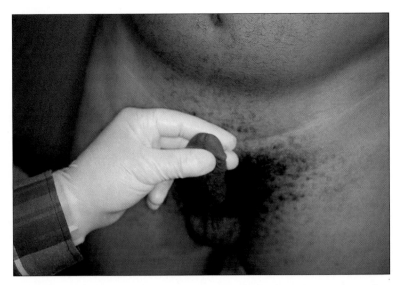

FIGURE 1-14 Urethral stripping to elicit discharge. Approximately 5% to 10% of men with gonorrhea are asymptomatic, and about half of asymptomatic infections may be identified clinically by urethral stripping during the physical examination. After stripping the urethra, smaller amounts of discharge may be visualized.

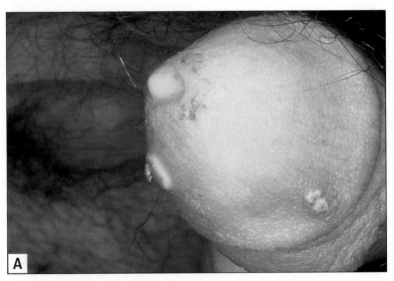

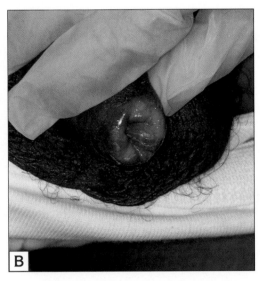

FIGURE 1-15 Pyoderma. Pyoderma is a well-recognized complication of gonococcal urethritis and is seen more frequently in cases in which treatment was delayed and in uncircumcised men. **A,** Gonococcal urethritis with pyoderma. **B,** Gonococcal urethritis causing ulcerative pyoderma of the prepuce. (Panel 15B *courtesy of* M.F. Rein, MD.)

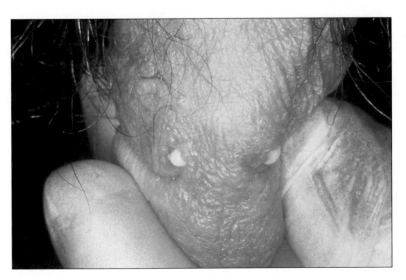

FIGURE 1-16 Gonococcal tysonitis. Gonococcal tysonitis, inflammation of the periurethral Tyson's glands (glandulae preputiales), results in a purulent discharge from the glands. These glands normally secrete a sebaceous material that contributes to smegma. (*Courtesy of* the Centers for Disease Control and Prevention.)

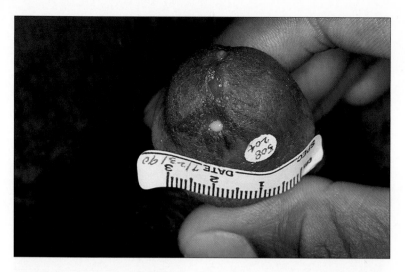

FIGURE 1-17 Gonococcal urethritis in a patient with hypospadias. Hypospadias is the most common congenital abnormality of the lower genitourinary tract. This case demonstrates that susceptibility to gonococcal infection occurs in areas where there is columnar epithelium.

Clinical Manifestations in Women

Common signs and symptoms of gonorrhea in women		
	Symptoms	**Signs**
Genital infection	Vaginal discharge	Mucopurulent cervical
	Lower abdominal	discharge
	pain	Cervical friability
	Dysuria	Cervical edema
	Dyspareunia	Cervical erythema
	Increased menstrual	
	flow	

FIGURE 1-18 Common signs and symptoms of gonorrhea in women. In women, cervicitis is the most common syndrome. Symptoms of gonococcal cervicitis include increased cervical discharge, lower abdominal pain, cervical-vaginal tenderness, dysuria, and dyspareunia. Dyspareunia and abdominal pain may be symptoms of early pelvic inflammatory disease. Approximately 50% of women with gonococcal cervicitis are asymptomatic. When symptoms do occur, they are usually more pronounced during the menses.

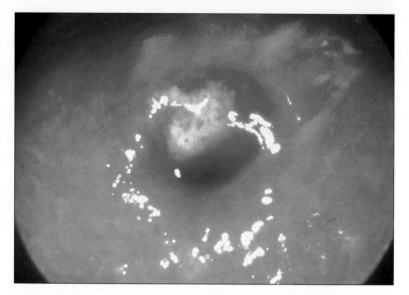

FIGURE 1-19 Mucopurulent gonococcal cervicitis. On physical examination, the typical appearance of gonococcal infection in women includes cervical edema, erythema, and mucopurulent discharge, yielding mucopurulent cervicitis. The differential diagnosis of mucopurulent cervicitis includes gonococcal cervicitis, chlamydial cervicitis, herpetic cervicitis, chronic dysplastic changes due to human papillomavirus disease, and cervical inflammation due to chronic vaginitis.

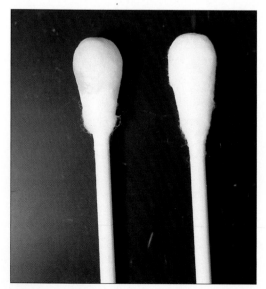

FIGURE 1-20 Swab test for mucopurulent cervicitis. Mucopurulent cervicitis can be diagnosed clinically by the swab test. A swab is inserted into the endocervix and then examined in good light. In a normal examination, it should remain white or be covered with clear cervical mucus (*right panel*). In the setting of mucopurulent cervicitis, purulent cervical discharge imparts a yellow color to the swab (*left panel*). Fifty percent to 60% of women with gonococcal cervicitis also have positive urethral cultures for *Neisseria gonorrhoeae*. More of these women have urethral symptoms, the most pronounced being dysuria. Gonococcal urethritis is occasionally seen as part of the dysuria-pyuria syndrome. On physical examination, urethral discharge is occasionally visible.

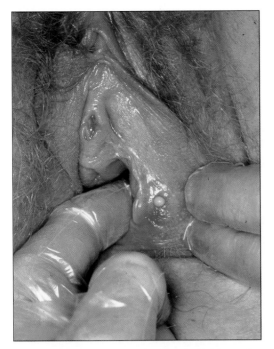

FIGURE 1-21 Bartholinitis. Bartholinitis and inflammation of the labial glandular structures are occasionally seen in women with gonococcal infection. These conditions manifest as acute painful swelling of the labial folds, and often, a discrete mass can be visualized on physical examination. In bartholinitis, purulent discharge can be expressed from the duct by applying pressure to the gland. The swollen gland itself is visible in this slide, but normally Bartholin's glands are neither palpable nor visible.

Microorganisms associated with bartholinitis

Neisseria gonorrhoeae
Anaerobes
Chlamydia trachomatis
Ureaplasma urealyticum
Escherichia coli
Proteus mirabilis
Streptococcus spp
Herpes simplex virus
Staphylococcus aureus (rarely)
Haemophilus influenzae (rarely)

FIGURE 1-22 Other nonsexually transmitted disease microorganisms are occasionally associated with bartholinitis.

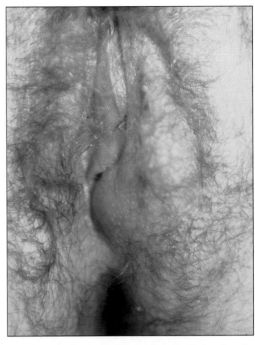

FIGURE 1-23 Gonococcal Bartholin's gland abscess. The left Bartholin's gland is visibly enlarged in this patient. Although gonococcal bartholinitis usually can be treated with standard regimens for anogenital gonococcal infections, some workers have recommended extending the regimen to 3 days. Failure to respond to antimicrobial treatment alone necessitates surgical drainage.

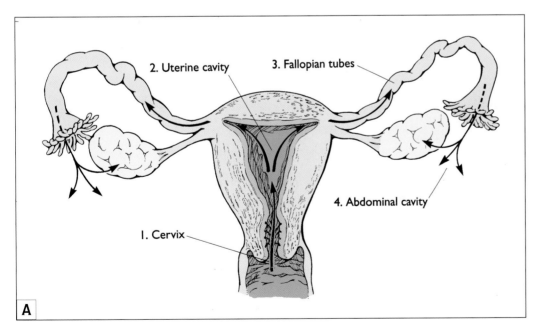

A

FIGURE 1-24 Pelvic inflammatory disease. Pelvic inflammatory disease (PID) occurs in approximately 30% of women who have untreated gonococcal infection. PID is seen more commonly during the menstrual period, in women who douche, and in women who have had a previous episode of PID. Its complications are infertility (approximately 10% incidence for each episode of PID) and an increased incidence of ectopic pregnancy. Clinically, PID presents as lower abdominal pain, adnexal tenderness, and cervical tenderness. **A,** Sequence of extension in PID. Pathologically, PID includes inflammation of any or all of the upper genital tract structures, producing endometritis, salpingitis, pelvic peritonitis, or tubo-ovarian abscess. (*continued*)

B. Clinical features of pelvic inflammatory disease

Peritonitis
  Nausea, emesis, abdominal distention, rigidity, tenderness
  Pelvic or abdominal cavity abscess may form
Endocervicitis
  May be asymptomatic
  Vaginal discharge, cervical inflammation or infection, local
    tenderness
Endosalpingitis
  Constant bilateral lower quadrant pain aggravated by body
    motion
  Tenderness in one or both adnexal areas
  Abscess may form
Endometritis
  Menstrual irregularity

FIGURE 1-24 (*continued*) **B,** Clinical features of PID. (Panel 24A *courtesy of* M.F. Rein, MD.)

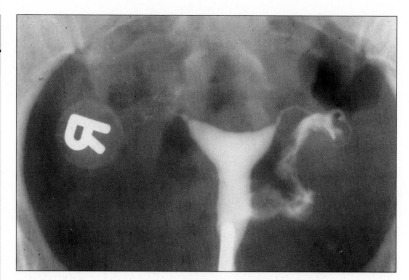

FIGURE 1-25 Radiographic view of pelvic inflammatory disease. A hysterosalpingogram, produced by instilling radiopaque dye into the uterine cavity, is performed as part of a workup for involuntary infertility. In this patient, the dye outlines the uterine cavity and reveals the lumen of the fallopian tube on the left; dye then spills into the peritoneal cavity. On the right, there is complete obstruction of the fallopian tube secondary to salpingitis. (*Courtesy of* the Centers for Disease Control and Prevention.)

FIGURE 1-26 Gonococcal ophthalmia neonatorum. Ophthalmia neonatorum is a purulent conjunctivitis caused by inoculation of gonococci during vaginal delivery through an infected birth canal. The incubation period is usually about 3 days but may be prolonged if an ineffective conjunctival prophylaxis has been used. The condition is largely preventable with the use of antimicrobial eye drops instilled at birth. It is usually bilateral. (*Courtesy of* the Centers for Disease Control and Prevention.)

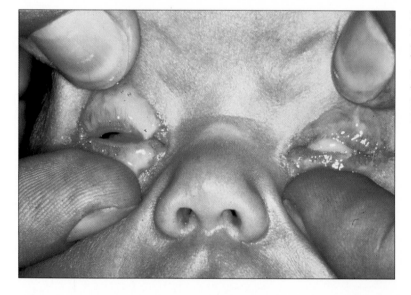

Extragenital and Disseminated Gonococcal Infection

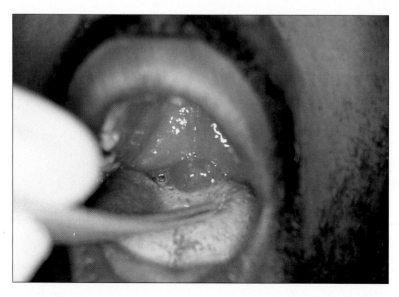

FIGURE 1-27 Gonococcal pharyngitis. Gonococcal pharyngitis is seen in both men and women who have had oral sexual exposure. Gonococcal pharyngitis is symptomatic in approximately 50% of cases only and is impossible to differentiate clinically from bacterial pharyngitis due to other causes, such as group A streptococci, or viral pharyngitis. Left untreated, gonococcal pharyngitis spontaneously resolves within 6 weeks. Diagnostic tests for gonococcal pharyngitis should include a bacterial culture on selective media. (*Courtesy of* E. Sawada, MD.)

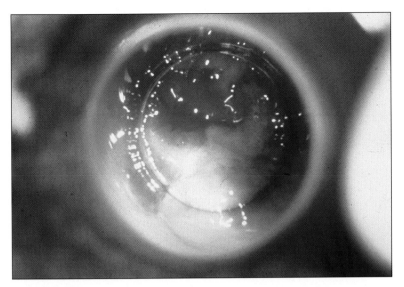

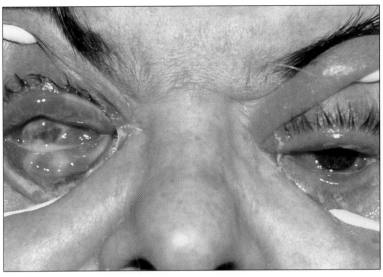

FIGURE 1-28 Gonococcal proctitis. Gonococcal proctitis is seen in two settings. In homosexual men or heterosexual women who practice receptive anal intercourse, gonococcal proctitis is accompanied by inflammation, which includes symptoms of rectal discharge, tenesmus, and constipation. Upon anoscopy, rectal discharge is commonly seen, as well as purulent inflammation of the mucosal surfaces. In these settings, symptoms are present in only 50% of cases; therefore, it is imperative that individuals who have had receptive anal intercourse have routine cultures for gonococcal disease as part of an evaluation for sexually transmitted diseases. In heterosexual women, asymptomatic gonococcal rectal infection is seen in 10% to 15% of women with cervical infection, usually without gross evidence of mucosal inflammation. These infections are thought to occur secondary to tracking of infected secretions across the perineal surface from a primary genital site.

FIGURE 1-29 Gonococcal conjunctivitis in an adult. Gonococcal ophthalmia is an uncommon but devastating complication of gonococcal disease. In the developing world, gonococcal ophthalmia is still a major cause of blindness. Despite the institution of gonococcal screening programs and neonatal prophylaxis, gonococcal ophthalmia is still occasionally seen in developed countries. Adult cases are usually due to self-inoculation or unusual sexual practices. Gonococcal ophthalmia initially presents as an acute purulent conjunctivitis.

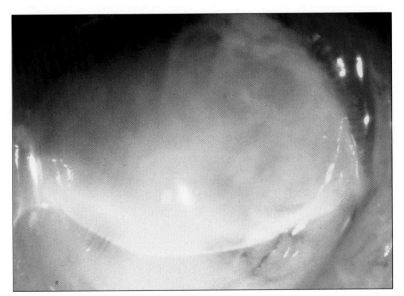

FIGURE 1-30 Gonococcal ophthalmia with corneal opacification. Left untreated, gonococcal ophthalmia can rapidly progress to inflammation of other anatomical structures within the eye, especially the cornea (keratitis). Progression can be extremely rapid, within 24 hours; therefore, rapid diagnostic and therapeutic intervention with systemic antibiotics is critical. (*Courtesy of* S. Ullman, MD.)

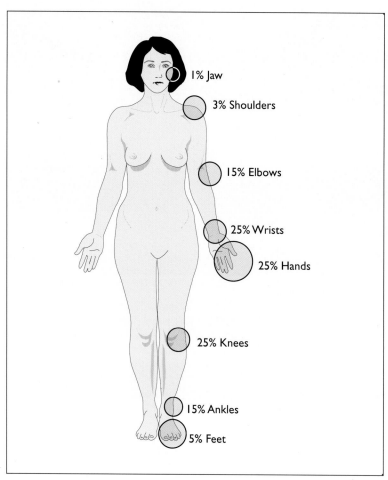

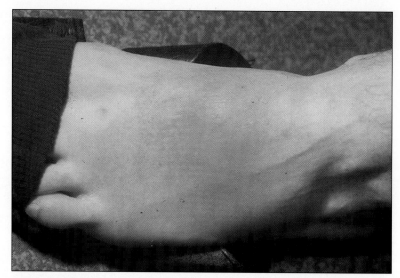

FIGURE 1-32 Gonococcal tenosynovitis. The arthritis of disseminated gonococcal infection is often accompanied by inflammation of the overlying tendons. This finding helps differentiate gonococcal arthritis from other infections. The tenosynovitis is sometimes visible as erythema overlying the tendons. (*Courtesy of* the Centers for Disease Control and Prevention.)

FIGURE 1-31 Distribution of affected joints in disseminated gonococcal infection. A small (0.5%) proportion of patients with mucosal gonorrhea develops disseminated gonococcal infection (DGI). DGI represents gonococcal sepsis and manifests as a complex syndrome. The classic syndrome consists of fevers, joint pains, and rash. The rheumatologic symptoms usually consist of tenosynovitis of the large joints (oligoarthritis). A subset of patients develops frank septic arthritis, usually of the large joints. Aspiration of the joint yields purulent synovial fluid. Culture of the fluid is positive in only 50% of cases. The percentages on this figure indicate the percentage of patients with involvement of each joint (monoarticular or biarticular).

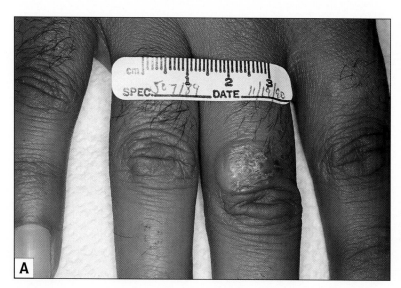

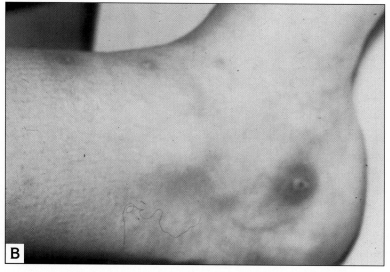

FIGURE 1-33 Rash of disseminated gonococcal infection. The rash of disseminated gonococcal infection manifests as a sparse distribution of papular, vesicular, or pustular lesions, usually on the extensor surfaces of the extremities. **A,** Pustular lesion of disseminated gonococcal infection on the right middle finger.

B, Pustular lesion of disseminated gonococcal infection on the heel. Disseminated gonococcal infection is easily treated with appropriate antibiotics, such as quinolones or third-generation cephalosporins. Current recommendations call for a full week of antibiotic treatment.

DIAGNOSIS

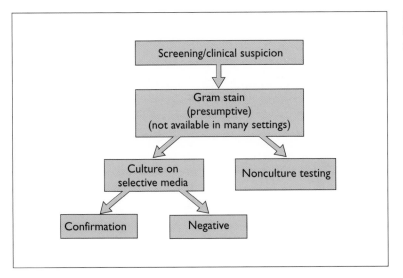

FIGURE 1-34 Diagnosis of *Neisseria gonorrhoeae* infection. Gram stain is a rapid, inexpensive test that may obviate the need for culture in some settings.

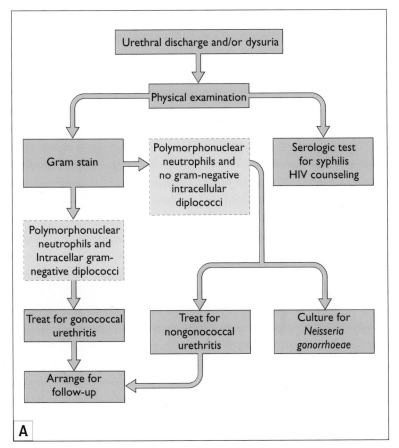

A

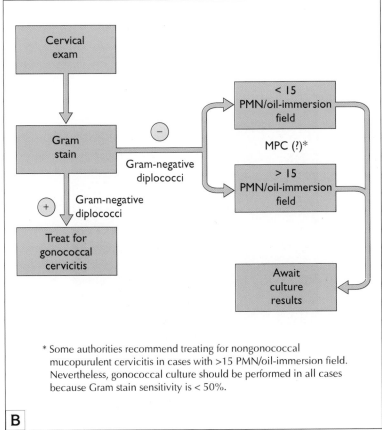

B

* Some authorities recommend treating for nongonococcal mucopurulent cervicitis in cases with >15 PMN/oil-immersion field. Nevertheless, gonococcal culture should be performed in all cases because Gram stain sensitivity is < 50%.

FIGURE 1-35 A, Practical approach to diagnosis and management of a male patient with urethritis. Management of gonococcal urethritis should include treatment for possible coincident chlamydial infection. **B,** Practical approach to diagnosis and management of a female patient with cervical discharge. Over 50% of women with nongonococcal cervicitis do not present with any symptoms. (MPC—mucopurulent cervicitis; PMN—polymorphonuclear neutrophils).

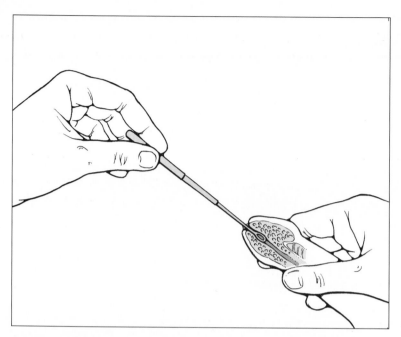

FIGURE 1-36 Specimen collection from men. From men, if a discharge is present, sterile loops can be used to obtain a discharge specimen; if no discharge is present, intraurethral swabbing is recommended, as illustrated.

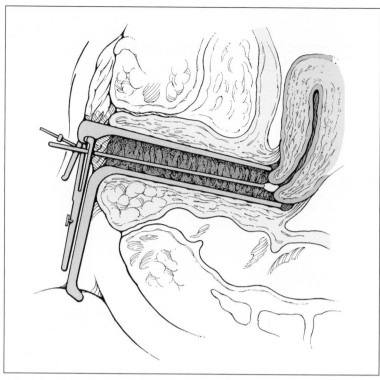

FIGURE 1-37 Specimen collection from women. In women, cervical cultures are taken from the endocervical canal after ectocervix is cleaned of mucosal debris. Rectal and pharyngeal specimens may also be plated directly onto the supplemented selective media.

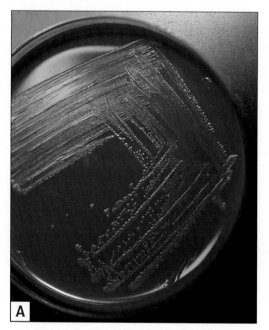

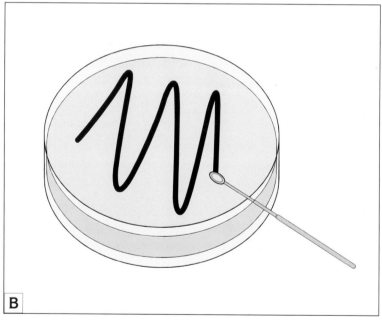

FIGURE 1-38 Culture of *Neisseria gonorrhoeae* on selective media. Diagnosis of gonococcal infection from nonsterile mucosal sites uses supplemented selective (*ie*, antibiotic-containing) media to isolate the organism. The most common media formulations are supplemented chocolate agar to which low concentrations of vancomycin, colistin, trimethoprim, and an antifungal are added. **A**, After 24 to 48 hours of incubation at 35° C in a 5% carbon dioxide environment, typical round, gray colonies are seen. **B**, It is common practice to cross-streak the culture plates immediately after the specimen is obtained to enhance the opportunity for isolation of single colonies.

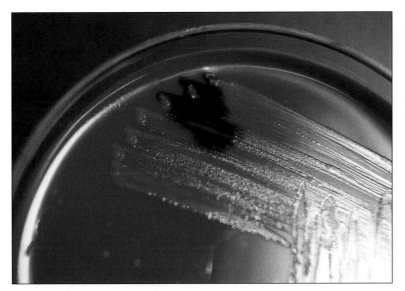

FIGURE 1-39 Oxidase reaction test for *Neisseria gonorrhoeae*. A presumptive diagnosis of *N. gonorrhoeae* infection is made after isolation of characteristic colonies followed by a positive oxidase reaction. Tetramethyl-*p*–phenylene diamine hydrochloride (0.5%) is applied to the colonies, and a purple color develops in 10 to 15 seconds. Alternatively, the dimethyl compound (1%) may be used in the same manner, which results in development of a black color, as illustrated here. This test demonstrates that the organism is a member of the *Neisseria* family and, in many clinics, is sufficient for a presumptive diagnosis of gonococcal infection. The specificity is about 93% to 99%. Confirmatory tests required for microbiologic confirmation include fluorescent antibody techniques and sugar fermentation. *N. gonorrhoeae* ferments glucose but not maltose, lactose, or sucrose. Confirmation should be performed on all nongenital isolates (*eg*, pharynx, conjunctiva, synovium) and on all isolates from cases of rape or potential medicolegal situations.

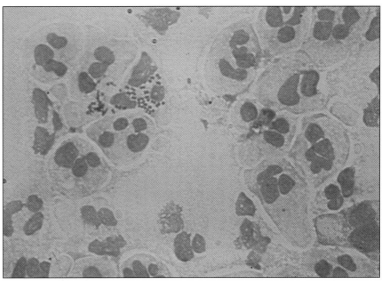

FIGURE 1-40 Positive Gram stain of urethral smear. In the clinic setting, the Gram stain usually is used for presumptive diagnosis of gonococcal infection. Urethral Gram stain in symptomatic men has a sensitivity and specificity of > 95%. Gonococcal urethritis is demonstrated by the presence of > 5 leukocytes/oil-immersion field and observation of gram-negative intracellular diplococci. Some men, particularly those who have recently urinated, have smaller numbers of leukocytes.

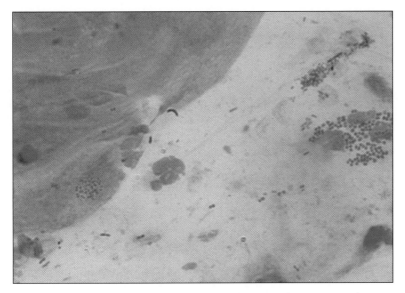

FIGURE 1-41 Endocervical gram-stained smear. In women, the sensitivity of Gram stain for gonococcal cervicitis is lower. Cervical inflammation is defined as > 15 leukocytes/oil-immersion field. Gram-negative intracellular diplococci are the *sine qua non* of gonococcal cervicitis. Because the normal vagina and cervix contain commensal *Neisseria* and other gram-negative species, intracellular diplococci (as opposed to extracellular organisms, which are normal flora) are an essential element for the Gram stain diagnosis of gonococcal cervicitis. Gram-negative intracellular diplococci are observed to the right of the field. The sensitivity of the endocervical smear is only about 50%, and a negative smear does not rule out cervicitis.

Gram stain diagnosis of gonorrhea

Specimen	Sensitivity	Specificity
Urethral	95%–98%	96%–99%
Cervical	50%–70%	90%–95%

FIGURE 1-42 Sensitivity and specificity of Gram-stain diagnoses. Gram stain is widely used for bedside clinical diagnosis of presumptive gonococcal infection, especially in sexually transmitted diseases clinics. In men, the Gram stain is highly sensitive and specific. Sensitivity in women is lower because of the presence of commensal organisms and the nonhomogeneity of cervical inflammation.

New diagnostic techniques for gonorrhea			
	Specimens	Sensitivity	Specificity
DNA hybridization (genetic probe)	Genital	90%–95%	95%–98%
Polymerase chain reaction	Genital	98%–100%	99%–100%
Ligase chain reaction	Urine (male and female)	95%–99%	99%–100%

FIGURE 1-43 Newer diagnostic techniques. In the last 5 years, newer techniques for the diagnosis of gonococcal infection have been developed. Genetic probe techniques based on DNA hybridization have been used successfully and are widely available in many clinical settings. DNA amplification techniques are under development and should be approved by late 1995. These noncul-ture techniques are based on the amplification and identification of *Neisseria gonorrhoeae*–specific DNA sequences. Because these techniques are not based on organism viability, but rather the detection of DNA subcomponents, the techniques will be useful in field settings or other situations in which gonococcal culture is not routinely available because of logistic considerations.

TREATMENT

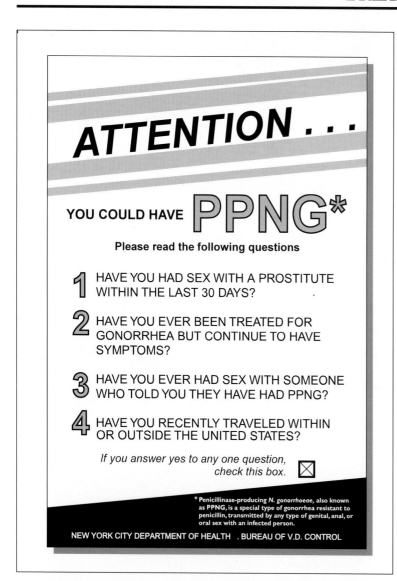

FIGURE 1-44 Antibiotic resistance in *Neisseria gonorrhoeae*. Detection of antibiotic resistance has been a concern since the early 1980s. This poster, by the New York City Department of Health, represents an attempt to control penicillin-resistant gonorrhea by targeting "risk groups." These types of interventions succeeded initially but were costly. However, once resistant strains become endemic, interventions for eradication do not work. (PPNG—penicillinase-producing *N. gonorrhoeae*.)

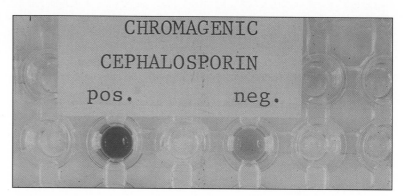

FIGURE 1-45 Colorimetric detection of antibiotic-resistant *Neisseria gonorrhoeae*. β-Lactamase resistance to penicillin is easily detectable by colorimetric techniques. For example, if a suspension of β-lactamase–producing *N. gonorrhoeae* is mixed with a chromogenic cephalosporin, the molecule is hydrolyzed and changes color from yellow to red (*left*). Further definition of antibiotic resistance requires the determination of minimum inhibitory concentrations by standardized agar dilutions. In this technique, agar plates are prepared with varying dilutions of the antibiotic to be tested, and the ability of organisms to grow on these agar plates is evaluated. (*Courtesy of* the Centers for Disease Control and Prevention.)

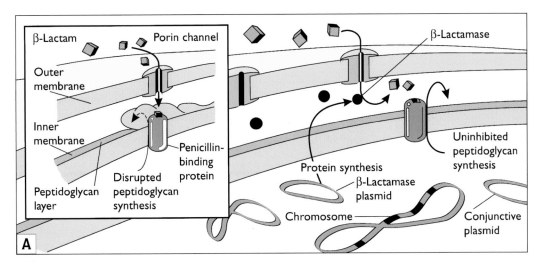

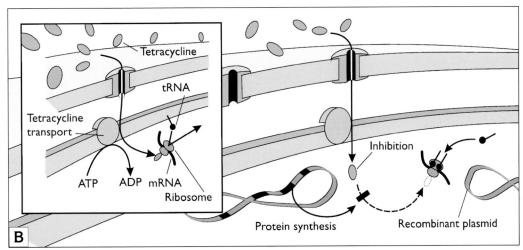

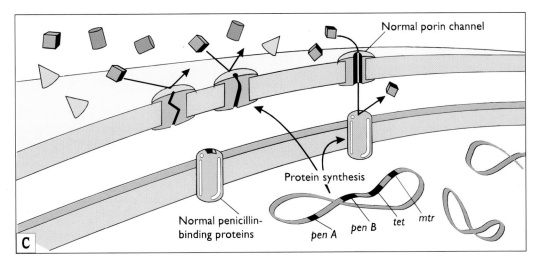

Figure 1-46 Mechanisms of antibiotic resistance in *Neisseria gonorrhoeae*. There are two major types of antibiotic resistance in *N. gonorrhoeae*: plasmid and chromosomally mediated resistance. Plasmids are transferable pieces of DNA that are present in multiple copies within the organism. Therefore, plasmid-mediated resistance (for example, to penicillin and tetracycline) is easily widely disseminated and generally results in very high levels of antibiotic resistance, usually causing treatment failure. Conversely, chromosomally mediated resistance is based on the slower development of mutations within the organism. These mutations, in turn, code for absorption properties of the penicillin-binding proteins, porins, and other membrane structures that mediate antibiotic transport and absorption. **A,** Plasmid-mediated penicillin resistance. In penicillin-susceptible strains (*left panel*), β-lactam binds to penicillin-binding protein on the inner membrane of *N. gonorrhoeae*, resulting in disrupted peptidoglycan synthesis. In resistant strains (*right panel*), transferable plasmids mediate the production and export of TEM-1 β-lactamase, which hydrolyzes penicillins. **B,** Plasmid-mediated tetracycline resistance. Tetracyclines operate by interacting with ribosomal messenger RNA (mRNA) in the bacteria, blocking the binding of transfer RNA (tRNA) to the ribosome-mRNA complex (*left panel*). Plasmid-mediated tetracycline resistance occurs as a result of the *tet M* resistance determinant integrated into a gonococcal transferable plasmid. The *tet M* determinant mediates the blocking of tetracycline at the tRNA of bacteria (*right panel*). **C,** Chromosomally mediated resistance. A variety of chromosomal mutations can confer resistance in the gonococcus. These mutations may be additive. The most common mechanisms involve either inhibition of absorption of antibiotics through the cell membrane or alteration of the outer membrane penicillin-binding proteins. (*Adapted from* Zenilman JM: Gonorrhea: Clinical and public health aspects. *Hosp Pract* 1993, 28(2A):29–50; with permission.)

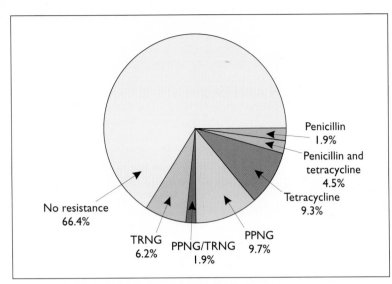

FIGURE 1-47 Distribution of antimicrobial resistance in gonococcal isolates. The surveillance of antibiotic resistance is a major concern of the Centers for Disease Control and Prevention (CDC). In the late 1980s, the CDC established the Gonococcal Isolate Surveillance Project, which systematically evaluates gonococcal resistance in the United States. These results have been invaluable in helping assess treatment protocols. For example, in 1992, the Project demonstrated that antibiotic resistance was widespread and was of multiple types. (PPNG—penicillinase-producing *Neisseria gonorrhoeae*; TRNG—tetracycline-resistant *N. gonorrhoeae*.) (*Courtesy of* the Centers for Disease Control and Prevention.)

Oral therapy for gonorrhea

Quinolones	Ciprofloxacin	500 mg once
	Ofloxacin	400 mg once
	Norfloxacin	800 mg once
	Enoxacin	400 mg once
Cephalosporins	Cefixime	400 mg once
	Cefuroxime axetil	1 g once

FIGURE 1-48 Oral therapies for gonorrhea. Successful treatment of gonococcal infection requires the use of antibiotics that are effective against all types of organism resistance. The antibiotics that are currently widely used include the quinolones and third-generation cephalosporins. Cephalosporins and penicillin act by inhibiting peptidoglycan cross-linking during cell replication. Penicillin-binding proteins are an important mediator of the process. Quinolones act by inhibiting cellular topoisomerae, which mediates DNA coiling during replication and protein synthesis. Both of these drug classes have been widely effective and can be used in single-dose oral therapies. *All patients treated for gonococcal disease also should be cotreated for chlamydia, as confection rates are high.* Partners of individuals with gonococcal infection or pelvic inflammatory disease should be referred for diagnosis and treatment. Current public health practice calls for the presumptive treatment of known sexual contacts of an individual with gonorrhea. In addition, patients evaluated for sexually transmitted disease, including gonococcal infection, should be counseled and tested for HIV infection.

Therapy for disseminated gonococcal infections

Parenteral phase	Ciprofloxacin	400 mg every 12 hrs
	Ofloxacin	400 mg every 12 hrs
	Ceftriaxone	1 g every 24 hrs
	Cefotaxime	1 g every 8 hrs
Oral phase	Ciprofloxacin	500 mg twice daily
	Ofloxacin	400 mg twice daily
	Cefixime	400 mg twice daily

FIGURE 1-49 Therapy for disseminated gonococcal infections (DGI). Treatment of DGI is predicated on the concept of gonococcal septicemia. Parenteral treatment is given until defervescence, followed by oral therapy to complete a full week of antimicrobial administration.

Interaction of HIV and gonococcal infection

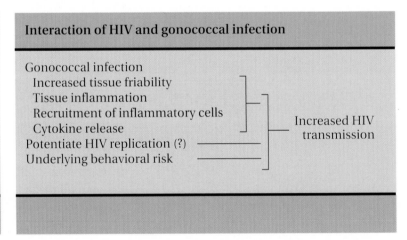

Gonococcal infection
  Increased tissue friability
  Tissue inflammation
  Recruitment of inflammatory cells   Increased HIV
  Cytokine release   transmission
Potentiate HIV replication (?)
Underlying behavioral risk

FIGURE 1-50 Interactions between gonorrhea and HIV infection. Aggressive treatment of gonorrhea and other exudative sexually transmitted diseases may affect HIV prevention activities. Gonococcal infection is increasingly seen as a cofactor for the transmission of HIV. Prospective studies in Africa and retrospective studies performed in the United States have demonstrated that individuals infected with *Neisseria gonorrhoeae* are three to five times more likely to become infected with HIV than individuals without gonococcal infection. From a pathophysiologic standpoint, gonococcal inflammation—*ie*, the recruitment of inflammatory cells to the mucosal site, and the associated increased friability of the inflamed mucosa and consequent vascular access to a potential pathogen—is the operational hypothesis. Confirmation of these data awaits further experimental verification.

SELECTED BIBLIOGRAPHY

Centers for Disease Control and Prevention: Surveillance for sexually transmitted disease. *MMWR* 1993, 42(SS-3):1–13.

Centers for Disease Control and Prevention: 1993 Sexually transmitted diseases treatment guidelines. *MMWR* 1993, 42(RR-14):1–102.

Schwarcz SK, Zenilman JM, *et al.*: National surveillance of antimicrobial resistance in *Neisseria gonorrhoeae*. *JAMA* 1992, 264:1413–1417.

Tramont EC, Boslego JW: *Neisseria gonorrhoeae*. *In* Gorbach S, Bartlett J, Blacklow N (eds.): *Infectious Diseases*. Philadelphia: W.B. Saunders; 1992:1443–1551.

Zenilman JM: Gonorrhea: Clinical and public health aspects. *Hosp Pract* 1993, 28:29–50.

CHAPTER 2

Chlamydial Infections

Robert B. Jones

ETIOLOGY

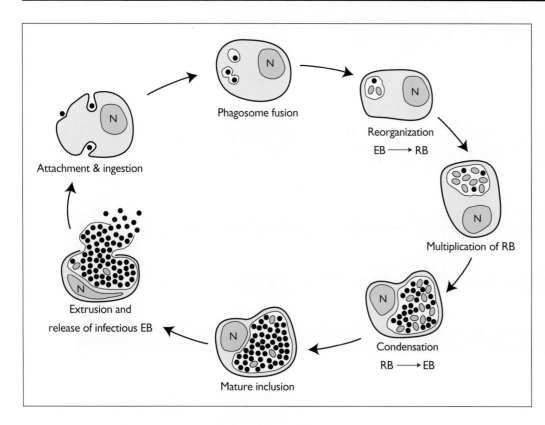

Phagosome fusion

Reorganization
EB ⟶ RB

Attachment & ingestion

Multiplication of RB

Extrusion and
release of infectious EB

Condensation
RB ⟶ EB

Mature inclusion

FIGURE 2-1 Life cycle of *Chlamydia trachomatis*. Chlamydiae are obligate intracellular parasites. The extracellular, metabolically inactive elementary bodies (EBs) attach to and invade host cells, remaining a membrane-bound vesicle that avoids phagosome–lysosome fusion. EBs undergo transformation into the intracellular, replicative form, the reticulate body (RB). The RBs are osmotically fragile and unable to exist outside the protected environment of the inclusion. They replicate by binary fission. RBs condense to form the infectious EBs, which are then released from the host cell. The entire cycle takes 48 to 72 hours in tissue culture. (N—nucleus.) (Moulder JW: Interaction of chlamydiae and host cells *in vitro. Microbiol Rev* 1991, 55:143–190.) (*From* Jones R: *Chlamydia trachomatis. In* Mandell GR, Bennett JE, Dolin R (eds.): *Principles and Practice of Infectious Diseases*, 4th ed. New York: Churchill Livingstone; 1995:1680; with permission.)

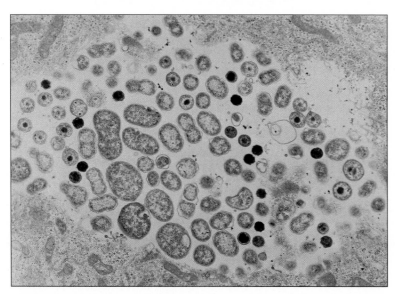

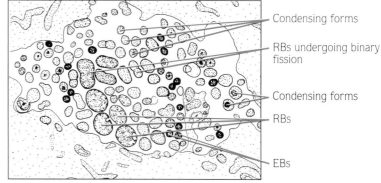

Condensing forms

RBs undergoing binary fission

Condensing forms

RBs

EBs

FIGURE 2-2 Thin-section electron photomicrograph of an inclusion containing *Chlamydia trachomatis*. Elementary bodies (EBs) are highly electron dense and very regular in shape. Reticulate bodies (RBs) are less dense, with dispersed chromatin, and are larger than EBs. In this photomicrograph, several RBs are undergoing binary fission. Forms intermediate between RBs and EBs are also present, which are RBs in the process of condensation to EBs. These forms are smaller, and an increase in electron density can be seen in their centers. (Original magnification, × 10,000.) (*Courtesy of* B.A. Collett, MD.)

Infectious serotypes of *Chlamydia trachomatis* and associated diseases	
Strain	**Disease**
L_1, L_2, L_3	Lymphogranuloma venereum
	Cervicitis
	Proctitis
A, B, Ba, C	Ocular trachoma (in endemic areas)
D–K	Oculogenital disease in adults and children (worldwide)

FIGURE 2-3 Infectious serotypes of *Chlamydia trachomatis* and associated diseases. Studies using monoclonal antibody typing and DNA sequencing of the gene for the major outer-membrane protein of *C. trachomatis* have delineated at least 15 serotypes (strains) of the organism. Serovars L_1, L_2, and L_3 are more invasive than the other serovars and produce disease in lymphatic tissue, including lymphogranuloma venereum, cervicitis, and proctitis (primarily in homosexual men). Other strains characteristically produce superficial infection involving the columnar epithelium of the eye, genitalia, or respiratory tract. Serovariants of these strains, particularly for serovars D and I, have been described, and undoubtedly others exist.

DIAGNOSTIC TECHNIQUES

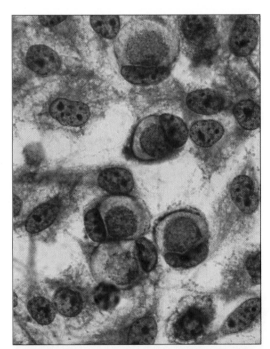

FIGURE 2-4 Giemsa strain of cultured McCoy cells infected with *Chlamydia trachomatis* and stained at 72 hours after inoculation. Infected cells have a large inclusion that fills most of the cytosol, pushing the nucleus to one side. Individual elementary bodies can be barely appreciated as fine dots at this magnification ($\times$ 750). The apparent condensation of the inclusion away from the host cell membrane is an artifact of fixation. Giemsa staining allows better evaluation of the morphology of the inclusions than other staining techniques, but it is relatively insensitive for their detection after inoculation with clinical specimens. The morphology of *C. trachomatis* inclusion differs from that of the other two species of *Chlamydia* in that there is usually only one inclusion per host cell and they are large with diffuse contents. In contrast, the inclusions of *Chlamydia psittaci* and *Chlamydia pneumoniae* are frequently multiple but much smaller, resembling large granules in the cytoplasm of the infected cell.

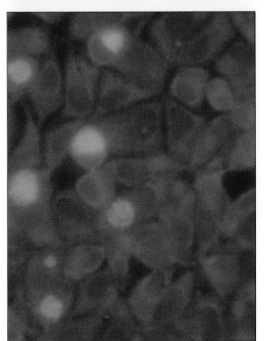

FIGURE 2-5 Indirect immunofluorescent staining of cultured McCoy cells inoculated with *Chlamydia trachomatis* and stained at 72 hours after inoculation. Indirect immunofluorescent staining uses a mouse monoclonal antibody specific for chlamydial lipo-oligosaccharide, followed by a fluorescein isothiocyanate–conjugated goat anti-mouse IgG antibody. This technique demonstrates antibody-binding organisms contained within a cellular inclusion. It is one of the most sensitive methods for detecting inclusions in tissue culture. Other diagnostic techniques include antigen detection by enzyme-linked immunoassay, direct fluorescent antibody staining (*see* Fig. 2-7), nucleic acid hybridization, and nucleic acid amplification. (Original magnification, $\times$ 400.)

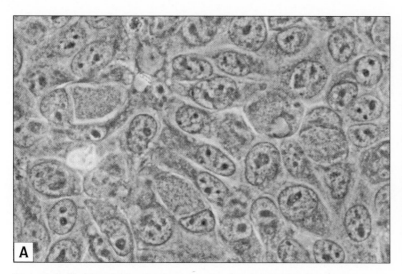

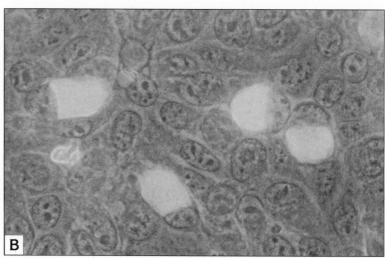

FIGURE 2-6 Phase photomicrograph of cultured McCoy cells infected with *Chlamydia trachomatis* observed at 72 hours after fixation. **A**, Four single inclusions are observed. The apparent condensation of the inclusion away from the host cell membrane is an artifact of fixation. The nuclei are pushed to the side of the cell by the inclusion. **B**, The same field treated with a fluorescein-labeled polyclonal rabbit antibody is observed with a combination of phase and fluorescence microscopy, defining the inclusions. (*Courtesy of* M.F. Rein, MD.)

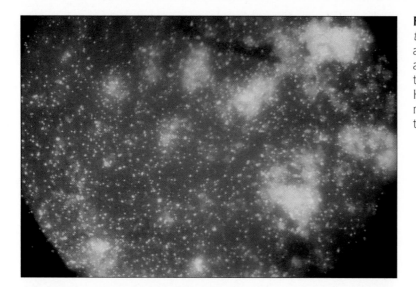

FIGURE 2-7 Direct fluorescent antibody staining of *Chlamydia trachomatis*. Direct fluorescent antibody staining was done using a fluorescein isothiocyanate–tagged monoclonal antibody directed against the major outer-membrane protein of *Chlamydia*. Elementary bodies can be seen as bright apple-green, round organisms. Host cells are counterstained orange to provide contrast. This technique is approved for clinical diagnosis, although this many elementary bodies rarely are seen in a clinical specimen.

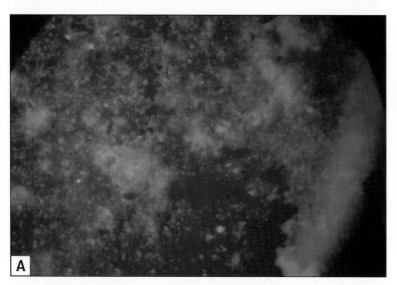

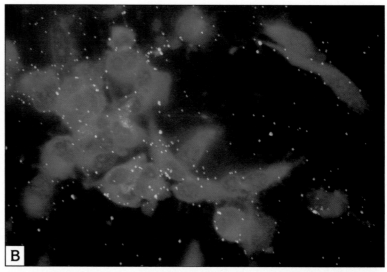

FIGURE 2-8 Microimmunofluorescent detection of human serum antibody directed against *Chlamydia trachomatis*. Purified elementary bodies suspended in a 10% yolk sac preparation are allowed to adhere to a glass slide. These yolk sac dots are then incubated with human serum, followed by mouse anti-human IgG or IgM conjugated to fluorescein isothiocyanate (FITC). **A**, Negative control. In the absence of human antibody to *Chlamydia*, the FITC-conjugated antibody to human IgG does not bind. The yolk sac preparation absorbs an orange counterstain that provides contrast. **B**, Positive study. Human serum containing antibody to *C. trachomatis* binds to the elementary bodies in the yolk sac preparation and also binds the FITC anti-human antibody. The elementary bodies are seen as small fluorescent green dots. Serologic testing for *Chlamydia* is of value for population-based studies but generally is not useful in the diagnosis of active infection.

Laboratory diagnosis of uncomplicated *Chlamydia trachomatis* infection

	Sensitivity, %	Specificity, %
Culture	52–92	99–100
Antigen detection or nucleic acid hybridization	50–70	95–99
Rapid tests	48–75	95–98
PCR	65–95	> 99
LCR	85–95	> 99
Serology	85–100	< 65

LCR—ligase chain reaction; PCR—polymerase chain reaction.

FIGURE 2-9 Laboratory diagnosis of uncomplicated *Chlamydia trachomatis* infection. Although culture remains the gold standard for diagnosis of chlamydia infection, antigen detection or nucleic acid hybridization techniques have been developed that may be used instead. These include enzyme-linked immunosorbent assays, direct fluorescent antibody tests, and nucleic acid hybridization. Rapid tests refer to kits designed for office use and are based on an immunosorbent or nucleic acid hybridization assay. Both the polymerase chain reaction and the ligase chain reaction appear to be more sensitive than culture by 30% or more. However, both have problems with inhibitors causing falsely negative results at some body sites (particularly the endocervix) and cross-contamination in inexperienced laboratories. Both tests have been used successfully to detect genital infection using urine as a primary specimen and may offer a means for noninvasive screening in the future. Serologic evaluation, including complement fixation and microimmunofluorescence tests, is useful in population-based studies but, because of its low specificity, is not useful in the diagnosis of current (as opposed to past) infection in individuals. (Schachter J: Diagnosis of *Chlamydia trachomatis* infection. *In* Orfila J, Byrne GI, Chernesky MA, *et al.* (eds.): *Chlamydial Infections: Proceedings of the Eighth International Symposium on Human Chlamydial Infections.* Bologna, Italy: Società Editrice Esculapio; 1994:293–302.)

CLINICAL MANIFESTATIONS

Clinical spectrum of *Chlamydia trachomatis* infections

Men	Women
Trachoma	Trachoma
Acute inclusion conjunctivitis	Acute inclusion conjunctivitis
LGV	LGV
Urethritis	Urethritis
Epididymitis	Cervicitis
Proctitis	Pelvic inflammatory disease
	Acute
	Chronic asymptomatic

LGV—lymphogranuloma venereum.

FIGURE 2-10 Clinical spectrum of *Chlamydia trachomatis* infections. Trachoma is a chronic conjunctivitis and an important preventable cause of blindness in endemic areas (parts of Africa, the Middle East, Asia). Adult inclusion conjunctivitis occurs in both men and women worldwide and frequently is associated with a concurrent genital tract infection. Lymphogranuloma venereum also affects both men and women and is endemic in areas of Asia, Africa, South America, and the Caribbean, with sporadic cases occurring elsewhere. Genital infections caused by *C. trachomatis* represent the most common bacterial sexually transmitted diseases in the United States, with an estimated 3 to 4 million cases annually. Gonorrhea and chlamydiae are the most frequent causes of urethritis in men less than 35 years of age, with epididymitis occurring in approximately 5% of cases of untreated nongonococcal urethritis. Proctitis has been recognized primarily in homosexual men engaging in anal intercourse. In women, approximately 20% of cases of acute pelvic inflammatory disease (PID) are associated with *C. trachomatis* infections, and it is estimated that one third of women with untreated chlamydial infection of the genital tract will develop acute PID. However, chronic asymptomatic or "silent" PID is a more frequent outcome. Both can lead to sequelae of infertility, ectopic pregnancy, or chronic pelvic pain syndrome.

Nongonococcal Urethritis

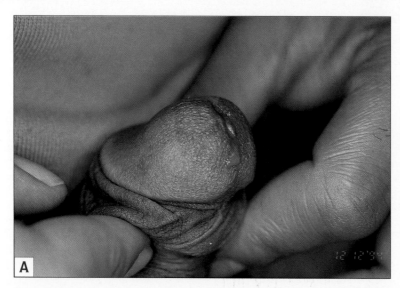
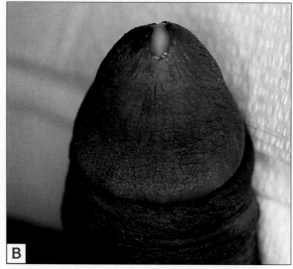

FIGURE 2-11 Urethral discharge in urethritis. **A.** Urethral discharge from a man with chlamydial urethritis. **B.** Urethral discharge from a man with gonococcal urethritis. There is considerable overlap between signs and symptoms of gonococcal and chlamydial urethritis. However, in newly acquired chlamydial urethritis, the discharge tends to be scant, thin, and watery, whereas in gonococcal urethritis, it is usually more copious and purulent. The incubation period usually is longer in chlamydial urethritis (7–10 days) than in gonococcal urethritis (3–5 days).

Clinical features of gonococcal and nongonococcal urethritis in men

	Gonorrhea	Nongonococcal urethritis
Incubation	1–7 days	3–21 days
Onset	Abrupt	Gradual
Symptoms	Prominent	Milder
Dysuria only	2%	27%
Discharge only	27%	47%
Both	71%	38%
Discharge	Purulent (91%)	Mucoid (58%)

FIGURE 2-12 Clinical features of gonococcal and nongonococcal urethritis in men. *Chlamydia trachomatis* urethritis is generally less severe than gonococcal urethritis, although there is sufficient overlap between the signs and symptoms so that in an individual patient, these two forms of urethritis cannot be differentiated solely on clinical grounds. Nongonococcal urethritis is diagnosed by documentation of a leukocytic urethral exudate and by exclusion of gonorrhea by Gram stain or culture. At least one third of men with chlamydial urethral infection have no signs or symptoms of urethritis. (Jacobs NF, Kraus SJ: Gonococcal and nongonococcal urethritis in men: Clinical and laboratory differentiation. *Ann Intern Med* 1975, 82:7–12.)

Management of urethritis in men

Evaluate for presence of urethral discharge:
  Strip the urethra and look for discharge
  Obtain an intraurethral swab specimen for gonorrhea culture and Gram stain
If Gram stain shows ≥ 5 PMN/oil-immersion field (× 1000), then patient has urethritis
If Gram stain shows GNID, then patient has gonorrhea and should be treated for both gonorrhea and possible coinfection with chlamydia
If patient has urethritis but no GNID, then patient should be treated for chlamydial infection only
If < 5 PMN/oil-immersion field, evaluate further for cause of symptoms, including Gram stain of urine sediment from first-void urine

GNID—gram-negative intracellular diplococci; PMN—polymorphonuclear leukocytes.

FIGURE 2-13 Management of urethritis in men. In a man with urethral discharge, the presence of five or more polymorphonuclear leukocytes per oil-immersion field on Gram stain establishes a diagnosis of urethritis. The absence of organisms with the morphology of *Neisseria gonorrhoeae* (gram-negative intracellular diplococci) and subsequent failure to culture *N. gonorrhoeae* establish a diagnosis of nongonococcal urethritis. All scenarios should include testing for both gonorrhea and *Chlamydia trachomatis*.

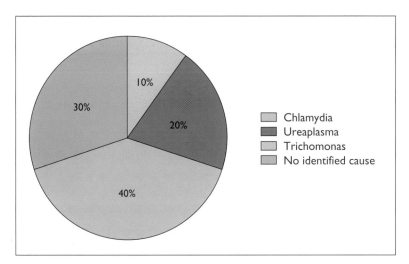

FIGURE 2-14 Etiologic agents of nongonococcal urethritis. *Chlamydia trachomatis* is the cause of 30% to 50% of symptomatic cases of nongonococcal urethritis. Another 10% to 20% of cases are due to *Ureaplasma urealyticum* and 10% to *Trichomonas vaginalis*. The proportions in this figure are approximate and are based on results of multiple studies. The rate given for *T. vaginalis* infection is based on culture rather than wet mount and is higher than the rate many investigators report.

Treatment of uncomplicated *Chlamydia trachomatis* genital infections

Doxycycline	100 mg 2 times a day × 7 days
Azithromycin	1.0 g × 1 dose
Alternatives:	
Erythromycin base	500 mg 4 times a day × 7 days
Ethylsuccinate	800 mg 4 times a day × 7 days
Ofloxacin	300 mg 2 times a day × 7 days
Amoxicillin	500 mg 3 times a day × 7–10 days

FIGURE 2-15 Treatment of uncomplicated *Chlamydia trachomatis* genital infections. For several years, standard therapy for uncomplicated genital tract infection has been doxycycline, with erythromycin as a first alternative. Azithromycin is as effective as doxycycline and has the advantage of single-dose therapy with administration at the time of diagnosis, thus obviating potential problems with compliance. However, it is more expensive than doxycycline. Amoxicillin is recommended only for pregnant women who cannot tolerate erythromycin. (Centers for Disease Control and Prevention: Recommendation for the prevention and management of *Chlamydia trachomatis* infections, 1993. *MMWR* 1993, 42:1–39.)

Indications for empiric therapy for *Chlamydia trachomatis* infections in men

Urethritis (gonococcal or nongonococcal)
Epididymitis (age < 35 years)
Contact to a partner with known chlamydial infection

FIGURE 2-16 Indications for empiric therapy for *Chlamydia trachomatis* infections in men. Clinical conditions in which the likelihood of a chlamydial infection is high enough to warrant presumptive treatment include urethritis and epididymitis. For both, therapy should include agents directed against both *C. trachomatis* and *Neisseria gonorrhoeae*.

Epididymitis

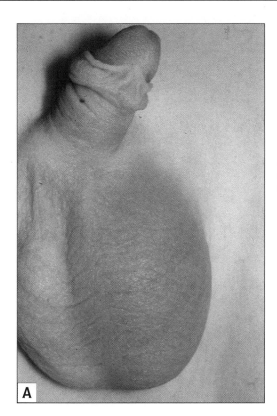

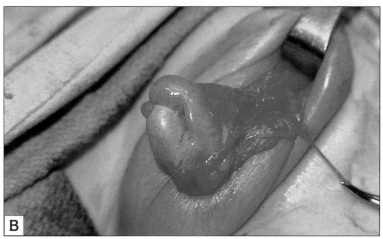

FIGURE 2-17 Epididymitis. **A**, Enlarged, erythematous scrotum of a patient with epididymitis. **B**, Scrotum contents viewed at surgery. The epididymis is erythematous and edematous in contrast to the relatively normal appearing testes. Epididymitis occurs in approximately 5% of cases of untreated chlamydial urethritis. In men under age 35 years, *Chlamydia trachomatis* and *Neisseria gonorrhoeae* are the most frequent causes. In older men, the Enterobacteriaceae must also be considered as possible causes. The presence of a urethral discharge or inguinal lymphadenopathy favors the diagnosis of chlamydial or gonococcal disease. (*Courtesy of* J.J. Mulcahy, MD.)

Evaluation of suspected epididymitis

Rule out testicular torsion

Gram stain of urethral exudate or intraurethral swab specimen for *Neisseria gonorrhoeae* and nongonococcal urethritis

Culture of urethral exudate or intraurethral swab specimen for *Neisseria gonorrhoeae*

Test of intraurethral swab specimen for *Chlamydia trachomatis*

Culture and Gram stain smear of uncentrifuged urine for gram-negative bacteria

FIGURE 2-18 Evaluation of suspected epididymitis. The primary differential diagnostic consideration is usually testicular torsion.

Treatment of epididymitis

Empiric treatment indicated before culture results are available

Recommended regimen:

Ceftriaxone	250 mg intramuscularly × single dose
and	
Doxycycline	100 mg orally 2 times a day × 10 days

Alternative therapy:

Ofloxacin	300 mg orally 2 times a day × 10 days

FIGURE 2-19 Treatment of epididymitis. Empiric treatment of epididymitis is indicated before culture results are available. Treatment includes agents directed against both *Chlamydia trachomatis* and *Neisseria gonorrhoeae*, the major pathogens of epididymitis. (Centers for Disease Control and Prevention: 1993 Sexually transmitted diseases treatment guidelines. *MMWR* 1993, 42(RR-14):81–82.)

Cervicitis

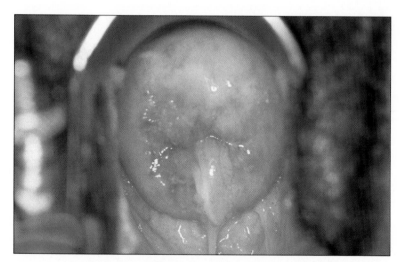

FIGURE 2-20 Mucopurulent cervicitis photographed at colposcopy. Mucopurulent cervicitis is a clinical diagnosis made during a speculum examination of the cervix. The diagnosis depends on the presence of yellow-green discharge in the endocervical os (although the color is better assessed against the white background of a swab). Mucopurulent cervicitis is highly associated with infection with *Neisseria gonorrhoeae* and *Chlamydia trachomatis*, but especially with the latter. Recovery of *C. trachomatis* also is associated in a linear fashion with the number of polymorphonuclear leukocytes detected per high-power field in a Gram stain of the endocervical exudate. (*Courtesy of* D. Soper, MD.)

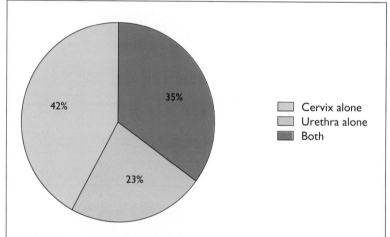

FIGURE 2-21 Rates of isolation of *Chlamydia trachomatis* from the cervix and urethra of infected women. Approximate proportions are reported based on recovery of organisms from women attending a sexually transmitted diseases clinic. Urethral culture (in addition to endocervical culture) increases the identification of infected women. Most women infected at the urethra probably also are infected at the endocervix, but the organism is not recovered from both sites because of the lack of sensitivity of culture. (Jones RB, Katz BP, *et al.*: Effect of blind passage and multiple sampling on recovery of *Chlamydia trachomatis* from urogenital specimens. *J Clin Microbial* 1986, 24:1029–1033.)

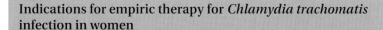

Evaluation of suspected cervicitis

Diagnosis depends on color of endocervical exudate (*ie*, yellow-green color against white swab tip)

Gram stain of endocervical exudate to evaluate inflammatory cells can be performed

If mucopurulent cervicitis is diagnosed:

1. Perform diagnostic testing for gonorrhea and chlamydia, and base treatment on test results

    or

2. Empiric therapy for both gonorrhea and chlamydia (test to facilitate management of partners)

Notify and treat partners

FIGURE 2-22 Evaluation of suspected cervicitis. About 70% of women with endocervical *Chlamydia trachomatis* infection are asymptomatic or have only mild symptoms of vaginal discharge, bleeding, mild abdominal pain, or dysuria. Dysuria may reflect concurrent urethral infection. Diagnosis depends on detection of a yellow-green endocervical exudate. Gram stain of this exudate can be done to detect inflammatory cells, but interpretation of Gram stain results is controversial, as ≥ 10 polymorphonuclear leukocytes has been correlated with the presence of both gonococcal and chlamydial infections.

Indications for empiric therapy for *Chlamydia trachomatis* infection in women

Contact of a man with urethritis (gonococcal or nongonococcal)

Contact of a partner with known chlamydial infection

Gonorrhea or pelvic inflammatory disease

Mucopurulent cervicitis (?)

FIGURE 2-23 Indications for empiric therapy for *Chlamydia trachomatis* infection in women. Because of the possibility of asymptomatic infection, women who are contacts of a man with urethritis or a partner with known chlamydial infection should receive empiric therapy. Patients with documented or suspected infection with *Neisseria gonorrhoeae* also should receive presumptive treatment for chlamydial infection. Mucopurulent cervicitis is an indication for either testing or treatment (*See* Fig. 2-22).

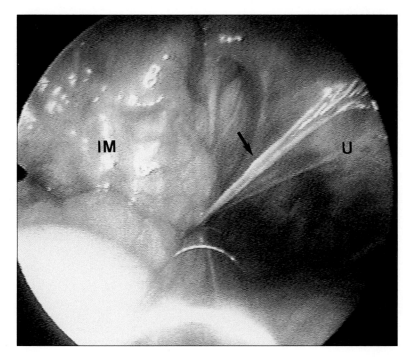

FIGURE 2-24 Chronic pelvic inflammatory disease at laparoscopy in a women being evaluated for infertility. The left fallopian tube is encased in an inflammatory mass (*IM*) with adhesion (*arrow*) between the mass and uterus (*U*). The patient was 25 years of age and had no prior history of pelvic inflammatory disease (PID). However, she did have high serum titers (1:512) of antibody to *Chlamydia trachomatis*, indicative of past or current infection with the organism. Approximately 20% of women with PID have *C. trachomatis* recovered from the urogenital tract. PID associated with chlamydiae may range from acute, severe disease with perihepatitis and ascites, to asymptomatic or "silent" salpingitis. (Cates W Jr, Rolfs RT Jr, Aral SO: Sexually transmitted diseases, pelvic inflammatory disease, and infertility: An epidemiologic update. *Epidemiol Rev* 1990, 12:199–220.) (*Courtesy of* M.K. Shepard, MD.)

Other Infections

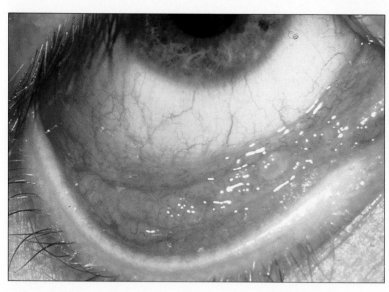

Figure 2-25 Inclusion conjunctivitis in an adult. Pronounced lymphoid follicle formation is evident in the palpebral conjunctiva. Some hyperemia also is present. Approximately one half of patients with this condition have concurrent genital tract infection with *Chlamydia trachomatis* and, in all cases, require systemic rather than topical therapy. (*Courtesy of* R.D. Deitch, Jr, MD.)

Clinical characteristics associated with Reiter's syndrome

Urethritis or cervicitis
Polyarticular arthritis
Sacroiliitis
Conjunctivitis
Balanitis/vulvovaginitis
Stomatitis
Keratoderma blennorrhagica

Figure 2-26 Clinical characteristics associated with Reiter's syndrome. Approximately 1% of men with nongonococcal urethritis develop an acute septic arthritis syndrome referred to as sexually reactive arthritis, with one third developing full Reiter's syndrome. The syndrome occurs less frequently in women with chlamydial infections. Reiter's syndrome is strongly associated with the HLA-B27 haplotype as well as with preceding mucosal infection with *Chlamydia trachomatis*, *Shigella flexneri*, *Salmonella*, *Yersinia enterocolitica*, or *Campylobacter*. An exaggerated cell-mediated and humoral immune response to chlamydial antigens is thought to underlie the inflammation at involved target organs in these genetically predisposed persons. (*From* Hansfield HH, Pollock PS: Arthritis associated with sexually transmitted diseases. *In* Holmes KK, *et al.* (eds.): *Sexually Transmitted Diseases*, 2nd ed. New York: McGraw-Hill; 1990:737–751; with permission.)

Clinical characteristics of proctitis due to *Chlamydia trachomatis*

Anorectal pain, tenesmus, bloody mucopurulent discharge, fever, abdominal pain, diarrhea

Diffusely friable, hemorrhagic rectal mucosa with discreet ulcerations on sigmoidoscopy

Chlamydial serologic tests frequently diagnostic, with organisms identified by culture or immunofluorescent staining of swab specimens

Diffuse inflammation with crypt abscess, granulomas, and giant cells in biopsy (resembles Crohn's disease)

Progresses to fistulas, perirectal abscess, or rectal strictures

Figure 2-27 Clinical characteristics of proctitis due to *Chlamydia trachomatis*. Both adults and infants may have asymptomatic carriage of *C. trachomatis*, but in homosexual men who engage in receptive anal intercourse, *C. trachomatis* is a fairly common cause of proctitis and proctocolitis. As outlined in the figure, infection with serovars of the lymphogranuloma venereum biovar (especially L_2) produces a severe, ulcerative disease that may be confused clinically with herpes simplex proctitis or histologically with Crohn's disease. Infection with the trachoma serovars D to K is associated with a milder form of disease.

Lymphogranuloma Venereum

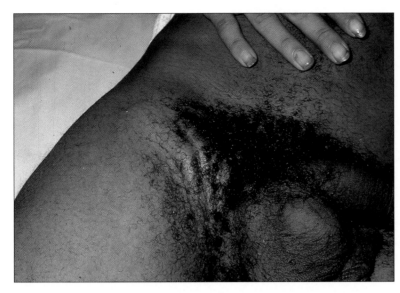

Natural history of lymphogranuloma venereum

Initial manifestations: nongonococcal urethritis, vesicle, papule, or ulcer 3–12 days after exposure
Regional lymphadenopathy and constitutional symptoms 2–24 weeks after exposure
Suppurative lymphadenitis
Sequelae: multiple draining fistulae, rectal strictures, chronic ulcerations, and elephantiasis of external genitalia

FIGURE 2-28 Unilateral inguinal and femoral lymphadenopathy in a man with lymphogranuloma venereum. The inguinal and femoral nodes on the patient's right are enlarged with overlying erythema, and they are divided by the inguinal ligament (groove sign). A vesicular primary lesion is evident near the base of the penile shaft. Untreated, the involved nodes would continue to enlarge with periadenitis to form a firm mass or bubo. Over time, the buboes may become fluctuant and drain spontaneously or involute. (*Courtesy of* A. Hood, MD.)

FIGURE 2-29 Natural history of lymphogranuloma venereum. Lymphogranuloma venereum is a sexually transmitted disease caused by the L_1, L_2, and L_3 serovars of *Chlamydia trachomatis*. It is endemic in areas of Africa, India, southeast Asia, South America, and the Caribbean and occurs in sporadic cases elsewhere (with 277 cases in the United States in 1990). The disease progresses through three stages. Following infection, a primary lesion forms on the genital mucosa, where they usually go unnoticed. The secondary stage involves regional lymphadenopathy, typically of the inguinal nodes, and systemic symptoms including fever, headache, and myalgias. The involved nodes continue to enlarge with periadenitis to form a bubo, which ultimately ruptures to drain or involutes.

Relationship between site of primary infection and subsequent lymph node involvement in lymphogranuloma venereum

Site of primary infection	Affected lymph nodes
Penis, anterior urethra	Superficial and deep inguinal
Posterior urethra	Deep iliac, perirectal
Vulva	Inguinal
Vagina, cervix	Deep iliac, perirectal, rectocrural, lumbosacral
Anus	Inguinal
Rectum	Perirectal, deep iliac

FIGURE 2-30 Relationship between site of primary infection and subsequent lymph node involvement in lymphogranuloma venereum. The secondary stage of lymphogranuloma venereum involves lymphadenopathy of the nodes draining the site of the primary lesion. Inguinal lymph nodes are characteristically involved in men, but the site of lymphadenopathy varies with the site of infection. The lymphadenopathy is usually unilateral.

Perinatal Infections

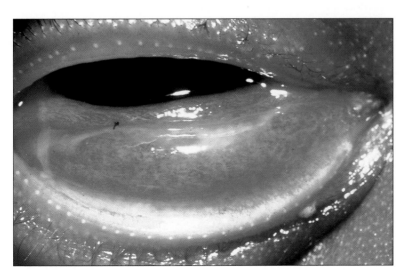

FIGURE 2-31 Neonatal inclusion conjunctivitis due to *Chlamydia trachomatis*. Marked conjunctival erythema and edema and a watery ocular discharge typically appear in infants with neonatal conjunctivitis. This condition occurs in approximately 30% of infants born to infected women and usually is acquired during passage through the infected birth canal. First manifestations appear between 5 and 12 days after birth. (*Courtesy of* R.D. Deitch, Jr, MD.)

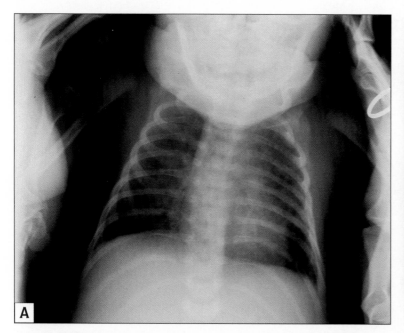
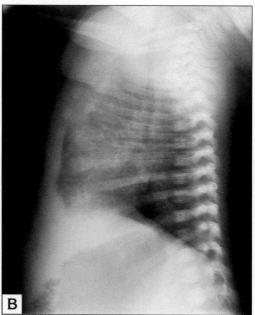

FIGURE 2-32 Infant chlamydial pneumonia. **A** and **B**, Posteroanterior and lateral chest radiographs reveal a diffuse interstitial infiltrate. Ten percent to 20% of infants delivered vaginally to infected mothers develop this complication, usually within the first 6 months of life. Clinical characteristics include listlessness, cough, hypoxemia, and a relatively prolonged course if untreated. The disease is rarely life-threatening but may predispose to reactive airways disease later in childhood. (*Courtesy of* J.W. Gaebler, MD.)

Incidence of chlamydial infection in infants born to infected mothers	
Seroconversion	60%–70%
Neonatal conjunctivitis	18%–50%
Infant pneumonia	11%–20%

FIGURE 2-33 Incidence of chlamydial infection in infants born to infected mothers. Infection is typically acquired during passage through an infected birth canal. (*From* Alexander ER, Harrison HR: Chlamydial infections in infants and children. *In* Holmes KK, *et al.* (eds.): *Sexually Transmitted Diseases*, 2nd ed. New York: McGraw-Hill; 1990:811–820; with permission.)

SURVEILLANCE AND PREVENTION

A. Prevalence of *Chlamydia trachomatis* infections in sexually active men	
Nongonococcal urethritis	≈ 40%
Gonorrhea	≈ 20%
Asymptomatic	10%–28%

B. Prevalence of *Chlamydia trachomatis* infections in sexually active women	
Gonorrhea	30%–50%
Contacts to partners with urethritis	33%–66%
Screening	
Family planning clinics	5.2%–9%
Adolescent clinics	9%–28%
College student health	8%–9%

FIGURE 2-34 Prevalence of *Chlamydia trachomatis* infections in sexually active men and women. **A**, Prevalence in men (with and without clinical disease). Rates of 10% are typical for men in active-duty military service in industrialized nations and for adolescent youth undergoing physical examinations for sports. Higher rates have been noted in inner city youths attending emergency rooms for non-genitourinary–related symptoms. Gonorrhea is a major risk factor for chlamydial infection in both men and women. **B**, Prevalence in women. Contacts to partners with urethritis include both gonococcal and nongonococcal urethritis.

Higher prevalence rates are seen in women who are contacts to men with documented chlamydial infection. (Hook EW III, Reichart CA, Upchurch DM, *et al.*: Comparative behavioral epidemiology of gonococcal and chlamydial infections among patients attending a Baltimore, Maryland, sexually transmitted disease clinic. *Am J Epidemiol* 1992, 136:662–672.)

Risk factors for chlamydial infection in women

Demographic	Behavioral
Age < 20 yrs	Recent partner change
Nonwhite race	Multiple partners
Single marital status	Inconsistent use of barrier contra-
Use of oral contraceptives	ceptives

FIGURE 2-35 Risk factors for chlamydia infection in women. Although most infected women are asymptomatic, it is women who suffer the most serious consequences of genital chlamydial infection. Risk factors vary in different population groups, but in most circumstances, being a sexual partner of a man with either gonococcal or nongonococcal urethritis confers a risk of infection in excess of 30%. (Cates W Jr, Wasserheit JN: Genital chlamydial infections: Epidemiology and reproductive sequelae. *Am J Obstet Gynec* 1991, 164:1771–1781.)

Indications for screening women for chlamydial infections

Special circumstances
  Admission to detention facility
  Presentation for induced abortion

Routine pelvic examination, including prenatal or family
  planning visit
Mucopurulent cervicitis
Sexually active < 20 years of age
20–24 years of age who either:
  1) admits inconsistent use of barrier contraceptives *or*
  2) has had a new or > one sex partner in the preceding 3
    months
> 24 years of age with both of above risk factors (1) and (2)

FIGURE 2-36 Indications for screening women for chlamydial infections. Programs that appear effective in reducing transmission of *Chlamydia trachomatis* include screening of high-risk populations for asymptomatic infection and partner notification and treatment. Women younger than 20 years who are sexually active should be screened for chlamydiae during all pelvic examinations, unless sexual activity has been limited to a single, mutually monogamous partner. Otherwise, annual testing is warranted. (Centers for Disease Control and Prevention: 1993 Sexually transmitted diseases treatment guidelines. *MMWR* 1993, 42(RR-14):50–56.)

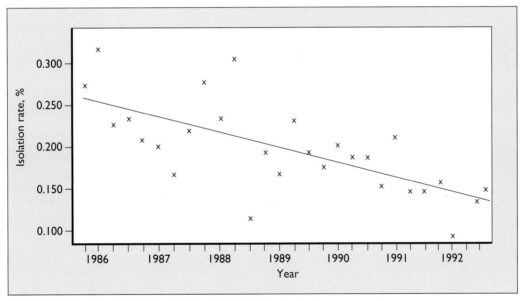

FIGURE 2-37 Effect of chlamydia surveillance and treatment program on prevalence of chlamydia isolated from adolescent women. The prevalence of *Chlamydia trachomatis* infections was determined by culture in women at their first visit to an adolescent clinic. A steady decrease has been seen since the institution of a chlamydial control program in 1984. Key elements of this program have included presumptive treatment of individuals at high risk for infection as well as active screening and partner-notification programs. (Ramstedt K, Forssman L, Giesecke J, Granath F: Risk factors for *Chlamydia trachomatis* infection in 6810 young women attending family planning clinics. *Int J STD AIDS* 1992, 3:117–122. Katz BP, Blythe MJ, VanDerpol B, Jones RB: Evaluation of a chlamydial control program among adolescent women. *In* Orfila J, Byrne GI, Chernesky MA, *et al.* (eds.): *Chlamydial Infections: Proceedings of the Eighth International Symposium on Human Chlamydial Infections.* Bologna, Italy: Società Editrice Esculapio; 1994:48–51.)

SELECTED BIBLIOGRAPHY

Batteiger BE, Jones RB: Chlamydial infections. *Infect Dis Clin North Am* 1987, 1:55–81.

Centers for Disease Control and Prevention: 1993 Sexually transmitted diseases treatment guidelines. *MMWR* 1993, 42(RR-14):1–56.

Holmes KK, Mårdh P-A, Sparling PF, Wiesner PJ (eds.): *Sexually Transmitted Diseases*, 2nd ed. New York: McGraw-Hill; 1990.

Jones RB: *Chlamydia trachomatis* (trachoma, perinatal infections, lymphogranuloma venereum, and other genital infections). *In* Mandell GL, Bennett JE, Dolin R (eds.): *Principles and Practice of Infectious Diseases*, 4th ed. New York: Churchill Livingstone; 1995:1679–1704.

CHAPTER 3

Infections Due to Genital Mycoplasmas

William M. McCormack
Michael F. Rein

CHARACTERISTICS AND DIAGNOSIS

Characteristics of mycoplasmas

Growth in cell-free media
No cell wall
Highly pleomorphic, 0.3–0.8 μm in diameter
Contain both DNA and RNA
Require sterols for growth
Resistant to antimicrobial agents that act on the cell wall
  (penicillins, other β-lactams)
Susceptible to tetracyclines, macrolides, and fluoroquinolones

FIGURE 3-1 Characteristics of mycoplasmas. Mycoplasmas are the smallest free-living agents and are distributed throughout nature. Their cell membrane contains sterols, a feature that is shared by fungi but not by bacteria or viruses. Because they lack a cell wall and are therefore deformable, mycoplasmas pass through filters that retain bacteria, and thus they were originally believed to be viruses. Their possession of both RNA and DNA and their ability to grow in cell-free media discriminate them from viral pathogens. Likewise, the presence of sterols in their cell membrane differentiates mycoplasmas from cell-wall deficient forms of bacteria (L-forms).

Mycoplasmal species isolated from humans

Oropharyngeal	Genital
Mycoplasma pneumoniae	*Ureaplasma urealyticum*
Mycoplasma salivarium	*Mycoplasma hominis*
Mycoplasma orale	*Mycoplasma genitalium*
Mycoplasma buccale	*Mycoplasma primatum*
Mycoplasma faucium	*Mycoplasma fermentans*
Mycoplasma lipophilum	*Mycoplasma pirum*
Acholeplasma laidlawii	*Mycoplasma penetrans*

FIGURE 3-2 Mycoplasmal species isolated from humans. *Mycoplasma pneumoniae*, the most important human pathogen, causes upper and lower respiratory tract infection. The other oropharyngeal species have not been convincingly associated with any human illness. *Ureaplasma urealyticum* and *Mycoplasma hominis* are common genital isolates that have been associated with human disease. *Mycoplasma genitalium* and *Mycoplasma primatum* are uncommon isolates of uncertain significance. *Mycoplasma fermentans*, *Mycoplasma pirum*, and *Mycoplasma penetrans* have been isolated from patients with HIV infection, although their role in HIV disease remains to be elucidated.

Differential characteristics of the genital mycoplasmas

	Mycoplasma hominis	*Ureaplasma urealyticum*
Growth	Aerobic	Anaerobic
Energy source	Arginine	Urea
Optimal pH	6.0	7.4
Colony size	100 μm	10–20 μm
Antibiotic susceptibility	Clindamycin	Erythromycin

FIGURE 3-3 Differential characteristics of the genital mycoplasmas, *Mycoplasma hominis* and *Ureaplasma urealyticum*. These characteristics allow identification of the organisms in the diagnostic microbiology laboratory.

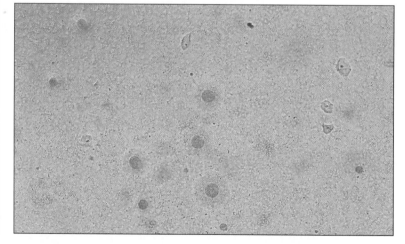

FIGURE 3-4 Colonies of *Mycoplasma hominis* growing on solid medium. *M. hominis* colonies grow with a distinctive "fried egg" appearance.

FIGURE 3-5 Growth of *Ureaplasma urealyticum* in liquid medium. Urease activity results in an elevation of pH, causing a change in the color of the phenol red pH indicator from yellow to red.

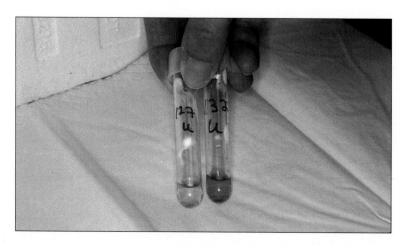

Techniques for isolation of genital mycoplasmas
1. Inoculate clinical specimens obtained from potentially infected sites into liquid holding media immediately 2. Hold at 4° C 3. Transport to the laboratory as soon as possible 4. Inoculate into isolation media at once or store at -70° C until examined

FIGURE 3-6 Techniques for isolation of genital mycoplasmas. The methods used for the collection and handling of clinical specimens that are to be examined for the genital mycoplasmas, *Mycoplasma hominis* and *Ureaplasma urealyticum*, are outlined.

Media for initial isolation of genital mycoplasmas
Beef-heart infusion (PPLO) broth (70%) Fresh yeast extract (10%) Horse serum (20%) Antibiotics to inhibit other microorganisms (penicillin, polymyxin B, amphotericin B) Antibiotics to differentiate *Mycoplasma hominis* and *Ureaplasma urealyticum* (clindamycin or erythromycin) Energy source (arginine or urea) pH indicator (phenol red)

PPLO—pleuro-pneumonia–like organisms.

FIGURE 3-7 Media for initial isolation of genital mycoplasmas. Mycoplasmas have exacting growth requirements and are often difficult to recover. Lipids are an important element in the media and are supplied by the horse serum. Because *Mycoplasma hominis* is susceptible to clindamycin, media containing this antibiotic are relatively selective for *Ureaplasma urealyticum*. Conversely, media containing erythromycin inhibit the growth of *U. urealyticum* but permit recovery of *M. hominis*. Furthermore, *M. hominis* utilizes arginine as an energy source, whereas *U. urealyticum* uses urea.

CLINICAL EPIDEMIOLOGY

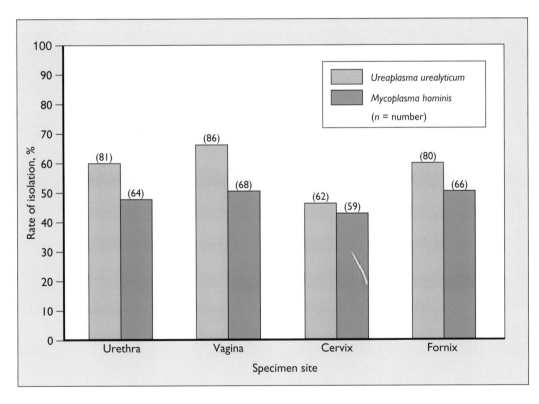

FIGURE 3-8 Isolation sites of the genital mycoplasmas, *Ureaplasma urealyticum* and *Mycoplasma hominis*, in 132 women. Specimens obtained from the vagina were more likely to yield positive cultures than were specimens obtained from the urethra, cervix, or fornix. (McCormack WM, Rankin JS, Lee YH: Localization of genital mycoplasmas in women. *Am J Obstet Gynecol* 1972, 112:920–923.)

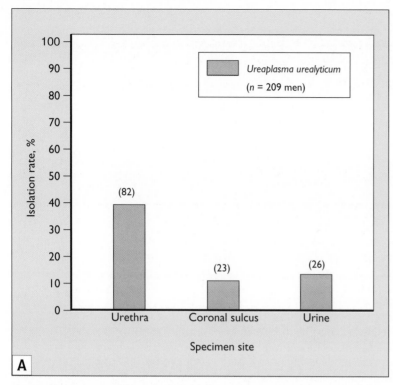

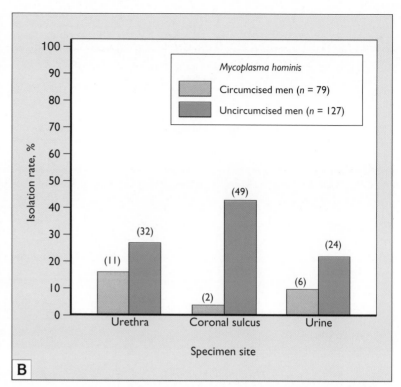

FIGURE 3-9 A and **B**, Optimal sites for obtaining specimens for detection of the genital mycoplasmas, *Ureaplasma urealyticum* (*panel 9A*) and *Mycoplasma hominis* (*panel 9B*), from men. The urethra, sampled with a calcium alginate swab, was the site most likely to yield a positive culture for *U. urealyticum* in all men and for *M. hominis* in circumcised men. For uncircumcised men, the coronal sulcus was the best culture site for *M. hominis*. Urine cultures were less sensitive than urethral cultures for identification of both species. (Tarr PI, Lee YH, Alpert S, *et al.*: Comparison of methods for the isolation of genital mycoplasmas from men. *J Infect Dis* 1976, 133:419–423.)

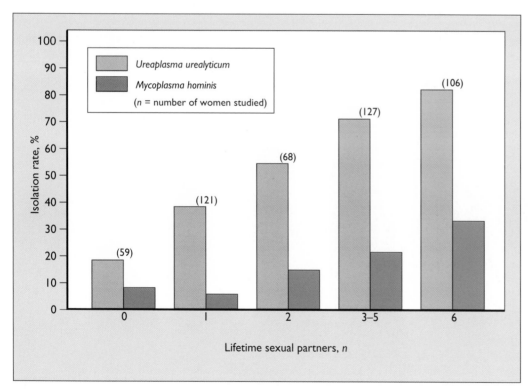

FIGURE 3-10 Sexual experience and vaginal colonization with genital mycoplasmas, *Mycoplasma hominis* and *Ureaplasma urealyticum*, in 481 normal women. Colonization was infrequent among sexually inexperienced women and rose in relation to the lifetime number of male sexual partners. (McCormack WM, Rosner B, Alpert S, *et al.*: Vaginal colonization with *Mycoplasma hominis* and *Ureaplasma urealyticum. Sex Transm Dis* 1986, 13:67–70.)

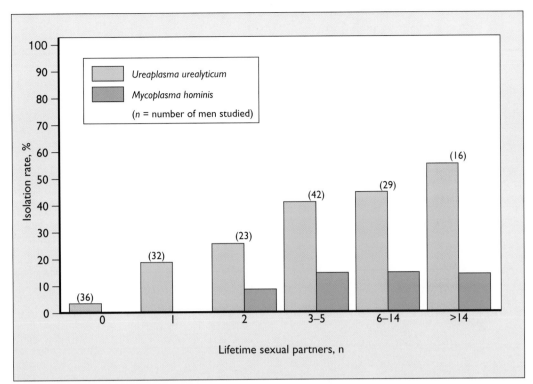

FIGURE 3-11 Sexual experience and colonization with genital mycoplasmas, *Mycoplasma hominis* and *Ureaplasma urealyticum*, in normal men. Colonization was infrequent among sexually inexperienced men and rose in relation to the number of lifetime female sexual partners. (McCormack WM, Lee Y-H, Zinner SH: Sexual experience and urethral colonization with genital mycoplasmas: A study in normal men. *Ann Intern Med* 1973, 78:696–698.)

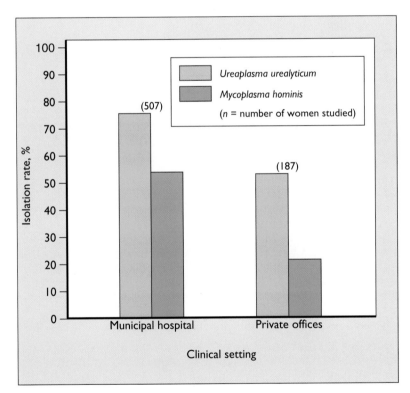

FIGURE 3-12 Colonization with genital mycoplasmas, *Mycoplasma hominis* and *Ureaplasma urealyticum*, among women seen in different clinical settings. Patients seen at the municipal hospital were more likely to be colonized with both species than were women seen in the offices of private obstetricians and gynecologists. (McCormack WM, Rosner B, Lee Y-H: Colonization with genital mycoplasmas in women. *Am J Epidemiol* 1973, 97:240–245.)

DISEASES OF MEN

Association between the genital mycoplasmas and diseases of men

	Evidence suggesting a causal role	
Clinical condition	*Mycoplasma hominis*	*Ureaplasma urealyticum*
Nongonococcal urethritis	None	Strong
Prostatitis	Weak	Weak
Epididymitis	None	None
Reiter's disease	None	None

FIGURE 3-13 Association between genital mycoplasmas, *Mycoplasma hominis* and *Ureaplasma urealyticum*, and diseases of men. Ureaplasmas and *M. hominis* have been associated with a large variety of clinical conditions in men and women but are considered a cause of only a few. In men, *U. urealyticum* is associated strongly with nongonococcal urethritis, although the proportion of total cases due to this agent is uncertain.

Differential clinical response of men with nongonococcal urethritis to sulfonamide or spectinomycin

	Pretreatment culture results		
Treatment	*C. trachomatis* positive, *U. urealyticum* negative	*C. trachomatis* negative, *U. urealyticum* positive	*P* value
Sulfonamide	7/7	5/19	P=0.0012
Spectinomycin	0/6	9/11	P=0.0023

FIGURE 3-14 Differential clinical response of men with nongonococcal urethritis to treatment with sulfonamide or spectinomycin. Ureaplasmas initially had difficulty in being accepted as a cause of nongonococcal urethritis (NGU). Some researchers inoculated themselves with *Ureaplasma urealyticum* and developed NGU. More convincing evidence for a true etiologic role came from differential treatment studies of naturally occurring disease. Men with NGU were tested by culture for ureaplasmas and chlamydiae and then were treated with an agent effective against only ureaplasmas (spectinomycin) or chlamydiae (sulfonamide). Statistically significant differences in cure rates were observed. The data are consistent with an independent etiologic role for both *Chlamydia trachomatis* and *U. urealyticum* (Taylor-Robinson D, Csonka GW, Prentice MJ: Human intraurethral inoculation of ureaplasmas. *Q J Med* 1977, 46:309–326. Bowie WR, Floyd JF, Miller, *et al.*: Differential response of chlamydial and ureaplasma-associated urethritis to sulfafurazole (sulfisoxazole) and aminocyclitols. *Lancet* 1976, ii:1276–1278.)

Treatment failures among men with nongonococcal urethritis with *Ureaplasma urealyticum* recovered from pretreatment cultures

Posttreatment *U. urealyticum*	Men studied	Treatment failures
Eliminated	57	5 (9%)
Persisted	21	7 (33%)

FIGURE 3-15 Treatment failures among men with nongonococcal urethritis who had *Ureaplasma urealyticum* recovered from pretreatment cultures. In a study evaluating tetracycline treatment of nongonococcal urethritis (NGU), treatment failures occurred more often if the ureaplasmas persisted after treatment. These data are consistent with an etiologic role for *U. urealyticum* in some cases of NGU. (Bowie WR, Yu JS, Fawcett A, *et al.*: Tetracycline in nongonococcal urethritis: Comparison of 2-g and 1-g daily for 7 days. *Br J Vener Dis* 1980, 56:332–336.)

DISEASES OF WOMEN

Association between genital mycoplasmas and diseases of women

	Evidence suggesting a causal role	
Clinical condition	*Mycoplasma hominis*	*Ureaplasma urealyticum*
Abscess of Bartholin's gland	Weak	None
Vaginitis	None	None
Pelvic inflammatory disease	Strong	Weak
Postabortal fever	Strong	None
Postpartum fever	Strong	None

FIGURE 3-16 Association between the genital mycoplasmas, *Mycoplasma hominis* and *Ureaplasma urealyticum*, and diseases of women. *M. hominis* has been cultured from the blood of approximately 10% of women with postabortal fever, and increased antibody titers are detected in approximately 50% of such women. Furthermore, the organism is isolated in anecdotal cases from women with postpartum fever. *M. hominis* has also been isolated from the fallopian tubes of women with salpingitis. Antibodies to *M. hominis* are more common in women with salpingitis than in others. (Taylor-Robinson D, McCormack WM: The genital mycoplasmas. *N Engl J Med* 1980, 302:1003–1010, 1063–1067. Weström L, Mårdh P-A: Acute salpingitis: Aspects of aetiology, diagnosis and prognosis. *In* Danielson D, Juhlin L, Mårdh P-A (eds.): *Genital Infections and Their Complications.* Stockholm: Almqvist and Wiskell; 1975:157–167. Mårdh P-A, Weström L: Antibodies to *Mycoplasma hominis* in patients with genital infections and in healthy controls. *Br J Vener Dis* 1970, 46:390.)

Association between antibody seroconversion and lochial colonization by *Mycoplasma hominis* in women with unexplained postpartum fever

	No. febrile women/No. studied
Antibody titer at delivery < 1:8	16/40 (40%)[*]
Seroconversion	
Yes	10/10 (100%)[†]
No	6/30 (20%)
Lochial *M. hominis*	
Yes	10/15 (67%)[‡]
No	6/25 (24%)
Antibody titer at delivery ≥ 1:8	7/50 (14%)[*]
Seroconversion	
Yes	4/26 (15%)
No	3/24 (12%)
Lochial *M. hominis*	
Yes	3/21 (14%)
No	4/29 (14%)

[*]*P*= < 0.01.
[†]*P* = < 0.001.
[‡]*P* = < 0.025.

FIGURE 3-17 Association between antibody seroconversion and lochial colonization by *Mycoplasma hominis* in women with unexplained postpartum fever. The presence of preexisting antibody to *M. hominis* protects again postpartum fever caused by *M. hominis*, even when the organism is present in lochia. This observation supports the role of the organism as a cause of postpartum fever. (Platt R, Lin J-SL, Warren JW, *et al.*: Infection with *Mycoplasma hominis* in postpartum fever. *Lancet* 1980, ii:1217–1221.)

TREATMENT

Treatment of infections due to genital mycoplasmas		
	Ureaplasma urealyticum	*Mycoplasma hominis*
Treatment of choice	Doxycycline	Doxycycline
Alternate	Erythromycin Azithromycin	Clindamycin

FIGURE 3-18 Treatment of infections due to genital mycoplasmas. Specific doses and durations of therapy depend on the site of infection.

Association between clinical response to tetracycline therapy in nongonococcal urethritis and persistence of *Ureaplasma urealyticum*		
	Posttreatment	
Pretreatment tetracycline MIC of ureaplasmas	Persistent ureaplasmas	Persistent NGU
≥ 128 µg/mL	6/6 (100%)	3/6 (50%)
≤ 32 µg/mL	1/76 (1%)	3/76 (4%)

MIC—minimal inhibitory concentration; NGU—nongonococcal urethritis.

FIGURE 3-19 Association between clinical response to tetracycline therapy in nongonococcal urethritis (NGU) and persistence of *Ureaplasma urealyticum*. Urethral infection with *U. urealyticum* resistant to the tetracyclines has been associated with treatment failure in NGU. In a study of 82 men having NGU and whose pretreatment cultures contained *U. urealyticum*, high tetracycline minimal inhibitory concentrations of ureaplasmas correlated with persistence of *U. urealyticum* and persistence of NGU after treatment with doxycycline. Such resistant cases are usually resolved by treatment with erythromycin, 500 mg four times a day for 7 days, to which the organisms are uniformly sensitive. *Trichomonas vaginalis* is a rarer cause of the syndrome of treatment failure in NGU (*see* Chapter 6). (Stimson JB, Hale J, Bowie WR, Holmes KK: Tetracycline-resistant *Ureaplasma urealyticum*: A cause of persistent nongonococcal urethritis. *Ann Intern Med* 1981, 94:192–194.)

SELECTED BIBLIOGRAPHY

Glatt AE, McCormack WM, Taylor-Robinson D: Genital mycoplasmas. Holmes KK, Mårdh P-A, Sparling PF, *et al.* (eds.): *Sexually Transmitted Diseases*, 2nd ed. New York: McGraw-Hill; 1990:279–293.

McCormack WM, Rein MF: Urethritis. *In* Mandell GL, Douglas RG, Bennett JE (eds.): *Principles and Practice of Infectious Diseases*, 4th ed. New York: Churchill Livingstone; 1995:1063–1074.

Taylor-Robinson D: *Ureaplasma urealyticum* (T-strain mycoplasma) and *Mycoplasma hominis*. *In* Mandell GL, Douglas RG, Bennett JE (eds.): *Principles and Practice of Infectious Diseases*, 4th ed. New York: Churchill Livingstone; 1995:1713–1718.

Taylor-Robinson D, McCormack WM: The genital mycoplasmas. *N Engl J Med* 1980, 302:1003-1010, 1063–1067.

CHAPTER 4

Bacterial Vaginosis

Sharon L. Hillier

CLINICAL PRESENTATION AND DIAGNOSIS

A. Diagnostic features of bacterial vaginosis: Symptoms

	Physiologic	Bacterial vaginosis
Vulvar irritation	0	0 to +
Dysuria	0	0
Odor	0	+ to +++
Discharge	+	0 to ++

B. Diagnostic features of bacterial vaginosis: Signs

	Physiologic	Bacterial vaginosis
Labial erythema	0	0
Vaginal tenderness	0	0 to ++
Discharge		
Consistency	Floccular	Homogeneous with bubbles
Color	White	Gray-white
Adherence	0	+ to +++
pH	≤ 4.5	> 4.5
Whiff test	0	+ to +++

C. Diagnostic features of bacterial vaginosis: Microscopic findings

	Physiologic	Bacterial vaginosis
Epithelial cells	Normal	Clue cells (20%–90%)
Flora	Rods	+++ coccobacilli; + motile curved rods

FIGURE 4-1 Diagnostic features of bacterial vaginosis. **A**, Symptoms. **B**, Signs. **C**, Microscopic findings. Most women presenting to their physicians with vaginal symptoms have a condition first described by Gardner and Dukes in 1955 and now known as bacterial vaginosis. Affected women are usually sexually active and complain chiefly of vaginal malodor and a mild to moderate discharge. Other vaginal infections may closely resemble bacterial vaginosis, and an accurate diagnosis depends on laboratory examination of genital specimens.

Diagnostic criteria for bacterial vaginosis

1. Homogenous discharge
2. Distinct fishy odor released immediately after mixing vaginal secretions with 10% KOH (amine whiff test)
3. Vaginal pH > 4.5
4. Clue cells and characteristic alterations of vaginal microflora on microscopy

KOH—potassium hydroxide.

FIGURE 4-2 Diagnostic criteria for bacterial vaginosis. Patients complaining of vaginal discharge and odor and having a grayish-white, thin, adherent, homogeneous discharge on speculum examination can be diagnosed with bacterial vaginosis with reasonable certainty if they meet three of the four criteria outlined in the table. Wet mount microscopy demonstrating many "clue" cells and Gram stain showing altered vaginal flora are the most specific criteria for establishing the diagnosis. (Holmes KK, Handsfield HH: Sexually transmitted diseases. *In* Isselbacher KJ, *et al.* (eds.): *Harrison's Principles of Internal Medicine*, 13th ed. New York: McGraw-Hill; 1994:538–539.)

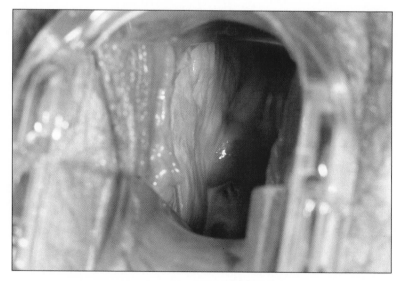

FIGURE 4-3 Speculum examination of a women with bacterial vaginosis. The discharge in bacterial vaginosis may often be subtle, presenting as a thin, homogeneous, milky discharge. Although many polymorphonuclear leukocytes can be seen in one third of women with bacterial vaginosis, there is usually no visible erythema on clinical examination. Vaginal odor is often the chief presenting complaint in affected women.

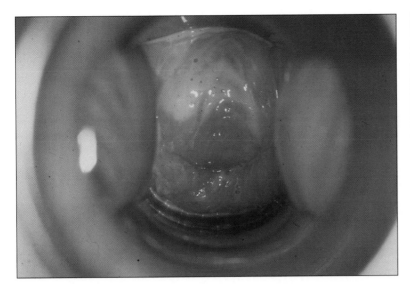

FIGURE 4-4 Speculum examination of a women with bacterial vaginosis showing adherent homogeneous discharge. Whereas the normal vaginal discharge is finely floccular, the discharge in bacterial vaginosis is homogeneous and often manifests small bubbles. The discharge is relatively thin, but, as here, it adheres to vaginal structures. An inflammatory response with erythema of the vaginal walls is usually absent. (*Courtesy of* H.L. Gardner, MD.)

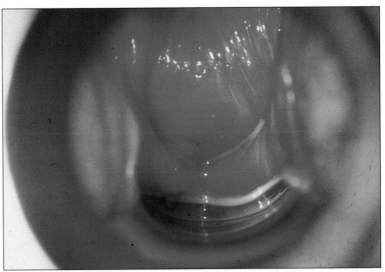

FIGURE 4-5 Speculum examination of a women with bacterial vaginosis showing little discharge. In many women, little discharge is present. Here, a very small amount of discharge has pooled in the posterior fornix. A characteristic bubble can be seen. Women with limited discharge may note vaginal odor as the only symptom of disease. The examiner should recognize that because of the adherent nature of the discharge, the discharge may be observed only as an increased light reflex returned from the vagina walls. (*Courtesy of* H.L. Gardner, MD.)

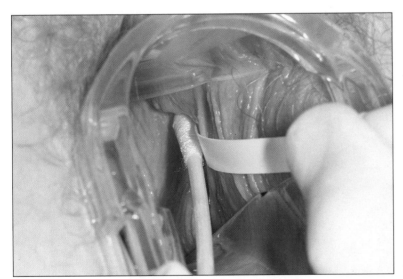

FIGURE 4-6 Measurement of vaginal pH from the lateral vaginal wall using pH paper. Measurement of vaginal pH is of clinical value because it provides an indirect measure of the number of lactobacilli present in the vagina. Vaginal lactobacilli ferment glucose to produce lactic acid, which acts to acidify the vagina and inhibit the growth of many vaginal and cervical pathogens. The pH should be measured on the vaginal wall or introitus in order to avoid contact with cervical mucus, which has a pH of 7.0. Normal vaginal pH is usually ≤ 4.5.

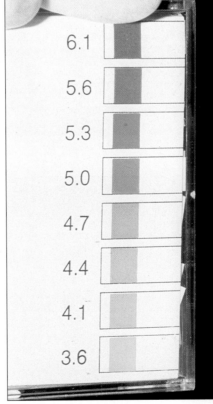

FIGURE 4-7 Measurement of vaginal pH for a women with a *Lactobacillus*-predominant vaginal flora (pH 4.1). Several types of pH paper suitable for use in the diagnosis of bacterial vaginosis are commercially available, but the most useful types are those having several gradations between pH 4 and 6. Women with bacterial vaginosis rarely have a vaginal pH < 4.7.

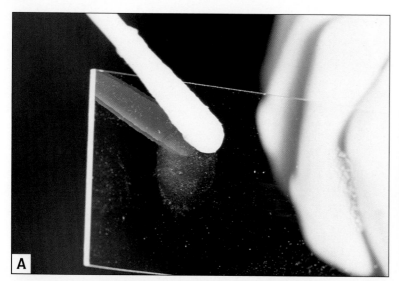

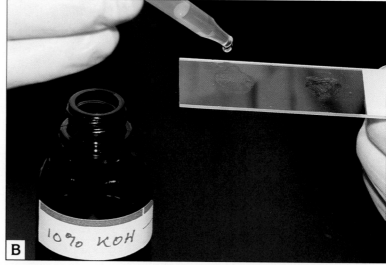

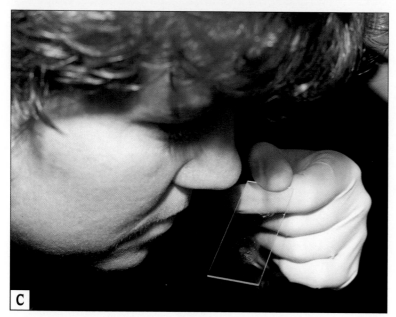

FIGURE 4-8 The amine odor test ("whiff test"). **A,** A vaginal swab is placed in 0.25 mL (250 µL) of saline to make a suspension of vaginal bacteria and cells. A drop of this saline suspension is then placed on a slide. **B,** A drop of 10% potassium hydroxide (KOH) is added to the slide, which increases the pH and results in volatilization of any amines that may be present in the vaginal fluid. **C,** The slide is sniffed for the characteristic fishy, amine odor. The volatile amines—putrescine, cadaverine, and trimethylamine—are produced by anaerobic bacteria in the vagina flora of women with bacterial vaginosis and released by KOH. A positive "whiff test" is indicative of an overgrowth of anaerobes in the vagina. A coverslip can be placed directly over the KOH wet mount for evaluation of fungal elements.

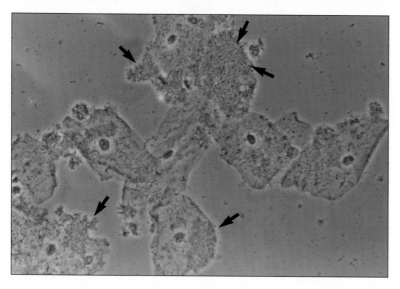

FIGURE 4-9 Microscopic examination for clue cells in vaginal fluid from a woman with bacterial vaginosis. A second wet mount preparation of vaginal fluid is examined under high-power (× 400) microscopy for clue cells (*arrows*). Clue cells are squamous epithelial cells having a granular appearance and indistinct cell borders obscured by adherent microorganisms. Clue cells are the single best clinical indicator of bacterial vaginosis and result from the attachment of *Gardnerella vaginalis*, anaerobic gram-negative rods, and gram-positive cocci to the cells. If at least one in five epithelial cells in the vaginal fluid is a clue cell, the specimen is categorized as clue cell positive. A few clue cells may be present in the vaginal fluid of women without bacterial vaginosis, caused by lactobacilli that bind to vaginal epithelial cells.

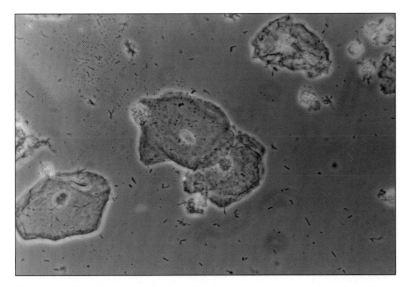

FIGURE 4-10 Microscopic examination of vaginal squamous epithelial cells from a women with normal vaginal flora. The small rods in the vaginal fluid are lactobacilli. The epithelial cell at the top of the field has edges that have turned back on themselves. These cells can be mistaken for clue cells when the microscope has not been properly focused. (Original magnification, × 400.)

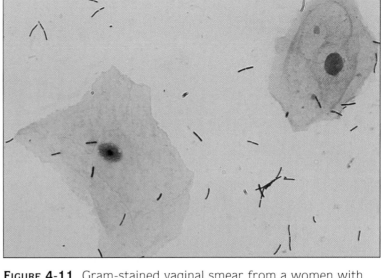

FIGURE 4-11 Gram-stained vaginal smear from a women with *Lactobacillus*-predominant vaginal flora. A normal *Lactobacillus*-predominant vaginal flora is composed of > 95% lactobacilli, which are generally present at concentrations of 10^6 organisms per gram of vaginal fluid. Other organisms, including staphylococci, coliforms, and anaerobes, are also usually present, but these organisms usually occur at 100- to 1000-fold lower concentrations than do the lactobacilli.

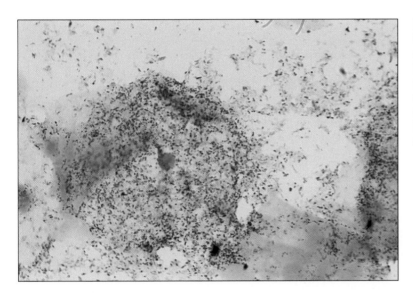

FIGURE 4-12 Gram-stained vaginal smear from a women with bacterial vaginosis. A large clue cell with edges covered by bacteria is visible in the center of the field. The *Lactobacillus* morphotypes have been replaced by small gram-negative anaerobic rods (*Prevotella, Porphyromonas, Bacteroides*) and small gram-variable rods (*Gardnerella vaginalis*). Mycoplasmas lack cells walls and therefore are not visible by Gram stain. The epithelial cell at the bottom of the field is a squamous epithelial cell without attached bacteria.

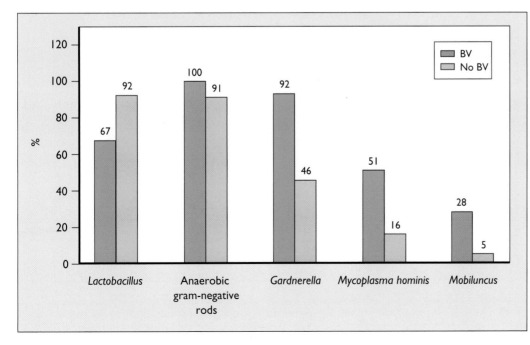

FIGURE 4-13 Frequency of vaginal microorganisms in women with and without bacterial vaginosis. The *orange bars* indicate women with bacterial vaginosis (BV), and the *yellow bars*, those without the condition. The microorganisms always present in women with clinical signs of bacterial vaginosis include anaerobic gram-negative rods (*Prevotella, Prophyromonas, Bacteroides,* and/or *Fusobacterium* spp) and *Gardnerella vaginalis*. *Mycoplasma hominis* is present in more than half of women with this condition, and *Mobiluncus* is present in 30% to 60% of women with bacterial vaginosis. By comparison, women with *Lactobacillus*-predominant flora are less likely to be colonized by these microorganisms, and when these microorganisms are present, they occur at lower concentrations than those observed in women with bacterial vaginosis.

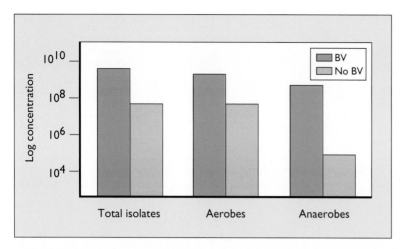

FIGURE 4-14 Concentration of aerobic and anaerobic bacteria in the vaginal flora of women with and without bacterial vaginosis. Whereas women without bacterial vaginosis (BV) usually have approximately 10^6 organisms per gram of vaginal fluid (*orange bars*), women with bacterial vaginosis usually have more than 10^9 organisms per gram of vaginal fluid (*red bars*). There is a 100-fold increase in the number of aerobic microorganisms, such as *Gardnerella vaginalis*, and a 10,000-fold increase in the concentration of anaerobic bacteria in women with bacterial vaginosis compared with women with *Lactobacillus*-predominant flora.

Standardized scoring criteria for Gram stain diagnosis of bacterial vaginosis

	Points assigned				
Morphotype	0	1	2	3	4
Lactobacillus	4+	3+	2+	1+	0
Anaerobic rods/*Gardnerella*	0	1+	2+	3+	4+
Mobiluncus	0	1–2+	3–4+	...	...

4+ = > 30 morphotypes/1000 × field 3+ = 6–30 morphotypes/1000 × field 2+ = 1–5 morphotypes/1000 × field 1+ = < 1 morphotypes/1000 × field	**Score** 0–3 = Normal 4–6 = Intermediate 7–10 = Bacterial vaginosis

FIGURE 4-15 Standardized scoring criteria for the Gram stain diagnosis of bacterial vaginosis. These criteria, developed by Nugent and colleagues, yield a score of 0 to 10 based on the relative prevalence of three bacterial morphotypes: large gram-positive rods (lactobacilli), small gram-negative to gram-variable rods (anaerobic rods and *Gardnerella*), and curved rods (*Mobiluncus*). (Nugent RP, Krohn MA, Hillier SL: Reliability of diagnosing bacterial vaginosis is improved by a standardized method of Gram stain interpretation. *J Clin Microbiol* 1991, 29:297–301.)

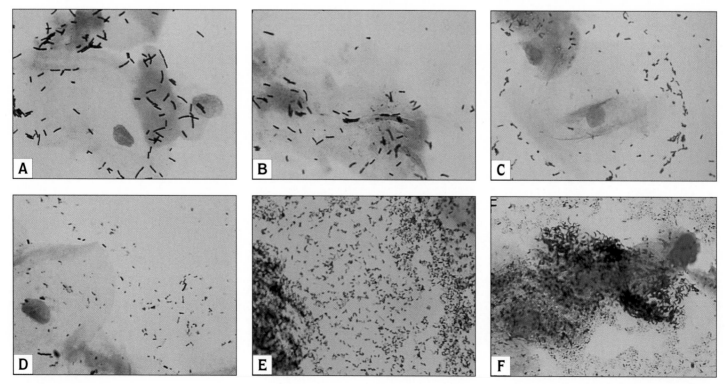

FIGURE 4-16 Gram-stained vaginal smears evaluated by the Nugent method. **A**, Normal smear; score 0. **B**, Normal smear; score 2. **C**, Intermediate smear; score 4. **D**, Intermediate smear; score 6. **E**, Bacterial vaginosis smear; score 8. **F**, Bacterial vaginosis smear; score 10. (Nugent RP, Krohn MA, Hillier SL: Reliability of diagnosing bacterial vaginosis is improved by a standardized method of Gram stain interpretation. *J Clin Microbiol* 1991, 29:297–301.)

PATHOPHYSIOLOGY

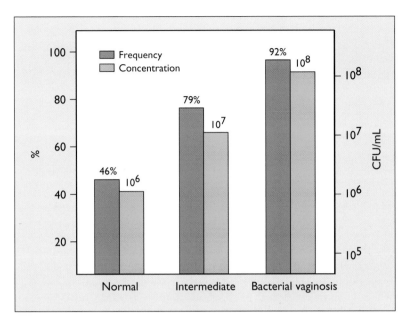

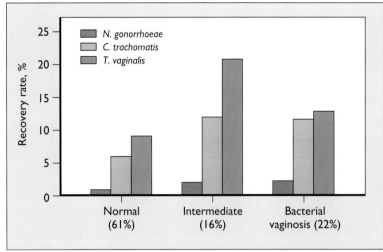

FIGURE 4-17 Frequency and concentration of *Gardnerella vaginalis* among women with normal, intermediate, or bacterial vaginosis vaginal Gram stains. Before the recognition of the importance of anaerobes in its etiology, bacterial vaginosis was called *Gardnerella vaginalis* vaginitis. This misconception has led to the erroneous assumption that all women with *G. vaginalis* have bacterial vaginosis. Although over 90% of women with bacterial vaginosis have > 10,000 colony-forming units (CFU) of *G. vaginalis* per gram of vaginal fluid, about half of sexually active women without this syndrome have high levels of this organism. For this reason, routine vaginal cultures for *G. vaginalis* have no clinical utility for the diagnosis of bacterial vaginosis. (Hillier SL, Krohn MA, Rabe LK, *et al.*: The normal vaginal flora, H_2O_2-producing lactobacilli, and bacterial vaginosis in pregnant women. *Clin Infect Dis* 1993, 16(suppl 4):S273–S281.)

FIGURE 4-18 Association of vaginal flora pattern with sexually transmitted disease pathogens. Gram-stained vaginal smears from 7918 pregnant women were evaluated by the Nugent method. Women with intermediate flora were more likely than women with normal flora to be infected with *Chlamydia trachomatis* (*orange bars*) or *Neisseria gonorrhoeae* (*red bars*). Women with intermediate vaginal flora were the most likely to be infected by *Trichomonas vaginalis* (*purple bars*). Asterisks indicate significant differences compared with normal ($P < 0.001$). (Hillier SL, Krohn MA, Nugent RP, Gibbs RS: Characteristics of three vaginal flora patterns assessed by Gram stain among pregnant women: Vaginal Infections and Prematurity Study Group. *Am J Obstet Gynecol* 1992, 166:938–944.)

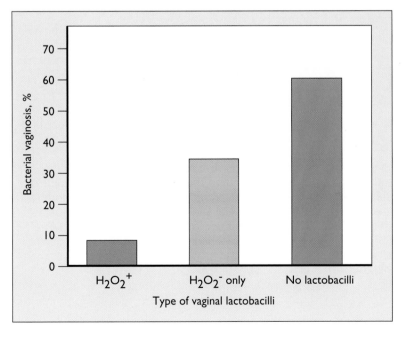

FIGURE 4-19 Association of vaginal flora pattern with vaginal colonization by hydrogen peroxide (H_2O_2)–producing lactobacilli. Women colonized by lactobacilli that produce H_2O_2 are the most likely to have a normal *Lactobacillus*-predominant vaginal flora, whereas one third of women having only H_2O_2-negative lactobacilli and 60% of women with no vaginal lactobacilli have bacterial vaginosis. (Hillier SL, *et al.*: The relationship of hydrogen peroxide–producing lactobacilli to bacterial vaginosis and genital microflora in pregnant women. *Obstet Gynecol* 1992, 79:369–373.)

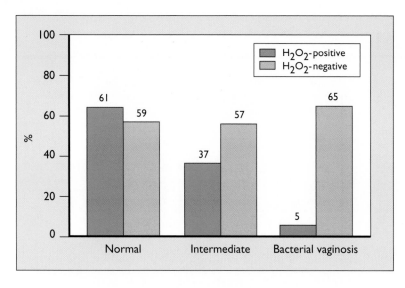

FIGURE 4-20 Prevalence of hydrogen peroxide (H_2O_2)–positive and –negative lactobacilli in women with different vaginal flora patterns. Almost two thirds of women having *Lactobacillus*-predominant smears are colonized by H_2O_2-producing lactobacilli, whereas only one in 20 women with bacterial vaginosis has H_2O_2-producing lactobacilli. (Hillier SL, Krohn MA, Rabe LK, *et al.*: The normal vaginal flora, H_2O_2-producing lactobacilli, and bacterial vaginosis in pregnant women. *Clin Infect Dis* 1993, 16(suppl 4):S273–S281.)

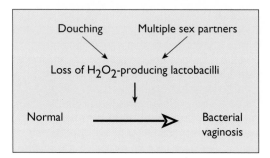

FIGURE 4-21 Pathogenesis of bacterial vaginosis. Although the mechanism is uncertain, it is known that women who douche routinely or have multiple sexual partners are at increased risk for loss of vaginal lactobacilli. These behaviors likely cause a disruption in the vaginal ecosystem, which may lead to loss of vaginal lactobacilli. Women with no lactobacilli or only hydrogen peroxide (H_2O_2)–negative lactobacilli are four to seven times more likely to develop bacterial vaginosis than are women colonized by H_2O_2-producing lactobacilli.

A. Support for sexual transmission of bacterial vaginosis	B. Arguments against an exclusively sexual transmission of bacterial vaginosis
1. BV is more prevalent among women with greater numbers of recent sexual partners. 2. BV is more prevalent in populations with a higher prevalence of other STDs. 3. Symptoms first develop in many women shortly after they become sexually active or have unprotected sex with a new partner. 4. Longitudinal studies have linked having multiple sexual partners to acquisition of bacterial vaginosis. 5. Vaginal recolonization with *Gardnerella vaginalis* is far more common in women reexposed to untreated male partners than to those who are not. 6. *G. vaginalis* is recovered from the urethras of > 80% of male sexual partners of infected women, and the isolates are almost always of the same biotype.	1. *Gardnerella vaginalis* and other organisms associated with BV can be isolated from prepubescent and sexually inactive women. 2. Syndrome of BV has been recognized in virgins. 3. Recurrences are observed in the absence of sexual reexposure. 4. Initial, simultaneous treatment of sexual partners cannot be shown to reduce recurrence rates. 5. Organisms associated with BV can be cultured from the rectum, from which site they might colonize the vagina.

BV—bacterial vaginosis.

BV—bacterial vaginosis; STD—sexually transmitted disease.

FIGURE 4-22 Role of sexual transmission in bacterial vaginosis. Bacterial vaginosis (BV) was initially described in sexually active women and is common in populations with a high prevalence of other sexually transmitted diseases, but the precise contribution of sexual transmission to acquisition of this condition remains controversial. Having multiple sexual partners is associated with acquiring BV, but this behavior may have a nonspecific effect on vaginal flora and predispose to BV by reducing the numbers of lactobacilli rather than transmitting specific organisms. Arguing against sexual transmission is that fact that BV occurs in virgins and sexually inactive women and that simultaneous treatment of sexual partners does not reduce recurrence rates. **A**, Support for sexual transmission of bacterial vaginosis. **B**, Arguments against an exclusively sexual transmission of bacterial vaginosis. (Bump RC, Buesching WJ III: Bacterial vaginosis in virginal and sexually active adolescent females: Evidence against exclusive sexual transmission. *Am J Obstet Gynecol* 1988, 158:935–939.)

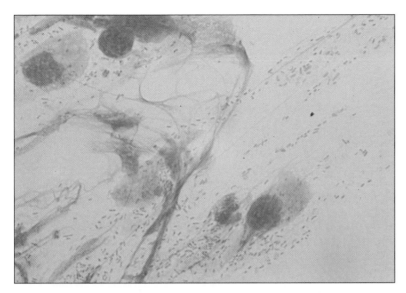

FIGURE 4-23 Gram-stained urethral smear from a man whose sexual partner had bacterial vaginosis. Men whose partners have bacterial vaginosis are sometimes heavily colonized in the urethra by anaerobic gram-negative rods, *Gardnerella*, and *Mobiluncus*. Nevertheless, treatment of the male sexual partner is rarely indicated because the recurrence of bacterial vaginosis is not decreased for women whose sexual partners are treated. (Lugo-Miro VI, Green M, Mazur L: Comparison of different metronidazole regimens for bacterial vaginosis. *JAMA* 1992, 268:92–95.)

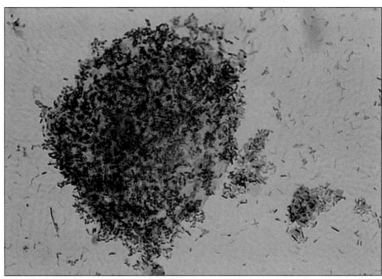

FIGURE 4-24 Gram-stained vaginal smear from a woman having bacterial vaginosis with a predominance of *Mobiluncus curtisii*. *Mobiluncus* ("moving hooks") are curved gram-variable rods that may be seen as rapidly motile forms in the saline wet mount. The clue cell in the center of the field is coated with *M. curtisii*, which tends to stain gram-positive. *Mobiluncus* is difficult to isolate from routine cultures because of the extreme oxygen sensitivity of this obligate anaerobe. This organism is rarely observed in women without bacterial vaginosis.

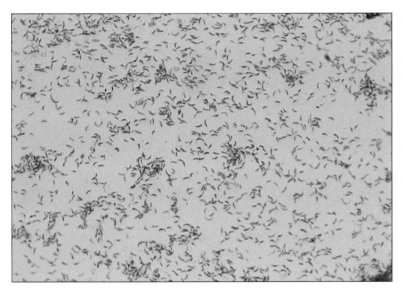

FIGURE 4-25 Gram stain of a pure culture of *Mobiluncus curtisii*. This organism is usually about 1 μm in length and has a curved diphtheroid appearance. *M. curtisii* is resistant to metronidazole *in vitro* but is usually eradicated following treatment of bacterial vaginosis with oral or vaginal metronidazole.

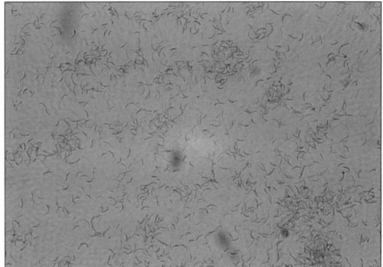

FIGURE 4-26 Gram stain of a pure culture of *Mobiluncus mulieris*. This species of *Mobiluncus* usually stains more gram-negative and is larger (2 to 2.5 μm) than *Mobiluncus curtisii*. This species is more susceptible to metronidazole than is *M. curtisii*, but success of therapy does not differ based on the species of *Mobiluncus* present in the vagina.

TREATMENT

Regimens for the treatment of bacterial vaginosis

Oral regimens
  Metronidazole 500 mg 2 times a day × 7 days
  Metronidazole 250 mg 3 times a day × 7 days
  Metronidazole 2 g as a single dose*
  Clindamycin 300 mg 2 times a day × 7 days[†]
  Cephalexin 250 mg 4 times a day × 7 days[‡]
  Cefadroxil 500 mg 2 times a day × 7 days[†]

Vaginal regimens
  Clindamycin 2% vaginal cream 5 g every night × 7 days
  Metronidazole 0.75% vaginal gel 5 g 2 times a day × 5 days

*Equivalence of this regimen to the 1-week courses remains controversial.
[†]Limited clinical data.
[‡]Principally anecdotal data.

FIGURE 4-27 Regimens for the treatment of bacterial vaginosis. Therapies for bacterial vaginosis are supported by varying amounts of data. Although a recent meta-analysis supported the use of single-dose oral metronidazole therapy, considerable data suggest that the failure rate is lower with a 1-week course. The use of cephalexin was originally described by Gardner and the value of cefadroxil is supported by a single study, but the precise mechanism for the efficacy of the first-generation cephalosporins remains undefined. Clindamycin has the advantage of demonstrated safety in pregnancy. The topical regimens are as effective as the oral ones. (Lugo-Miro VI, Green M, Mazur L: Comparison of different metronidazole regimens for bacterial vaginosis. *JAMA* 1992, 268:92–95. Gardner HL, Dukes CD: *Haemophilus vaginalis* vaginitis: A newly defined specific infection previously classified "nonspecific" vaginitis. *Am J Obstet Gynecol* 1995, 699:962. Wathne B, Hovelius B, Holst E: Cefadroxil as an alternative to metronidazole in the treatment of bacterial vaginosis. *Scand J Infect Dis* 1989, 21:585–586. Greaves WL, Chungfung J, Morris B, *et al.*: Clindamycin versus metronidazole in the treatment of bacterial vaginosis. *Obstet Gynecol* 1988, 72:799–802.)

Efficacy of clindamycin and metronidazole for treatment of bacterial vaginosis

Agent	Route	Dosage	Clinical efficacy
Clindamycin	V	5 g 2% once a day × 7 days	82%
	V	5 g 2% once a day × 3 days	82%
Metronidazole	O	500 mg 2 times a day × 7 days	80%
	V	5 g 0.75% 2 times a day × 5 days	71%–73%

O—oral; V—vaginal.

FIGURE 4-28 Efficacy of clindamycin and metronidazole for treatment of bacterial vaginosis. Oral metronidazole has been compared to intravaginal clindamycin cream in four double-blind placebo-controlled trials. In these four studies, 197 (82%) of 213 women who were treated with clindamycin cream and 161 (80%) of 202 metronidazole-treated women were cured after 1 month. One small study suggests that 3 days of intravaginal clindamycin is also 82% effective. Intravaginal metronidazole gel was 71% to 73% effective in two placebo-controlled trials. (Schmitt C, Sobel J, Meriwether C. Bacterial vaginosis: Treatment with clindamycin cream versus oral metronidazole. *Obstet Gynecol* 1993, 79:1020–1023. Andres FJ, Parker R, Hosein I, *et al.*: Clindamycin vaginal cream versus oral metronidazole in the treatment of bacterial vaginosis: A prospective, double-blind study. *South Med J* 1992, 85:1077–1080. Arrendondo JL, Higuero F, Hidalgo F, *et al.*: Clindamycin vaginal cream versus oral metronidazole in the treatment of bacterial vaginosis. *Arch AIDS STD Res* 1992, 6:183–195. Fischbach F, Petersen EE, Weissenbacker ER, *et al.*: Efficacy of clindamycin vaginal cream versus oral metronidazole in the treatment of bacterial vaginosis. *Obstet Gynecol* 1993, 82:405–410. Dhar J, Arya OP, Timmins DJ, *et al.*: Treatment of bacterial vaginosis with a three day course of 2% clindamycin vaginal cream: A pilot study. *Genitourin Med* 1994, 70:121-123. Hillier SL, Lipinski C, Briselden AM, *et al.*: Efficacy of intravaginal 0.75% metronidazole gel for the treatment of bacterial vaginosis. *Obstet Gynecol* 1993, 81:963–967. Livengood CH, McGregor JA, Soper DE, *et al.*: Bacterial vaginosis: Efficacy and safety of intravaginal metronidazole treatment. *Am J Obstet Gynecol* 1994, 170:759–764.)

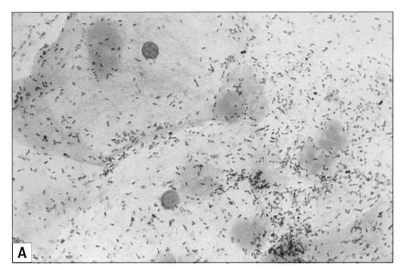

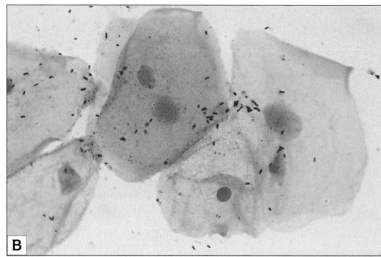

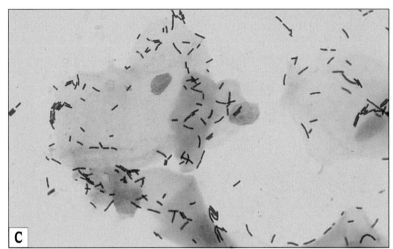

FIGURE 4-29 Effect of oral metronidazole treatment on the vaginal microflora of a women with bacterial vaginosis. **A,** Before treatment, this woman had an elevated vaginal pH, clue cells, and amine odor. Her vaginal smear had a score of 8, which was consistent with bacterial vaginosis. She was treated with 500 mg of oral metronidazole, twice daily for 7 days. **B,** After 2 days of therapy, anaerobic gram-variable and gram-negative rods had decreased in numbers, but lactobacilli had not become predominant. **C,** After 1 week of oral metronidazole therapy, a predominant vaginal *Lactobacillus* flora was restored, and the clinical signs of bacterial vaginosis had resolved.

Treatment of bacterial vaginosis with topical triple-sulfa cream

	Cures	
	8–10 days	21 days
Tinidazole + triple-sulfa	14/15 (93%)	8/8 (100%)
Tinidazole + base	15/15 (100%)	10/11 (91%)*
Placebo + triple-sulfa	12/16 (75%)	4/9 (44%)*
Placebo + base	4/11 (36%)	2/5 (40%)

*$P = 0.014.$

FIGURE 4-30 Treatment of bacterial vaginosis with topical triple-sulfa cream. Although triple-sulfa cream has been advertised extensively as treatment for bacterial vaginosis, a double-blind study has suggested otherwise. Women with bacterial vaginosis were treated with an oral imidazole (tinidazole) or placebo and vaginal triple-sulfa cream or placebo. When subjects were evaluated 21 days after treatment, there was a tendency toward a higher failure rate with the topical regimen. (Piot P, Van Dyck E, Godts P, *et al.*: A placebo-controlled, double-blind comparison of tinidazole and triple sulfonamide cream for the treatment of nonspecific vaginitis. *Am J Obstet Gynecol* 1983, 147:85–89.)

Ecologic treatment of bacterial vaginosis

	Cures*
0.92% acetic acid jelly, 5 mL 2 times a day	3/17 (18%)
100 µg/g dienestrol cream, 5 mg 2 times a day	1/16 (6%)
Yogurt, 5 mL 2 times a day	1/14 (7%)
Metronidazole, 500 mg by mouth 2 times a day	13/14 (93%)

*7 days of therapy, assessed at 4 wks posttreatment.

FIGURE 4-31 Treatment of bacterial vaginosis by replacing vaginal lactobacilli. Some investigators have attempted to treat bacterial vaginosis by replacing the lactobacillary flora. Lay publications have suggested the home remedy of yogurt douching, but an early study (shown here) suggested a lack of value for this approach. Topical treatment with microbiologically better-defined preparations of lactobacilli are under study. (Fredricsson B, Englund K, Weintraub L, *et al.*: Ecological treatment of bacterial vaginosis. *Lancet* 1987, 1:276. Neri A, Sabah G, Samra Z: Bacterial vaginosis in pregnancy treated with yoghurt. *Acta Obstet Gynecol Scand* 1993, 72:17–19.)

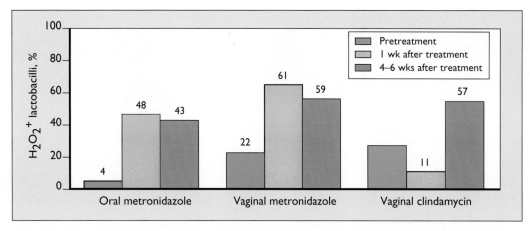

FIGURE 4-32 Effect of treatment regimens for bacterial vaginosis on vaginal colonization by hydrogen peroxide (H_2O_2)–producing lactobacilli. Metronidazole is not active against lactobacilli. Within 1 week after treatment of bacterial vaginosis with oral or vaginal metronidazole, there is a 48% increase in vaginal colonization by H_2O_2-producing lactobacilli. These H_2O_2-producing lactobacilli are still present at 4 to 6 weeks after therapy. Clindamycin is active against lactobacilli, and 1 week after intravaginal clindamycin therapy, there is a slight decrease in H_2O_2-producing lactobacilli, followed by an increase at 4 to 6 weeks after therapy. At 4 to 6 weeks after treatment, the number of women colonized by H_2O_2-producing lactobacilli is similar regardless of which therapy is used. (Agnew KJ, Hillier SL: The effect of treatment regimens for vaginitis and cervicitis on vaginal colorization by lactobacilli. *Sex Transm Dis* 1995, 22:No 5.)

Lack of efficacy of alternative treatments of bacterial vaginosis		
Class	**Form and use**	**Efficacy**
Disinfectant		
Chlorhexidine	Pessary	79%
Povidone-iodine	Pessary 2 times a day × 14 days	20%
Acidifier		
Lactic acid	Suppository; gel	20%–80%
Acetate	Gel; tampon	18%–38%
Yogurt		
Commercial, pH < 4.5	Douche, 10–15 mL 2 times a day × 14 days	88%
Commercial	Daily	7%
Lactobacillus		
Vivag (Pharmac-Vinci A/S, Denmark)	Suppository 2 times a day × 6 days	43%

FIGURE 4-33 Lack of efficacy of alternative treatments for bacterial vaginosis. Some patients with bacterial vaginosis have used therapies based on acid gels, *Lactobacillus* products, or disinfectants to avoid exposure to systemic antibiotics. Although this approach has been advocated by some authors, well-controlled clinical trials have found little benefit for these treatment modalities. Disinfectants and vaginal acidifiers can suppress the vaginal microorganisms that cause bacterial vaginosis, but these organisms are quickly reestablished in the vagina after use of the acidifier or disinfectant is discontinued. *Lactobacillus* in the form of suppositories or yogurt douches has had variable results. The lack of efficacy of *Lactobacillus* is probably attributable to the inability of these strains to colonize the vagina. (Neri A, Rabinerson D, Kaplan B: Bacterial vaginosis: Drugs versus alternative treatment. *Obstet Gynecol Surv* 1994, 49:809–813. Boeke AIP, Dekker JH, van Eijk JTM, *et al.*: Effect of lactic acid suppositories compared with oral metronidazole and placebo in bacterial vaginosis: A randomized clinical trial. *Genitourin Med* 1993, 69:388–392.)

CHAPTER 5

Pelvic Inflammatory Disease

Per-Anders Mårdh, Birger Möller,
Jorma Paavonen, Lars Weström

EPIDEMIOLOGY

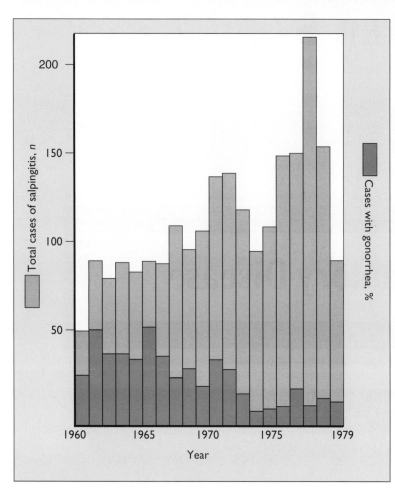

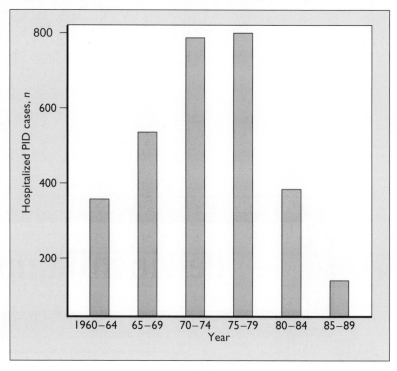

FIGURE 5-1 Annual number of gonococcal and nongonococcal cases of pelvic inflammatory disease (PID) hospitalized at a Swedish clinic between 1960 and 1979. The number of PID cases (confirmed by laparoscopy) increased during this period, despite a decrease in the absolute number of gonococcal cases. The nongonococcal PID cases were later found to be caused generally by *Chlamydia trachomatis*.

FIGURE 5-2 Annual number of hospitalized PID cases at a Swedish clinic between 1960 and 1989. Following a steady increase until the late 1970s, the number of PID cases has decreased rapidly in recent years. This decline is likely due to the decreased incidence of gonorrhea and, later, genital chlamydial infection seen in Sweden since that time. Gonorrhea is now a rare disease in this country. The prevalence of *Chlamydia trachomatis* is now in the range of 1% to 2% in young, sexually active groups.

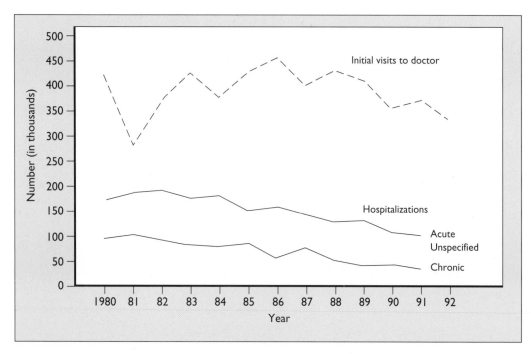

FIGURE 5-3 Annual number of cases of PID in women aged 15 to 44 years in the United States between 1980 and 1992. Current estimates from industrialized countries indicate an annual incidence of PID of 9.5 to 14 cases per 1000 women in their fertile years. In the United States, approximately 1 million women per year have an episode of symptomatic PID, with 250,000 to 300,000 being hospitalized. The number of hospitalized cases, which likely represents more severe cases, declined through the 1980s in the United States, but initial visits to physicians' offices (new episodes) remained steady. (*Adapted from* Division of STD/HIV Prevention: *Sexually Transmitted Disease Surveillance, 1992.* Atlanta: Centers for Disease Control and Prevention; 1993:26.)

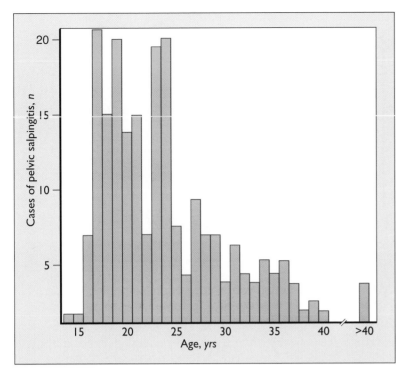

FIGURE 5-4 Age distribution of consecutive cases of salpingitis hospitalized at a Swedish gynecologic clinic. PID cases admitted to hospital are likely to represent cases with more severe disease. PID is a disease of young women, with 75% of cases occurring in women < 25 years of age. Many get their first PID episode during their teen years.

The woman at risk for PID		
	Risk indicator	Risk factor
Young age	+	+
Urban residence	+	-
Socioeconomic status	+	-
Substance abuse (including smoking)	+	+
Iatrogenic factors	-	+
Sex behavior	+	+
Douching	-	+
Acquisition of a sexually transmitted disease	-	+

FIGURE 5-5 Risk factors for PID. Important risk factors for the development of PID other than young age include multiple sexual partners or frequent intercourse with a single partner, as well as cigarette smoking or other substance abuse. Iatrogenic factors include invasive procedures involving the cervical canal, such as dilatation and curettage, insertion of an intrauterine device, or abortion, which open the upper genital tract to bacterial invasion. The acquisition of any sexually transmitted disease (STD) serves as a marker for acquisition of an STD specifically related to PID, such as gonorrhea, chlamydia infection, or bacterial vaginosis. (Rein MF: Therapeutic decisions in the treatment of sexually transmitted diseases: An overview. *Sex Transm Dis* 1981, 8:93–99.)

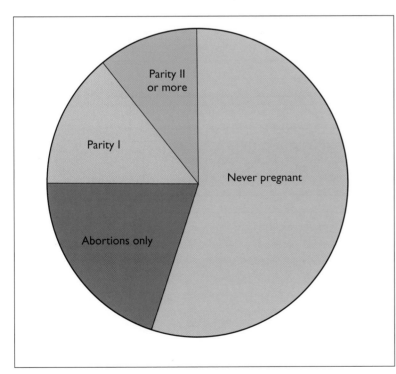

FIGURE 5-6 Parity at first episode of PID. Approximately 75% of women with salpingitis have never been pregnant. PID is very uncommon during pregnancy itself, but when present constitutes a medical/surgical emergency. PID during pregnancy is called *secondary salpingitis* and results from spread of infection from the intra-abdominal cavity to the fallopian tubes, not from the lower genital tract.

Severity of salpingitis (assessed laparoscopically) and duration of symptoms before seeking medical care, 1977–1984			
	Symptoms		
Severity	**≤ 2 days**	**> 3 days**	**Odds ratio**
None	56	232	Reference
Mild	39	131	0.81*
Moderate	34	168	1.2*
Severe	10	121	2.9*

*P for a trend < 0.01.

FIGURE 5-7 Severity of salpingitis (assessed laparoscopically) and duration of symptoms. Women with longer duration of symptoms before seeking medical care are more likely to have severe disease when assessed laparoscopically. Women often delay seeking medical care for symptoms of PID. Symptoms may be very mild or go unnoticed ("silent PID"), or their onset may be slow. In addition, mild or nonspecific symptoms may cause the physician to miss the diagnosis. Delay in treatment may place the woman at risk of severe complications, such as pelvic abscess formation.

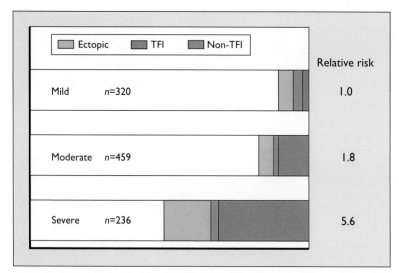

FIGURE 5-8 Severity of PID in women presenting with first-episode PID. In a series of 1015 women presenting with first-episode PID, the severity of disease was graded laparoscopically. Most women presented initially with moderately severe disease. Those with severe PID had a higher frequency of complications, including ectopic pregnancy, tubal factor infertility (TFI), and infertility related to other factors (non-TFI).

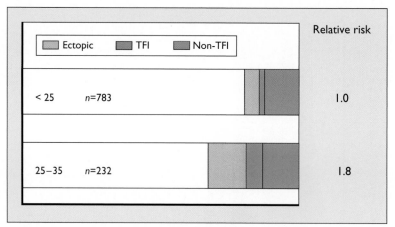

FIGURE 5-9 Age of patients presenting with first-episode PID. Of 1015 women presenting with their first episode of PID, three quarters were under age 25 years. Those over age 25 had a higher risk of presenting with complications, including ectopic pregnancy, tubal factor infertility (TFI), and infertility related to other factors (non-TFI).

PID and contraceptives

Method	Relative risk
None	1
Oral contraceptives	0.3
Intrauterine device	1.5
Barrier	0.6

FIGURE 5-10 Association between PID and contraceptive practice. The relative risk of PID in sexually active women, aged 20 to 29 years, using different contraceptive methods is outlined. The use of oral contraceptives may influence the course of both gonococcal and genital chlamydial infections. The pill may protect from ascending infection by *Chlamydia trachomatis*, but not by *Neisseria gonorrhoeae*. Whether the use of oral contraceptives increases the rate of acquisition of sexually transmitted diseases (STDs) (*ie*, by hormonal influence) or whether the increased rate of STDs with this method is related to sexual behavior (*ie*, by obviating the use of barrier contraceptives or by increasing the number of sexual partners) is unclear. Users of intrauterine devices (IUDs) have a higher risk of PID, especially in the first few months after insertion. The magnitude of this risk was previously overestimated but is now low with the modern IUDs currently available. Barrier contraceptives also decrease the risk of PID. (Juhlin L: Influence of contraceptive estrogen pills on sexual behavior and the spread of gonorrhea. *Br J Vener Dis* 1969, 45:321–324.)

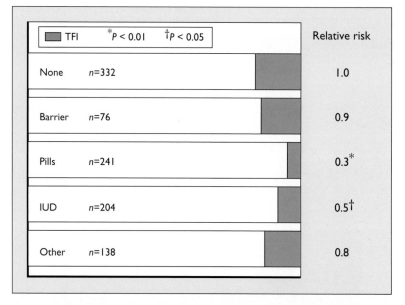

FIGURE 5-11 Contraceptive practice in women presenting with first-episode PID. Among 1015 women, users of oral contraceptives or intrauterine devices had a significantly greater risk of developing PID than users of barrier contraceptives. (IUD—intrauterine device; TFI—tubal factor infertility.)

Repeated episodes of PID	
Infections, *n*	% of women
1	80.9%
2	12.9%
≥ 3	6.2%

FIGURE 5-12 Recurrence of PID. Among a study population of patients hospitalized with PID, 20% had had more than one prior episode of PID. Reasons for recurrence include reinfection by the woman's sexual partner (failure to treat epidemiologically), inadequate therapy permitting relapse, postinfectious tubal damage rendering them more vulnerable to infection, and persistence of risk factors that placed the woman at risk initially.

CLINICAL PRESENTATION

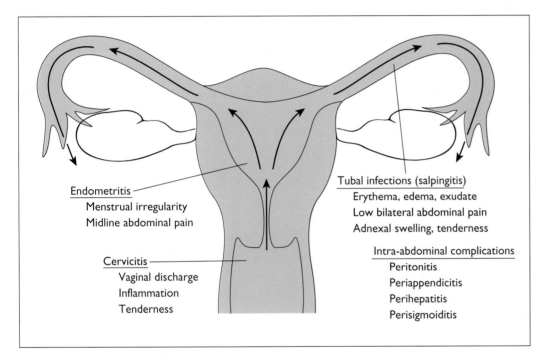

Endometritis
Menstrual irregularity
Midline abdominal pain

Cervicitis
Vaginal discharge
Inflammation
Tenderness

Tubal infections (salpingitis)
Erythema, edema, exudate
Low bilateral abdominal pain
Adnexal swelling, tenderness

Intra-abdominal complications
Peritonitis
Periappendicitis
Perihepatitis
Perisigmoiditis

FIGURE 5-13 Sequence of spread of PID. As infection ascends the genital tract, the evolution of symptoms classically proceeds from a mucopurulent discharge caused by cervicitis (possibly associated with dysuria or proctitis), to midline abdominal pain and abnormal vaginal bleeding caused by endometritis, to low bilateral abdominal and pelvic pain caused by salpingitis, with nausea and vomiting and abdominal tenderness due to direct spread of infection to the peritoneum and abdominal organs. This pattern of symptoms varies widely among patients, and disease may be symptomless. The preceding lower genital tract infection may be very slight or pass unnoticed. The onset of low, bilateral abdominal pain is usually regarded as the first symptom of ascending infection and salpingitis. Experimental data in animals confirm that organisms reach the fallopian tubes by ascending through the lumen of the genital tract rather than by hematogenous or lymphatic spread.

Cervicitis

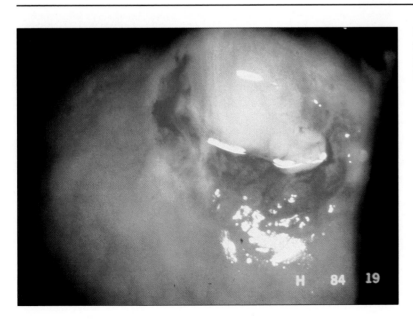

FIGURE 5-14 Colposcopic view of mucopurulent cervicitis in a woman with PID due to *Chlamydia trachomatis*. The findings include an endocervical mucopus, erythema, edema, and easily induced mucosal bleeding (friability).

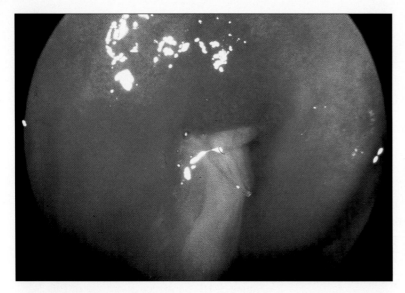

FIGURE 5-15 Colposcopic view of mucopurulent cervicitis in a patient with an intrauterine device (IUD). This patient was culture-positive for *Chlamydia trachomatis* and *Neisseria gonorrhoeae*. The insertion of an IUD increases the risk of PID in high-risk women. The association of IUDs with PID has made previous episodes of PID or a pattern of sexual behavior involving multiple partners a relative contra-indication to use of this method of contraception. IUDs have also been associated with actinomycotic infection of the fallopian tubes, although the precise risk related to IUD use remains unclear. (Scully RE, Mark EJ, McNeely WF, McNeely BU: Case records of the Massachusetts General Hospital: Case 10-1992. A 41-year-old woman with a swollen left knee, pelvic mass, and bilateral hydronephrosis. *N Engl J Med* 1992, 326:692–699.)

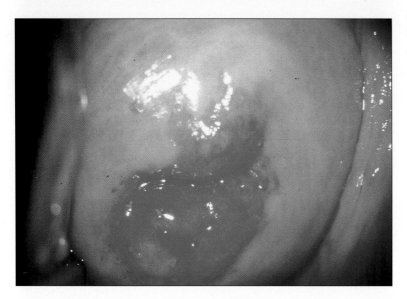

FIGURE 5-16 Severe cervical edema and friability in a patient with chlamydial cervicitis. In this patient, mucopurulent cervical discharge is not observed.

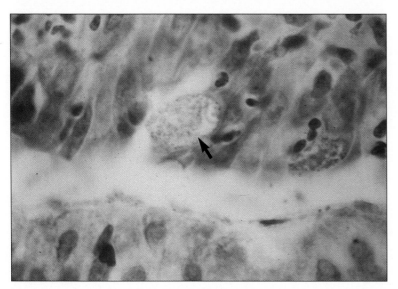

FIGURE 5-17 Histologic examination of cervical canal in cervicitis. The finding of chlamydial inclusions (*arrow*) in the columnar epithelium is pathognomonic.

Endometritis

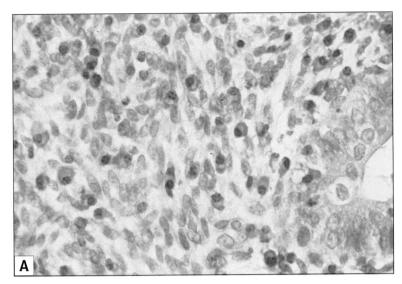

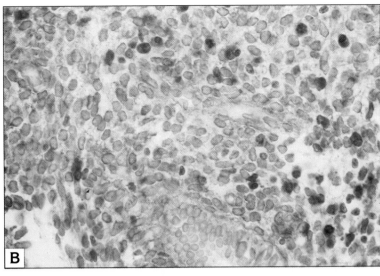

FIGURE 5-18 Histopathologic findings of plasma cell endometritis in PID. **A,** Hematoxylin-eosin staining. **B,** Immunoperoxidase staining (brown) showing IgG-positive plasma cells. The high number of plasma cells indicates severe endometritis. Studies have shown a good correlation between the presence of plasma cell endometritis and laparoscopically proven PID.

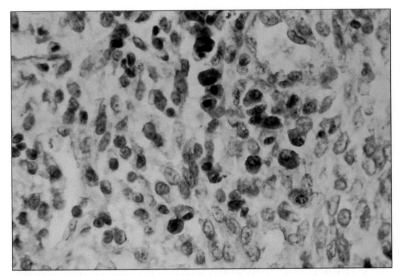

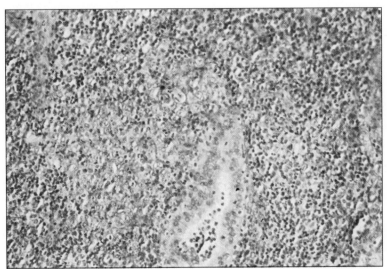

FIGURE 5-19 Chlamydial endometritis showing intense plasma cell infiltration. Endometrial biopsy shows plasma cell endometritis in a woman infected by *Chlamydia trachomatis*. Plasma cells are generally scarce in the genital tracts of healthy women. It was previously believed that plasma cell endometritis was a typical finding for gonococcal endometritis, but at that time, chlamydial infection was unknown and thus double-infection by chlamydia and gonococci was not recognized.

FIGURE 5-20 Histopathologic findings in severe endometritis. A severe inflammatory cell infiltrate, hyperplastic germinal centers, and intraepithelial and intraglandular inflammation are evident.

Salpingitis

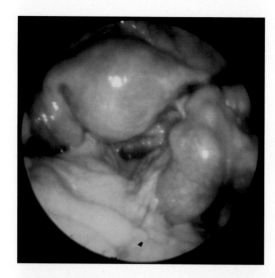

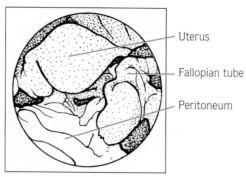

FIGURE 5-21 Laparoscopic view of uterus and swollen fallopian tubes in PID. Inflamed fallopian tubes, with or without lower genital tract infection, are typical in early or mild PID. In mild or doubtful cases, the presence of an infectious exudate confirms the diagnosis, although there is no correlation between symptoms and signs and the severity of PID. Laparoscopy markedly increases the specificity of the diagnosis of PID. Some under- and overdiagnosis, however, may occur.

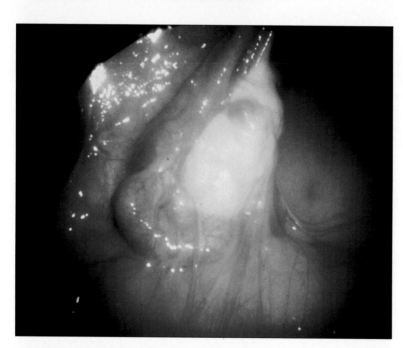

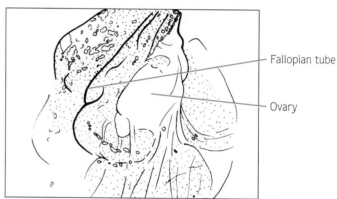

FIGURE 5-22 Laparoscopic view of moderately severe PID, showing distended, inflamed fallopian tube and ovary. The fallopian tube is slightly distended and hyperemic. Purulent exudate, exiting the fimbriated end of the tube, covers the ovary. Laparoscopy provides the opportunity to examine the fallopian tubes, appendix, liver, and other intra-abdominal organs, as well as to grade the severity of salpingitis. Intra-abdominal spread may occur in up to one fourth of chlamydial PID cases.

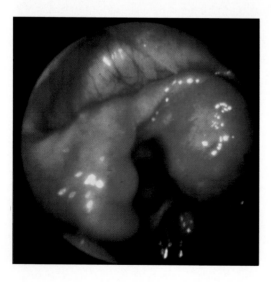

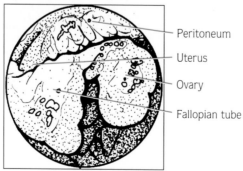

FIGURE 5-23 Laparoscopic view of chronic PID with severe tuboovarian adhesions and an occluded fallopian tube. The ovary is dramatically enlarged and has some exudate on its surface. The highly vascular peritoneum is visible above the fallopian tube. The presence of adhesions restricts the mobility of intra-abdominal organs, leading to the characteristic cervical motion tenderness on manipulation and to chronic pelvic pain.

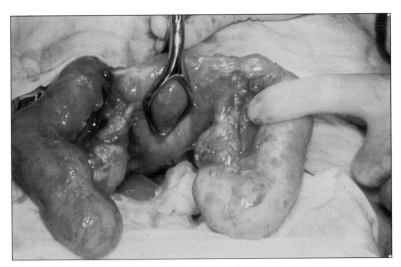

FIGURE 5-24 Severe PID at laparotomy. Bilateral tuboovarian abscesses can be seen. (*Courtesy of* D. Eschenbach, MD.)

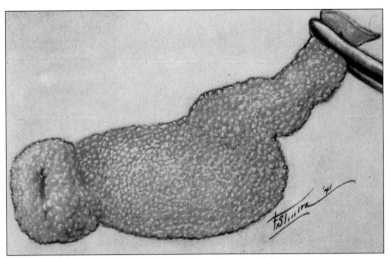

FIGURE 5-25 Tuberculous salpingitis. A pathology drawing from the previous century shows the nodular appearance of the enlarged fallopian tube. Tuberculosis of the genital tract became rare in many industrialized countries during the last decades, but with increased immigration and the increased incidence of tuberculosis in relation to HIV infection and AIDS, genital tuberculosis has once again come into focus. Tuberculous salpingitis generally results from hematogenous spread, not genital contact, in persons with prior tuberculosis. It begins in the fallopian tube and spreads to the uterus in 50% of cases, ovaries in 30%, cervix in 10%, and vagina in 1%. The disease should be considered in cases of PID not responsive to standard therapy, although regimens containing aminoglycosides or fluoroquinolones may alleviate the mycobacterial infection. (Carter JR: Unusual presentations of genital tract tuberculosis. *Int J Gynecol Obstet* 1990, 33:171–176.)

Intra-abdominal Manifestations of Pelvic Inflammatory Disease

Extragenital intra-abdominal spread in different grades of salpingitis			
	Grade I (*n* = 47)	Grade II (*n* = 100)	Grade III (*n* = 54)
Perihepatitis	0	5	4
Periappendicitis	1	4	4
Perisigmoiditis	0	1	4
Periappendicitis and perisigmoiditis	0	2	2

FIGURE 5-26 Number of extragenital intra-abdominal manifestations in 201 cases of PID of differing severity. Chlamydial infections may spread to the abdominal cavity causing periappendicitis, perihepatitis, peritonitis, perisplenitis, and, possibly, perisigmoiditis. Infected material may track up the right pericolic gutter to surround the liver, producing perihepatitis, the Fitz-Hugh Curtis syndrome. (Lopez-Zeno JA, Keith LG, Berger GS: The Fitz-Hugh Curtis syndrome revisited: Changing perspectives after half a century. *J Reprod Med* 1985, 30:567–582.)

A. Clinical findings in six cases of chlamydial periappendicitis: Physical findings				
Patient no.	Low abdominal pain (right/left)	Adnexal tenderness (right/left)	Vaginal discharge	Abnormal bleeding
1	+/+	+/+	+	–
2	–/+	+/–	–	+
3	+/+	+/+	+	+
4	+/–	+/–	+	+
5	+/+	+/+	–	–
6	+/+	+/+	+	+

FIGURE 5-27 Clinical findings in six cases of chlamydial periappendicitis. **A**, Physical findings. (*continued*)

B. Clinical findings in six cases of chlamydial periappendicitis: Laboratory findings

Patient no.	ESR, *mm/h*	Leukocyte count, $\times 10^{10}/L$	Rectal temperature, °C	MIF IgG antibody titer to *Chlamydia trachomatis* Acute	Convalescent
1	28	18.1	38.1	ND	32
2	34	8.4	37.7	256	256
3	62	8.3	37.6	512	ND
4	28	8.9	37.8	8	64
5	30	8.4	37.8	128	512
6	90	10.3	37.5	1024	4096

ESR—erythrocyte sedimentation rate; MIF—microimmunofluorescent; ND—not done.

FIGURE 5-27 (*continued*) **B,** Laboratory findings. Patients with chlamydial periappendicitis present with both signs of cervicitis and PID. They often have a high erythrocyte sedimentation rate, a comparatively minor rise in the leukocyte count, and low-grade fever. Cervical discharge is usually present.

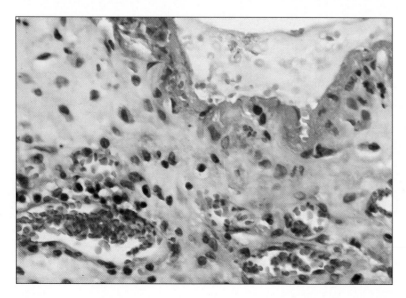

FIGURE 5-28 Laparoscopic view of liver surface with fibrin deposits in chlamydial perihepatitis. Perihepatitis in women with chlamydial PID is significantly more common in women *not* using oral contraceptives. In a series of women with laparoscopically proven chlamydial PID who were using the pill, perihepatitis occurred in 5%, but it was found in 27% of age-matched nonusers.

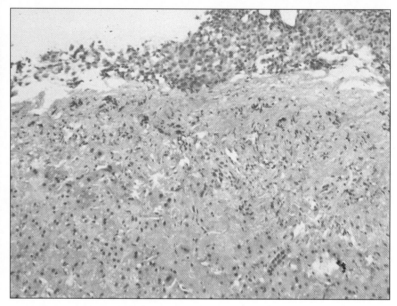

FIGURE 5-29 Histopathologic findings in chlamydial perihepatitis. There is inflammatory cell infiltration of the liver capsule in the absence of signs of true hepatitis. Although perihepatitis for years was believed to be a complication of gonococcal PID, in recent studies most cases have been associated with *Chlamydia trachomatis* (probably due to repeated episodes).

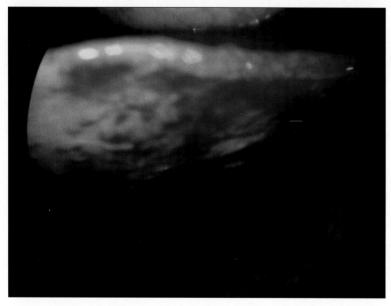

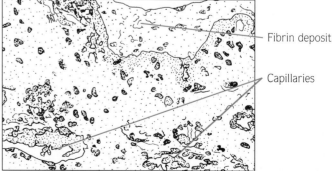

FIGURE 5–30 Histologic section of liver capsule in chlamydial perihepatitis showing fibrin deposition and a minor inflammatory response. Only a minimal inflammatory response is found adjacent to capillaries in the capsule. Hepatic enzymes are generally not increased or only very slightly elevated in cases of chlamydial perihepatitis. (Hematoxylin-eosin stain.)

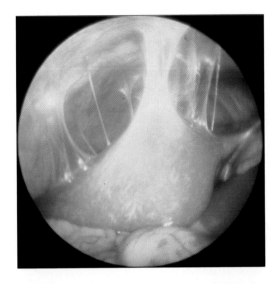

FIGURE 5-31 Violin-string adhesions in chlamydial PID and perihepatitis. The role of the violin-string adhesions in the pathogenesis of chronic abdominal pain is uncertain. Some gynecologists recommend resolving the adhesions to improve mobility of structures in the abdominal cavity. Before chlamydiae were known to be genital tract pathogens, these adhesions were considered typical for intra-abdominal gonococcal infection.

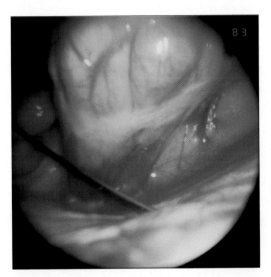

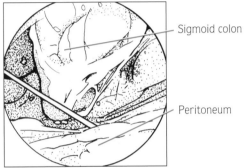

Sigmoid colon

Peritoneum

FIGURE 5-32 Laparoscopic view of perisigmoiditis in chlamydial PID. In addition to the fallopian tubes, the surface of the liver, intestines, and spleen may show inflammatory signs.

CLINICAL SYNDROMES

Gonococcal Pelvic Inflammatory Disease

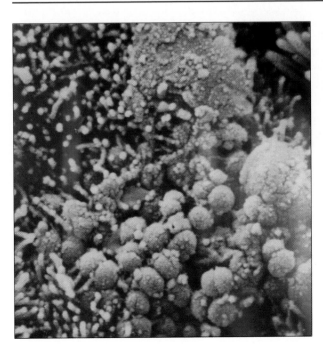

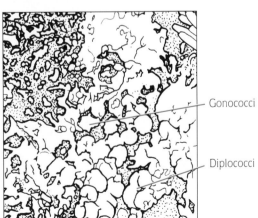

Gonococci

Diplococci

FIGURE 5-33 Scanning electron micrograph of gonococci on the surface of fallopian tube endoepithelium. A microcolony of gonococci can be seen. Many of the organisms have the classic diplococcal form of *Neisseria gonorrhoeae*.

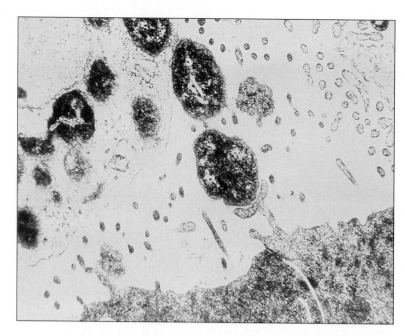

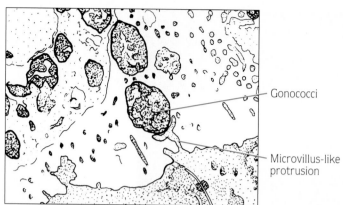

FIGURE 5-34 Electron micrograph of a gonococcus attached to a protrusion of fallopian tube epithelial cell. Extracellular blebs contain gonococcal endotoxin. Endotoxin gives signals to the epithelium to produce microvillus-like protrusions, the tips of which can meet tips of gonococcal pili. This minimizes the electrostatic forces acting between the cell and organism, thereby facilitating contact between organism and cell as the first step in the infectious process.

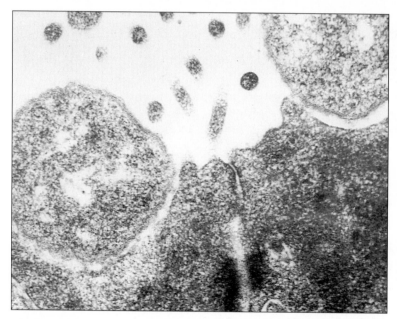

FIGURE 5-35 Electron micrograph of gonococci attached to endotubal epithelium, showing "pillow phenomenon." After contact is established between the gonococci and fallopian tube, the organisms appear to sink into the epithelial cell surface, like a head resting on a soft pillow.

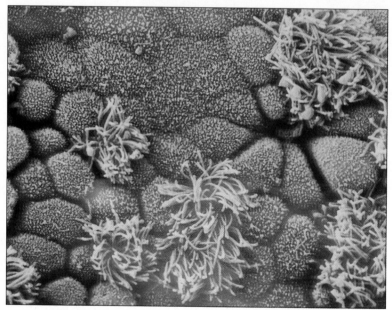

FIGURE 5-36 Scanning electron micrograph of healthy fallopian tube showing ciliated and nonciliated cells. Infection of the fallopian tubes damage the ciliated cells, which are important for transporting bacteria and sperm. The infection can interfere with the mucociliary wave activity of ciliated cells, resulting in an increased risk for extrauterine (tubal) pregnancy.

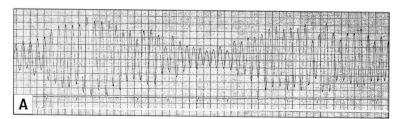

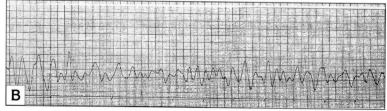

FIGURE 5-37 Mucociliary wave pattern of fallopian tube endothelial cells after gonococcal infection. **A**, Wave pattern from cultured fallopian tube epithelial cells from a healthy woman. **B**, Wave pattern from cultured epithelial cells from the same fallopian tube after infection by gonococci. The lipopolysaccharide of the gonococcal cell wall (endotoxin) may interfere with mucociliary wave activity in experimental infections of cell cultures.

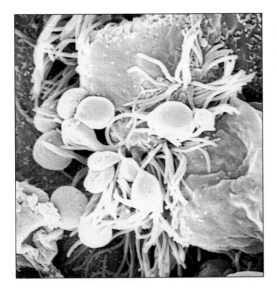

FIGURE 5-38 Scanning electron micrograph of experimental gonococcal infection of a fallopian tube epithelial cell culture. Attachment of organisms to ciliated cells is demonstrated. Microbial attachment to epithelial surfaces is the first stage of many infections, and one theoretical approach to vaccine prevention is to identify and generate local antibodies to those surface bacterial proteins responsible for attachment.

Clinical differences between patients with gonococcal and nongonococcal PID			
	Gonococcal PID	Nongonococcal PID	*P* value
Rectal temp > 38.0° C	48.0%	29.4%	< 0.001
Palpable adnexal swelling	51.5%	44.7%	< 0.05
Urethritis symptoms	21.1%	7.6%	< 0.001
Nulliparae	79.4%	63.5%	< 0.001
Onset of abdominal pain at menstrual bleeding	46.1%	22.9%	< 0.001

FIGURE 5-39 Clinical differences between patients with gonococcal and nongonococcal PID. In gonococcal salpingitis, the typical patient is young and of a lower socioeconomic group. She often has a short period of abdominal pain (< 3 days) before seeking medical attention. More often than in nongonococcal cases, she has a fever (> 38.0° C), urethritis symptoms (dysuria), and palpable adnexal swelling. The salpingitis becomes symptomatic at or shortly after menstruation.

Chlamydial Pelvic Inflammatory Disease

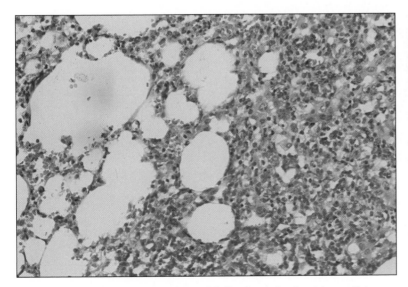

FIGURE 5-40 Histologic section of fallopian tube in chlamydial PID, showing massive inflammatory cell reaction. Intracytoplasmic chlamydial inclusions in columnar epithelium (not shown) and plasma cell infiltrates are typical of infection with *Chlamydia trachomatis*.

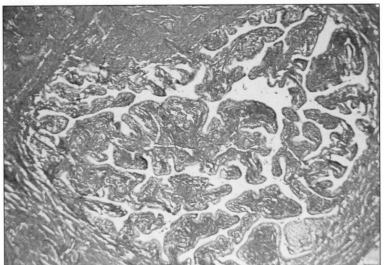

FIGURE 5-41 Histologic cross-section of infected fallopian tube in severe salpingitis due to *Chlamydia trachomatis*. The mucosa of the lateral portions of the tube (infundibulum and ampulla) display many tall folds yielding an irregular lumen. In this diseased specimen, the folds are markedly distorted and thickened.

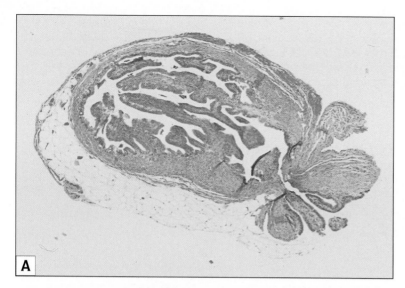

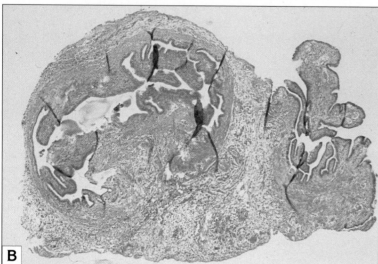

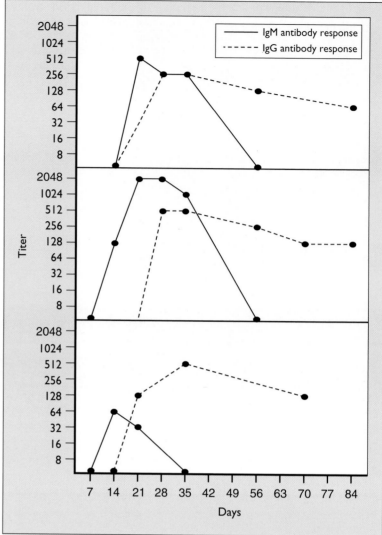

FIGURE 5-43 Titer of IgM and IgG antibodies to *Chlamydia trachomatis* in three grivet monkeys with experimentally induced PID. Experimental infection by *C. trachomatis* in these monkeys caused a conventional antibody response, with an IgM antibody response (*solid lines*) detectable within 1 to 2 weeks, followed by a switch to an IgG antibody response (*dashed lines*) with various patterns of persistence. In addition to the humoral antibody response, the development of cellular immunity to *C. trachomatis* can also be shown in experimental animals and in humans with naturally occurring PID. (Ripa RT, Möller B, Mårdh P-A, *et al.*: Experimental acute salpingitis in grivet monkeys provoked by *Chlamydia trachomatis*. *Acta Path Microbiol Scand* 1979, 87B:65–70.)

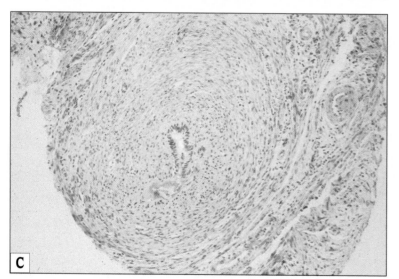

FIGURE 5-42 Salpingitis experimentally induced by inoculation of *Chlamydia trachomatis* in grivet monkeys. **A–C.** Sections of fallopian tubes taken at different days after infection show progressive damage, proving the etiologic role of *C. trachomatis* in salpingitis. Grivet monkeys have been long used as an *in vivo* model of PID.

Clinical differences between patients with chlamydial and nonchlamydial PID

	Chlamydial PID (n=84)	Nonchlamydial PID (n=39)	P value
Age < 30 yrs	9	11	0.05
Abdominal pain			
1–3 days	15	17	0.01
≥ 4 days	33	8	0.05
Rectal temp > 38.0° C	19	17	0.05
ESR ≥ 30 mm/h	50	8	0.001

ESR—erythrocyte sedimentation rate.

FIGURE 5-44 Clinical differences between patients with chlamydial and nonchlamydial, nongonococcal PID. Like gonococcal PID, chlamydial salpingitis is most often seen in young patients, but these women generally have a milder clinical picture, with a longer period of abdominal symptoms (7–9 days) before seeking medical care and rare fever. The erythrocyte sedimentation rate is generally elevated (up to 30–50 mm/h). Laparoscopy in these patients reveals more pronounced inflammatory reactions of the fallopian tubes, resulting in more tubal damage.

Mycoplasmal Pelvic Inflammatory Disease

Isolation of *Mycoplasma hominis* from cervical and tubal specimens in PID

	Women, n	M. hominis isolated	
		Cervix	Tubes
Healthy	50	2	0
PID	50	31	4

FIGURE 5-45 Rates of isolation of *Mycoplasma hominis* from cervix and fallopian tube specimens in healthy women and patients with salpingitis. In women from whom this mycoplasma species was isolated from the tubes, a significant antibody response was

demonstrated, indicating true infection rather than colonization with the organism. The epidemiology of PID associated with *M. hominis* is somewhat different from that associated with other organisms, in that it occurs more frequently among older women than does gonococcal or chlamydial PID and is associated with a longer hospital stay and prolonged elevation of the erythrocyte sedimentation rate. (Miettinen A, Saikku P, Jansson E, Paavonen J: Epidemiologic and clinical characteristics of pelvic inflammatory disease associated with *Mycoplasma hominis*, *Chlamydia trachomatis*, and *Neisseria gonorrhoeae*. *Sex Transm Dis* 1986, 13:24–28.)

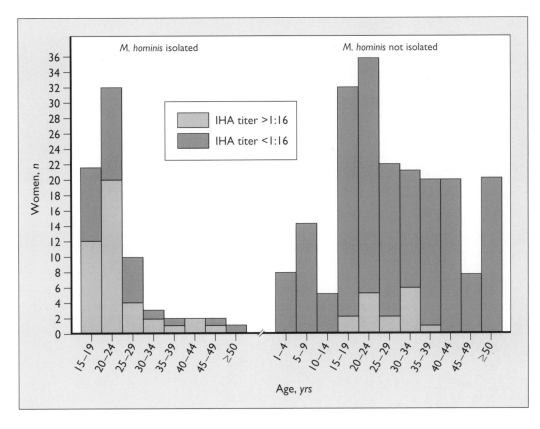

FIGURE 5-46 Prevalence of antibodies to *Mycoplasma hominis* in culture-negative and culture-positive women, by age. The prevalence of *M. hominis* antibodies was significantly higher in culture-positive (*left*) than in culture-negative cases (*right*). The usual antibiotic therapy (eg, tetracyclines or erythromycin) for upper respiratory tract and other infections may have eradicated the organism in women with persistent occurrence of *M. hominis* antibodies but negative cultures.

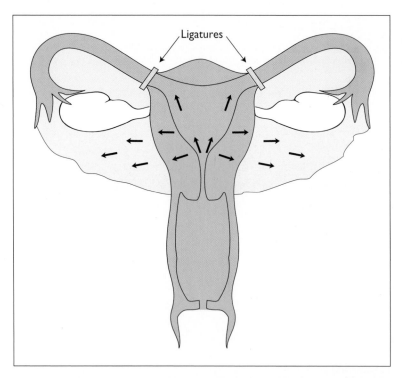

FIGURE 5-47 Lymphatic and hematogenous spread of *Mycoplasma hominis* to the upper genital tract. After ligatures were applied to the isthmus of the fallopian tubes, spread of the organism by lymphatic vessels to the parametrium was found in women; *M. hominis* was isolated from biopsy specimens from the upper genital tract. With gonococci and chlamydia, if the tubes are closed by a ligature at the isthmus, the woman will not develop PID, as proven in a large series of women studied decades ago.

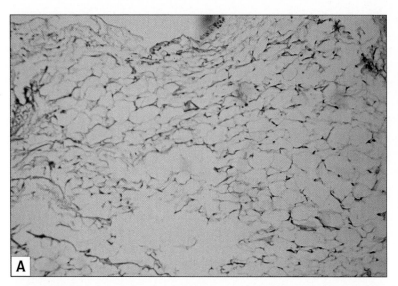

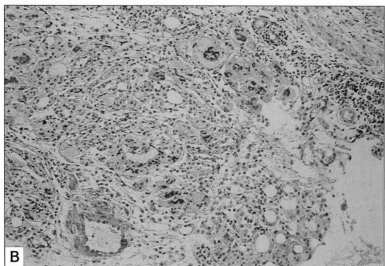

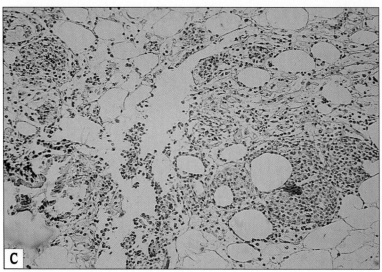

FIGURE 5-48 Parametritis experimentally produced in grivet monkeys by inoculation with *Mycoplasma hominis*. **A**, At time of inoculation (day 0). **B**, Day 14. **C**, Day 28. Parametritis was produced by inoculating *M. hominis* directly into the fallopian tubes of grivet monkeys, an *in vivo* model of PID. The sequence demonstrates progressive inflammation and destruction of the normal lacy tissue architecture. Such studies indicate that *M. hominis*, by itself, can establish genital infection. In histologic examinations in grivet monkeys experimentally infected with *M. hominis*, the findings correspond to nongonococcal salpingitis as described in older gynecologic textbooks. The so-called gonococcal salpingitis (before the chlamydia era) may have been double-infection by *Chlamydia trachomatis* and *Neisseria gonorrhoeae*. Up to 25% of PID cases have been demonstrated to be double-infected with gonococci and chlamydia. (Möller BR, *et al.*: Experimental infection of the genital tract of female grivet monkeys by *Mycoplasma hominis*. *Infect Immun* 1978, 20:248.)

SEQUELAE OF PELVIC INFLAMMATORY DISEASE

Chronic Pelvic Pain

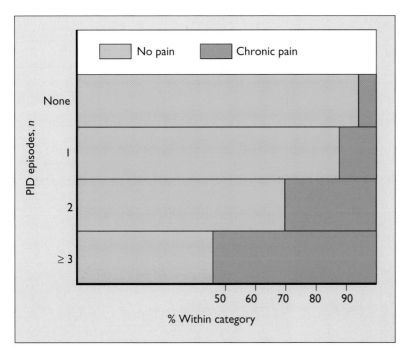

FIGURE 5-49 Chronic pelvic pain after PID, related to number of episodes. Chronic pain of > 6 months' duration was seen in 18% of women in a follow-up study of PID, compared with 5% of normal controls. The prevalence of pain increased with the number of prior episodes of PID. The cause of the pain may relate to increased intraovarian pressure and adhesions surrounding the ovaries (*see* Fig. 5-31).

Infertility After Pelvic Inflammatory Disease

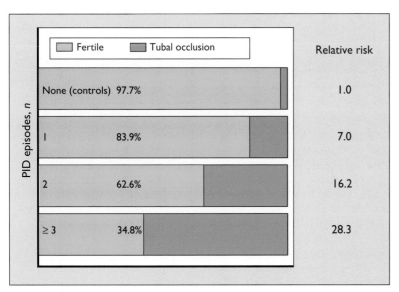

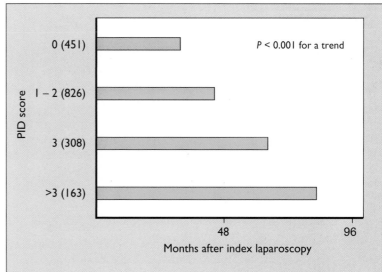

FIGURE 5-50 Fertility related to number of prior PID episodes. The frequency of tubal occlusion increases sharply with each recurrent episode of PID. Whether this tubal occlusion is due to adverse immune reactions in a previously challenged host or to repeated invasion of the tubes by chlamydia organisms is not known. On average, after a single episode of PID, approximately 12% of women become infertile. The rate increases to 25% after two episodes and to > 50% with three or more episodes. In this study of 1725 women, voluntarily infertile women excluded.

FIGURE 5-51 Mean time in months between index PID episode (assessed laparoscopically) and first pregnancy, by PID severity. The PID score, assessed via laparoscopy, relates to the severity of PID episodes (0, no PID; 1, mild PID; 2, moderately severe disease; 3, severe PID) and was totaled for any repeat episodes of PID following the index case (resulting in scores > 3). For women remaining fertile after PID, the mean time to successful pregnancy increases markedly with increasing severity of PID.

Tubal occlusion after PID, by severity of PID	
Salpingitis	**Tubal occlusion**
Mild	6.7%
Moderate	10.6%
Severe	28.1%

FIGURE 5-52 Tubal occlusion after PID, by severity of PID. The risk of tubal occlusion resulting in involuntary infertility increases with the severity of a single PID episode, but it also increases markedly with each subsequent episode of PID. PID is the major preventable cause of involuntary infertility in the United States.

Adjusted pregnancy rates after conservatively treated PID before and after the introduction of chemotherapy, 1930–1988

Antibiotic therapy	Studies, *n*	Patients, *n*	Adjusted pregnancy rate	Range
No	3	1026	27.9%	24%–43%
Yes	4	954	73.1%	24%–81%

FIGURE 5-53 Adjusted pregnancy rates after conservatively treated PID before and after the introduction of antibiotic chemotherapy between 1930 and 1988. In the preantibiotic era, rates of pregnancy following acute PID ranged from 24% to 43%, as assessed in three studies involving 1026 patients (clinical diagnosis in 94.8%). After antibiotic chemotherapy was introduced, the rates have improved to approximately 73%, as assessed in four studies of 954 patients (laparoscopic diagnosis in 81%).

Tubal factor infertility after one episode of PID, related to contraceptive method used at disease episode

Method	TFI, %	Relative risk	(95% CI)
None	11.8	1.0	
Barrier	10.5	0.9	(0.4–1.8)
Pill	3.7	0.3	(0.2–0.7)*
Intrauterine device	5.4	0.5	(0.2–0.9)†
Other	8.7	0.8	(0.4–1.4)

*$P < 0.01$.
†$P < 0.05$.
CI—confidence interval; TFI—tubal factor infertility.

FIGURE 5-54 Tubal factor infertility after one episode of PID, related to contraceptive method used at the time of the acute PID episode. The use of oral contraceptives may protect from ascending infection, and when infection does occur, there seems to be less severe inflammatory alterations in the tubes. Likewise, women on the pill in whom PID is diagnosed had a much better fertility prognosis than those not using such a contraception.

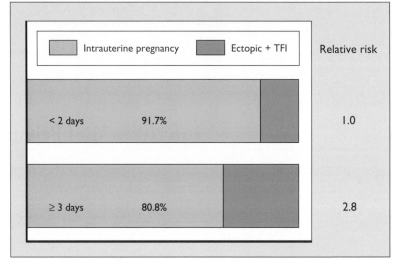

FIGURE 5-55 Influence of delayed care for PID on subsequent fertility rates. A delay in seeking medical care and receiving subsequent treatment of PID increases the risks of infertility. Rates of infertility after PID are also affected by patient age, severity of symptoms, contraception used, and number of PID episodes. This study followed 443 women after their first episode of PID until pregnancy developed and excluded women who were voluntarily infertile or had non–tubal factor infertility (TFI).

FIGURE 5-56 Proportion of fertile and infertile women with serum antibody to *Chlamydia trachomatis* (≥ 1:32). Serologic studies from eight studies indicate an association between infertility and infection by *C. trachomatis*. The pathogenic mechanisms by which *C. trachomatis* causes scarring and tubal occlusion are incompletely understood. (TFI—tubal factor infertility.)

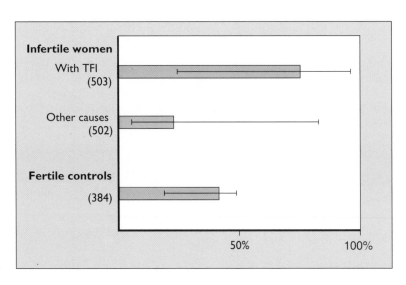

Ectopic (Tubal) Pregnancy

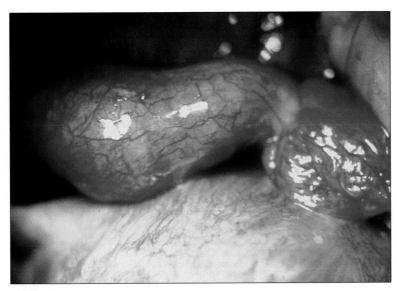

FIGURE 5-57 Laparoscopic view of an ectopic pregnancy. A swollen, edematous fallopian tube is pictured. A history of PID increases the risk of ectopic pregnancy approximately 10-fold.

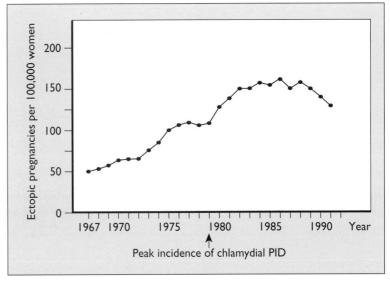

FIGURE 5-58 Number of ectopic pregnancies diagnosed in Turku, Finland between 1967 and 1992. After a steady increase until the mid-1980s, there has been a recent decrease in cases of ectopic pregnancy (as well as PID) in this population from the Turku, Finland, region. This decrease follows a decrease in prevalence of chlamydial infections in the general population of the sample area. Cases of extrauterine pregnancy are documented to occur approximately 7 years after an acute episode of PID. Once the prevalence of reported genital chlamydial infections began to decline in the early 1980s, then after a lag period of 7 years, the number of cases of ectopic pregnancies started to decrease. (*See also* Fig. 5-2.)

FIGURE 5-59 Infertility and first pregnancy in 1730 women followed after index PID episode. Following PID, the rate of ectopic pregnancy is 10-fold higher than that in women who never had the disease. The rate increases further with multiple episodes of PID.

Infertility and first pregnancy in 1730 women followed after the index PID

	PID episodes, *n*				
	0	**1**	**2**	**≥3**	**All PID**
Intrauterine pregnancy	433	852	124	24	1000
Ectopic pregnancy	6	61	24	15	100
TFI	4	79	46	30	155
Non-TFI	5	23	4	0	27
Total	448	1015	198	69	1282

TFI—tubal factor infertility.

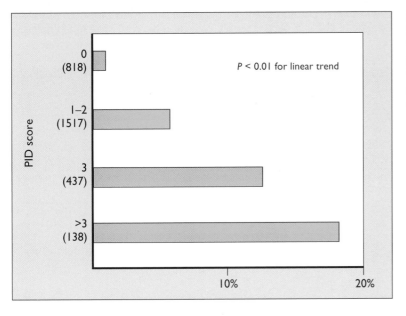

FIGURE 5-60 Percentage of all pregnancies that were ectopic after index PID episode, related to PID severity. Severity of PID symptoms also is correlated with the rate of postinfectious ectopic pregnancy. The PID score, assessed via laparoscopy, relates to the severity of PID episodes (0, no PID; 1, mild PID; 2, moderately severe PID; 3, severe PID) and was totaled for any repeat episodes of PID following the index case (resulting in scores > 3).

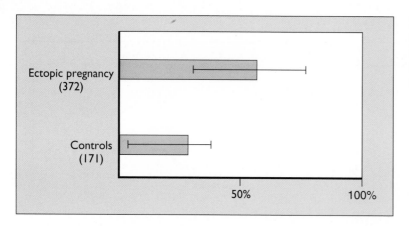

FIGURE 5-61 Proportion of women with serum antibody titers to *Chlamydia trachomatis* ≥ 1:32 in ectopic pregnancy and among healthy controls. Results from six studies seem to indicate that ectopic pregnancies often are seen in women who develop a significant antibody response to the agent.

DIAGNOSIS

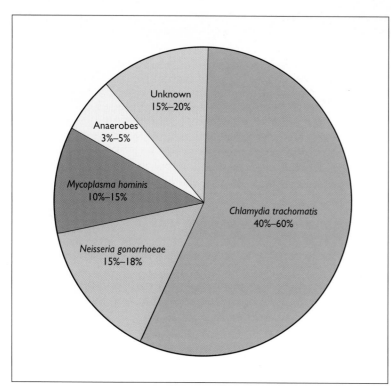

FIGURE 5-62 Etiological organisms in PID. The major etiologic agents of PID are *Neisseria gonorrhoeae* and *Chlamydia trachomatis*. The percentage of PID cases caused by either agent in a particular area depends on the prevalence of each agent. In Sweden, at the beginning of the 1970s, approximately 50% of PID cases were caused by *N. gonorrhoeae*, but in the middle of the 1990s, the corresponding rate was < 5%. Gonorrhea is less prevalent in Sweden than in the United States, accounting for the larger rate of *C. trachomatis* infection. Among the etiologic agents in PID, the most common anaerobic organisms found are *Bacteroides*, *Peptostreptococcus*, and *Peptococcus*, whereas the most common facultative bacteria include *Gardnerella vaginalis*, *Streptococcus*, *Escherichia coli*, and *Haemophilus influenzae*. *N. gonorrhoeae* and *C. trachomatis* are more often associated with initial episodes of PID, and other organisms appear in subsequent episodes, probably requiring tubal damage from prior gonococcal or chlamydial infection to facilitate their ascent and establishment in the upper genital tract. (*From* Weström L, Mårdh P-A: Salpingitis. *In* Holmes KK, *et al.* (eds.): *Sexually Transmitted Diseases*. New York: McGraw-Hill; 1984:620; with permission.)

Frequency of signs and symptoms of salpingitis vs lower genital tract infection

Symptom or sign	Acute salpingitis, % ($n = 623$)	LGTI only, normal tubes, % ($n=184$)
Low abdominal pain	100.0	100.0
Metrorrhagia	35.5	42.9
Urethritis symptoms	18.6	20.1
LGTI		
Purulent vaginal contents on microscopy	100.0	100.0
Symptom of discharge	54.6	56.5
Vomiting or nausea	10.3	9.2
Proctitis symptoms	6.9	2.7
Fever (> 38.0° C) at admission	32.9	14.1
Palpable adnexal swelling	49.4	24.5

LGTI—lower genital tract infection.

FIGURE 5-63 Frequency of signs and symptoms of salpingitis versus lower genital tract infection (LGTI). Acute salpingitis can vary from a symptomless disease to a severe condition with pelvic abscess formation, but the signs and symptoms are not specific. In a study of women presenting with assumed salpingitis based on clinical criteria, laparoscopic examination confirmed salpingitis in 65% but identified other pelvic disease in 12% and normal intrapelvic findings (LGTI only) in 23%. No single sign or symptom was pathognomonic. (Weström L, Mårdh P-A: Pelvic inflammatory disease: I. Epidemiology, diagnosis, clinical manifestations, and sequelae. *In* Holmes KK, Mårdh P-A (eds.): *International Perspectives on Sexually Transmitted Diseases: Impact on Venereology, Fertility, and Maternal and Infant Morbidity*. New York: McGraw-Hill; 1982.) (*From* Weström L, Mårdh P-A: Salpingitis. *In* Holmes KK, *et al.* (eds.): *Sexually Transmitted Diseases*. New York: McGraw-Hill; 1984:624; with permission.)

Laboratory test abnormalities in patients with suspected salpingitis

Test	Salpingitis	LGTI, normal tubes
ESR > 15 mm/h	75.9%	52.7%
Peripheral blood leukocytes > 10,000 mm³	59.1%	33.3%
Elevated antichymotrypsin, orosomucoid, and/or C-reactive protein level in serum	78.7%	24.0%
Genital isoamylases absent or decreased in peritoneal fluid	90.0%	20.0%

LGTI—lower genital tract infection.

Figure 5-64 Laboratory test abnormalities in patients with suspected PID. Among women presenting with assumed salpingitis based on clinical criteria, laparoscopy was used to confirm the diagnosis as salpingitis or lower genital tract infection. No single laboratory finding is both sensitive and specific for the diagnosis of PID (*ie*, none can both detect all cases of PID and exclude all women without PID). (*From* Weström L, Mårdh P-A: Salpingitis. *In* Holmes KK, *et al.* (eds.): *Sexually Transmitted Diseases*. New York: McGraw-Hill; 1984:624; with permission.)

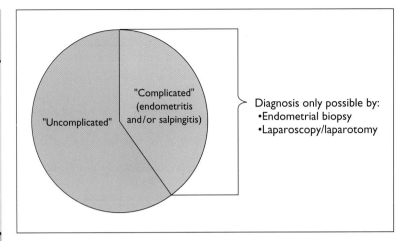

Figure 5-65 Uncomplicated versus complicated genital infection. Many "uncomplicated" genital infections are actually "complicated," and it is generally impossible to distinguish between them on solely clinical grounds. Up to 40% of all cases of genital chlamydial infection are, in fact, complicated genital infections (*ie*, endometritis and/or, less commonly, salpingitis). To determine whether a genital infection is complicated (*ie*, PID), one must perform an endometrial biopsy (may be done by aspiration through the cervical channel) or laparoscopy/laparotomy (which allows visual inspection of the fallopian tubes).

Diagnosis of PID based on any one of these procedures is uncertain

Visual inspection of the uterine tubes via laparoscopy or laparotomy

Office tests, such as ESR, leukocyte count, body temperature, and C-reactive protein

Increased leukocyte count and other signs of inflammation in transvaginal aspirates from pouch of Douglasi

Central laboratory tests, such as tests for acute phase reactants, interleukins and tumor markers, (*eg*, orosomucoid, CA 125)

Ultrasound

ESR—erythrocyte sedimentation rate.

Figure 5-66 Diagnostic uncertainty in PID. No single clinical or laboratory finding is pathognomonic for salpingitis, and a diagnosis of PID that is based on any one test is therefore uncertain. A variety of laboratory tests have been evaluated for their usefulness, including erythrocyte sedimentation rate, leukocyte count, body temperature, and C-reactive protein, as well as less-common serum measurements for cytokines and tumor markers; these tests may be useful in establishing the diagnosis when laparoscopy is unavailable.

Criteria for diagnosis of PID

All three minimum criteria must be present:
1. History of low abdominal pain and/or tenderness, with or without rebound
2. Cervical motion tenderness
3. Adnexal tenderness
   plus

One of these additional criteria must be present:
1. Culdocentesis that yields peritoneal fluid containing leukocytes and bacteria
2. Presence of inflammatory mass noted on pelvic exam or sonography
3. Elevated erythrocyte sedimentation rate
4. Evidence of *Neisseria gonorrhoeae* or *Chlamydia trachomatis* in endocervix:
   Gram stain from endocervix revealing gram-negative intracellular diplococci suggestive of *N. gonorrhoea*
   Monoclonal antibody-directed smear from endocervical secretions revealing *C. trachomatis*
   Mucopurulent endocervicitis
5. Presence of > 10 leukocytes/oil-immersion field on Gram stain of endocervical discharge

FIGURE 5-67 Criteria for diagnosis of PID. Early diagnosis and initiation of therapy are essential to limit spread of infection. In an attempt to improve the accuracy of clinical diagnosis, a combination of clinical and laboratory findings was assembled into standardized criteria. Patients presenting with all three "minimum" criteria plus at least one "additional" criterion should be considered to have PID, and therapy begun promptly; laparoscopy done in such patients shows objective evidence of PID in approximately 68%. In patients having the minimum criteria plus two additional criteria, the probability of PID rises to 90%, and with three additional criteria, it rises to 96% (although only 17% of patients with laparoscopy-confirmed PID have three additional findings). With PID, it is better to overtreat, and treatment should not be withheld from a patient with an equivocal diagnosis. (*Adapted from* Sweet RL: Pelvic inflammatory disease and tuboovarian abscess. *In* Gorbach SL, Bartlett JG, Blacklow NR (eds.): *Infectious Diseases.* Philadelphia: W.B. Saunders; 1992:867; with permission.)

Diagnostic tests in PID

Endometrial biopsy

Laparoscopy/laparotomy

Culture (tubal/endometrial)

Ultrasound

Supportive, *eg,* elevated erythrocyte sedimentation rate

FIGURE 5-68 Diagnostic tests in PID. Although not needed to justify a decision to treat, a definitive diagnosis of PID is made by either endometrial biopsy or laparoscopy/laparotomy. Histologic changes of endometritis are found in approximately 75% of women with laparoscopy-proven PID and in no women without PID. Laparoscopy or laparotomy allows direct visualization of the fallopian tubes and is the most specific method for diagnosing acute salpingitis; diagnostic criteria include 1) erythema of the fallopian tube, 2) edema of the fallopian tube, or 3) seropurulent exudate or fresh, easily lysed adhesions at the fimbriated end or serosal surface of the fallopian tube. An etiologic diagnosis is based on culture or other tests, including Gram stain, on endocervical swabs, endometrial biopsy, or culdocentesis. Ultrasound may help distinguish among the complications of PID, such as tuboovarian abscess, and other pelvic masses, such as ectopic pregnancy or ovarian cysts.

Advantages and disadvantages of sampling techniques in etiologic studies of acute salpingitis

Sampling site or technique	Advantages	Disadvantages
Endocervical swab	Generally applicable, easy to perform	Sampling remote from site of disease
Culdocentesis	Generally applicable, easy to perform	Risk of contaminating cul-de-sac by vaginal or bowel flora Sampling remote from site of disease
Fallopian tubes (endotubal swab or puncture of tube)	Sampling at site of disease	Requires laparoscopy or laparotomy Requires experienced investigator

FIGURE 5-69 Evaluation of sampling techniques in etiologic studies of acute salpingitis. A number of different sampling techniques and sites have been used to determine the specific etiology of PID. As with many infectious processes, samples taken from sites remote from the actual infection can give misleading results (such as in attempts to determine the etiology of osteomyelitis by culturing drainage from a sinus tract). Similarly, passing through a colonized area on the way to the site of infection risks obtaining spurious culture results (eg, passing through the vagina to access the cul-de-sac [pouch of Douglas] risks contamination with vaginal flora).

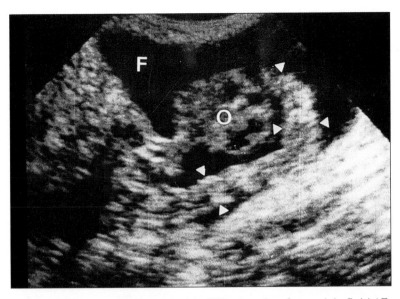

FIGURE 5-70 Vaginal ultrasound in PID, showing free pelvic fluid (*F*) and enlarged ovary (*O*). The fallopian tube (*arrowheads*) is thickened, the ovary is enlarged, and free fluid is seen in the peritoneum. Although not a diagnostic test, ultrasound is useful in distinguishing among the complications of PID, such as tuboovarian abscess, and other pelvic masses, such as ectopic pregnancy or ovarian cysts.

Differential diagnosis of acute salpingitis

Diagnosis after laparoscopy	Cases, *n*
Acute salpingitis	532
Normal findings	184
Acute appendicitis	24
Endometriosis	16
Corpus luteum bleeding	12
Ectopic pregnancy	11
Adhesion "chronic salpingitis"	6
Ovarian tumor	7
Mesenteric lymphadenitis	6
Miscellaneous	16

FIGURE 5-71 Differential diagnosis of PID. Other conditions presenting with low abdominal pain, pelvic mass, or vaginal bleeding must be distinguished from PID, and laparoscopy is of primary value in excluding these other surgical problems. The most common and serious surgical problems that may be confused with PID are unilateral. In one study, in patients who were diagnosed clinically as having salpingitis, subsequent laparoscopy found other intrapelvic disease in 12%, with acute appendicitis being the most common (false-positive diagnosis). In patients diagnosed clinically as having problems other than PID, subsequent laparoscopy sometimes identifies PID (false-negative diagnosis). (Jacobson L, Weström L: Objectivized diagnosis of acute pelvic inflammatory disease: Diagnostic and prognostic value of routine laparoscopy. *Am J Obstet Gynecol* 1969, 105:1088–1098.) (*From* Weström L, Mårdh P-A: Salpingitis. *In* Holmes KK, *et al.* (eds.): *Sexually Transmitted Diseases.* New York: McGraw-Hill; 1984:627; with permission.)

THERAPY

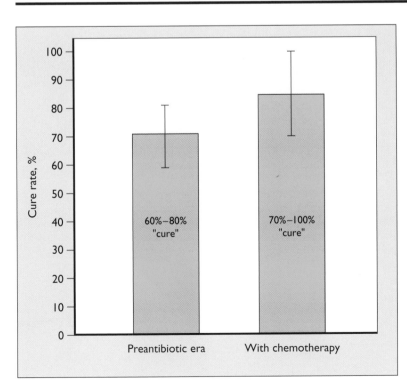

FIGURE 5-72 Clinical cure rates in conservatively treated PID. PID is a clinically self-limiting condition in most women, with total recovery even if untreated. In the preantibiotic era, however, persistence of microorganisms could be demonstrated in the fallopian tubes of patients after clinical recovery, and repeated flare-ups were common, indicating chronic infection. With proper antibiotic therapy, eradication of bacteria is possible, although a woman's fertility may be compromised by even a single PID episode.

Clinical and microbiologic endpoints in therapeutic PID studies

Patient's well-being
Normalization of inflammatory signs
Negative microbiologic tests
Normal second-look laparoscopy
Preserved fertility
Normal uterine passage tube tests

FIGURE 5-73 Endpoints for evaluating therapeutic trials in PID. The rational treatment of PID is hampered by a limited number of well-designed clinical trials. There are a number of difficulties in evaluating the results of treatment of PID, such as ensuring that the cases studied really have had an abdominal and/or tubal infection and finding a good endpoint for the trial (*eg*, relief of symptoms or preserved fertility). Excellent clinical studies should make use of objective and reproducible endpoints. Some endpoints require long-term follow-up.

Frequency of intrauterine pregnancies and tubal factor infertility after a single episode of PID, by antibiotic treatment

Antibiotic treatment	Women, *n*	Intrauterine pregnancy	Tubal factor infertility
Streptomycin + penicillin	56	85.8%	14.2%
Chloramphenicol + penicillin	211	89.6%	10.4%
Ampicillin	44	86.4%	13.6%
Doxycycline	106	85.8%	14.2%

FIGURE 5-74 Frequency of intrauterine pregnancies and tubal factor infertility after PID, by antibiotic treatment. Following a single episode of PID, the rate of infertility among women aged 15 to 34 years is approximately 13%, and the rate increases with the patient's age, duration of symptoms before treatment, severity of disease, and multiple episodes of PID. In a study of women treated between 1960 and 1974 with different antibiotic regimens, who had only one episode of laparoscopy-proven PID and who later exposed themselves to a chance of pregnancy, follow-up studies revealed similar rates of infertility (10%–14%) regardless of antibiotic treatment. These similar rates of infertility might indicate that not only the inflammatory process but also the repair process might cause later functional disturbance in the tubes. (Weström L, *et al.*: Infertility after acute salpingitis: Results of treatment with different antibiotics. *Curr Ther Res* 1979, 26:752.)

A. CDC treatment recommendations for acute PID: Outpatient management

Single dose of:*
  Cefoxitin 2 g intramuscularly
  plus
  Probenecid 1 g orally, given concurrently
      or
  Ceftriaxone 250 mg intramuscularly × 1 dose
      or
  Equivalent cephalosporin
Plus:
  Doxycycline 100 mg orally twice a day × 10–14 days
      or
  Tetracycline 500 mg orally 4 times a day × 10–14 days

*Follow-up in 72 hrs to ensure response.

FIGURE 5-75 The Centers for Disease Control and Prevention (CDC) treatment recommendations for acute PID. Optimal management requires prompt diagnosis and initiation of treatment, which consists of rest, avoidance of coitus, and antibiotics. The CDC in 1991 published recommendations for antibiotic regimens, but these regimens have not be evaluated in randomized clinical trials, and new agents and regimens are currently under review. Thus, the regimen of choice for treating PID has not yet been established. Any regimen used should provide broad coverage against organisms including *Chlamydia trachomatis*, *Neisseria gonorrhoeae*, anaerobes, gram-negative rods, and streptococci. **A**, Outpatient management. These empiric regimens are designed to provide broad coverage against the most common etiologic agents of PID. Patients who do not respond appropriately to therapy within 72 hours should be hospitalized. In rare patients unable to tolerate doxycycline or tetracycline, erythromycin (500 mg orally four times daily for 10 to 14 days) may be used. (*continued*)

B. CDC treatment recommendations for acute PID: Inpatient management

Regimen A*
Cefoxitin 2 g intravenously every 6 hrs
  or
Cefotetan 2 g intravenously every 12 hrs
plus
Doxycycline 100 mg orally or intravenously every 12 hrs
After discharge:
Doxycycline, 100 mg orally twice a day × 10–14 total days
Regimen B*
Clindamycin 900 mg intravenously every 8 hrs
plus
Gentamicin
  Loading dose: 2 mg/kg intravenously or intramuscularly
  Maintenance dose: 1.5 mg/kg every 8 hrs
After discharge:
Doxycycline 100 mg orally twice a day × 10–14 total days
  or
Clindamycin 450 mg orally 4 times a day × 10–14 total days

*Continue for at least 48 hrs after patient improves.

FIGURE 5-75 (*continued*) **B,** Inpatient management. Despite the prohibitive cost, some recommend treating all patients with PID in the hospital, where therapy can be monitored and adjusted more closely. In place of cefotetan, another cephalosporin that provides adequate coverage, such as ceftizoxime, cefotaxime, ceftriaxone, or other, may be used. Continuation of treatment after hospital discharge is important. (Centers for Disease Control and Prevention: Pelvic inflammatory disease: Guidelines for prevention and management. *MMWR* 1991, 40(RR-5):18–21.)

Criteria for hospitalization of women with acute PID

Uncertain diagnosis
Surgical emergency possible (*eg*, appendicitis, ectopic pregnancy)
Pelvic abscess suspected
Severe illness precluding outpatient management
Young adolescent patient
Unable to comply with or tolerate outpatient regimen
No response to outpatient therapy by 48–72 hrs
Clinical follow-up after 48–72 hrs cannot be arranged

FIGURE 5-76 Criteria for hospitalization of women with acute PID. Hospitalization should be considered for all patients with severe infection or an uncertain diagnosis. Hospitalization affords the opportunity to monitor and adjust therapy closely as well as the possibility to counsel the patient about sexually transmitted diseases and the long-term nature of PID and its sequelae, which is especially valuable in patients of young age. (Centers for Disease Control and Prevention: Pelvic inflammatory disease: Guidelines for prevention and management. *MMWR* 1991, 40(RR-5):18.)

Clinical cure rates in the treatment of acute PID

Treatment regimen	Patients, *n*	Clinical cure, *n* (%)	*P* value
Cefoxitin-doxycycline	75	73 (97)	
vs			NS
Clindamycin-tobramycin	73	70 (96)	
Cefotetan-doxycycline	33	30 (94)	
vs			NS
Cefoxitin-doxycycline	36	33 (92)	
Mezlocillin	32	30 (94)	
vs			NS
Cefoxitin-doxycycline	36	35 (97)	
Ampicillin-sulbactan	37	35 (95)*	
vs			NS
Cefoxitin-doxycycline	20	18 (90)	
Ciprofloxacin	33	31 (94)	
vs			NS
Clindamycin-gentamicin	35	34 (97)	

*Doxycycline added if *Chlamydia trachomatis* is identified.
NS—not significant.

FIGURE 5-77 Clinical cure rates with different antibiotic regimens in the treatment of PID. The CDC-recommended regimens of cefoxitin/doxycycline and clindamycin/gentamicin for inpatient therapy of acute PID have equal initial clinical efficacies and are recognized as the standards against which new regimens are tested. In general, combinations of either clindamycin and an aminoglycoside or a broad-spectrum cephalosporin plus doxycycline provide excellent initial clinical responses. Treatment with fluoroquinolones alone may result in posttreatment persistence of anaerobes in the endometrial cavity. (*From* Sweet RL: Pelvic inflammatory disease and tuboovarian abscess. *In* Gorbach SL, Bartlett JG, Blacklow NR (eds.): *Infectious Diseases.* Philadelphia: W.B. Saunders; 1992:868; with permission.)

Guidelines for patient care in PID

Diagnose and treat early; overtreat rather than undertreat

Provide supportive care as needed

Remove intrauterine device

Treat sex partners

Provide patient education about sexually transmitted diseases and PID

Follow-up at 48–72 hrs after initiating treatment

Avoid coitus for several weeks posttreatment

FIGURE 5-78 Guidelines for patient care in PID. Early diagnosis and prompt treatment are essential to avoid the complications of PID. Patients with equivocal diagnoses should receive treatment (overtreat) to ensure that a patient with PID does not go untreated. All patients being treated for PID require rest, and many will need supportive care with oral or intravenous hydration and nonsteroidal anti-inflammatory drugs or narcotics for pain relief. Intrauterine devices should be removed, because of the increased risk for PID that they impart as well as their possible interference in antibiotic action, and the patient should be educated about risk factors. Treatment of any patient is considered inadequate *unless the sex partners are properly evaluated and treated.* Follow-up includes evaluations at 48 to 72 hours to assess the patient's response to therapy, as well as posttreatment cultures to assess cure.

SELECTED BIBLIOGRAPHY

Cates W, Rolfs RT, Aral SO: Sexually transmitted diseases, pelvic inflammatory disease, and infertility: An epidemiologic update. *Epidemiol Rev* 1990, 12:199–220.

Centers for Disease Control and Prevention: Pelvic inflammatory disease: Guidelines for prevention and management. *MMWR* 1991, 40(RR-5):18.

Eschenbach DA, Buchanan RM, Pollock HM, *et al.*: Polymicrobial etiology of acute pelvic inflammatory disease. *N Engl J Med* 1975, 293:166–171.

Mårdh P-A, *et al.*: *Chlamydia trachomatis* infection in patients with acute salpingitis. *N Engl J Med* 1977, 296:1377.

Washington AE, Cates W Jr, Wasserheit JN: Preventing pelvic inflammatory disease. *JAMA* 1991, 266:2574–2580.

Weström L, Mårdh P-A: Acute pelvic inflammatory disease (PID). *In* Holmes KK, Mårdh P-A, Sparling PF, *et al.* (eds.): *Sexually Transmitted Diseases*, 2nd ed. New York: McGraw-Hill; 1990: 593–613.

CHAPTER 6

Trichomoniasis

John N. Krieger
Michael F. Rein

MICROBIOLOGY

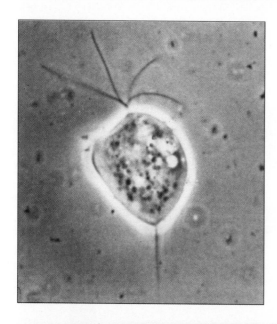

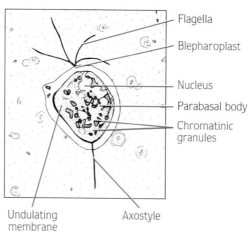

Flagella
Blepharoplast
Nucleus
Parabasal body
Chromatinic granules
Undulating membrane
Axostyle

FIGURE 6-1 Photomicrograph and diagram of *Trichomoniasis vaginalis*. Trichomoniasis is a specific infection with the protozoan *Trichomonas vaginalis*. The organism was first described in 1836 by M.A. Donné. In fresh preparations, the organism is typically pear-shaped and has average dimensions of 10 × 7 μm. It has four free anterior flagella, which appear to arise from a single stalk, and a fifth flagellum embedded in an undulating membrane. Rigidity is maintained by an axostyle, which traverses the cell and projects from the posterior end. (Kampmeier RH: Description of *Trichomonas vaginalis* by M.A. Donné. *Sex Transm Dis* 1978, 52:119–122. Krieger JN: Urologic aspects of trichomoniasis. *Invest Urol* 1981, 18:411–417.)

Laboratory characteristics of *Trichomonas vaginalis*

Size
Serotype
Surface carbohydrates
Surface proteins
Enzyme complement
Hemolytic activity
Experimental virulence

FIGURE 6-2 Laboratory characteristics of *Trichomonas vaginalis*. Strains of *T. vaginalis* have been shown to vary in several characteristics, some of which correlate with disease severity.

Site specificity of trichomonads infecting humans

Trichomonas vaginalis	Urogenital tract
Trichomonas tenax	Mouth, tonsils
Pentatrichomonas hominis	Gastrointestinal tract

FIGURE 6-3 Site specificity of trichomonads infecting humans. *Trichomonas vaginalis* is highly site specific, infecting only the urinary and genital tracts. Other trichomonads also infect or colonize humans at other sites. *Trichomonas tenax* resides in the mouth, being found in greater prevalence in those with periodontal disease, and *Pentatrichomonas hominis* is isolated from the lower gastrointestinal tract, often in association with diarrhea of varying severity. A pathogenic role for either species has not been established definitively. Trichomonads very rarely have been isolated from the lung and central nervous system. (Honigberg BM (ed.): *Trichomonads Parasitic in Humans*. New York: Springer-Verlag; 1990.)

EPIDEMIOLOGY

Prevalence of trichomoniasis

Asymptomatic women (Britain)	5%
Family planning clinics	3%–15%
Gynecology clinics	13%–23%
Pregnant women	20%–25%
Symptomatic women (Britain)	25%–50%
Vaginitis clinics	20%–46%
Venereal disease clinics	20%–30%
Prostitutes	50%–75%

FIGURE 6-4 Prevalence of trichomoniasis. Trichomoniasis is prevalent worldwide. *Trichomonas vaginalis* is sexually transmitted. Populations at high risk for other sexually transmitted infections traditionally have a high prevalence of trichomoniasis. A diagnosis of trichomoniasis should prompt the clinician to evaluate the patient for other sexually transmitted conditions. (*Courtesy of* the Centers for Disease Control and Prevention.)

Extragenital survival of *Trichomonas vaginalis*

Wet sponge	90 min
Urine	3 hrs
Wet cloth	Up to 24 hrs
Contamination after use by infected woman	
Bathtub	1%
Toilet seat	13%

FIGURE 6-5 Extragenital survival of *Trichomonas vaginalis*. Older studies have documented extragenital survival of *T. vaginalis*, suggesting the possibility of nonvenereal transmission, but such transmission must be extremely rare.

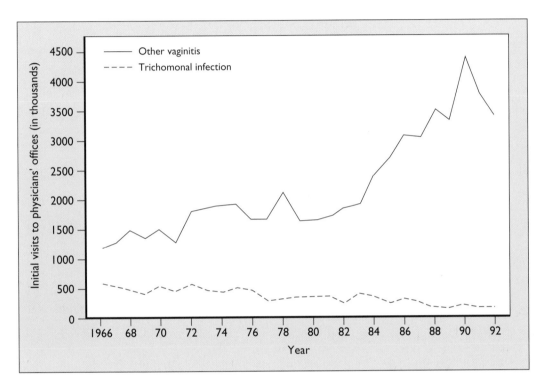

FIGURE 6-6 Incidence of trichomoniasis versus other vaginal infections in the United States between 1966 and 1992. The overall incidence of trichomoniasis seems to be decreasing in the United States, whereas the incidence of other forms of vaginitis is increasing. The decrease in trichomonal infection may be due to modifications in sexual behavior by individuals attempting to reduce their risk for other sexually transmitted diseases or, more likely, it may result from the increased use in sexually active populations of metronidazole as treatment for bacterial vaginosis. (*From* Division of STD/HIV Prevention: *Sexually Transmitted Disease Surveillance, 1992.* Atlanta: Centers for Disease Control and Prevention; 1993:29.)

CLINICAL PRESENTATION

Symptoms of women with vaginal trichomoniasis

None	9%–56%
Vaginal discharge	50%–75%
Malodorous	10%
Irritating, pruritic	23%–82%
Dyspareunia	10%–50%
Dysuria	30%–50%
Lower abdominal discomfort	5%–12%

FIGURE 6-7 Symptoms of women with vaginal trichomoniasis. Women with vaginal trichomoniasis classically complain of an irritating discharge. The incubation period ranges from about 5 to 28 days. Some women note that the symptoms begin or are exacerbated following menses. The clinical presentation of the infection is highly variable, however, and classic symptoms may not be present, with 25% of infected women being completely asymptomatic. Although abdominal discomfort is described by some women with trichomoniasis, its presence should prompt a careful evaluation for coincident endometritis or salpingitis of other etiologies. (Rein MF: *Trichomonas vaginalis. In* Mandell GL, Bennett JE, Dolin R (eds.): *Principles and Practice of Infectious Diseases*, 4th ed. New York: Churchill Livingstone; 1995:2497.)

Physical findings in women with vaginal trichomoniasis

None	15%
Diffuse vulvar erythema	10%–20%
Excessive discharge	50%–75%
Yellow, green	5%–20%
Frothy	10%–50%
Vaginal wall inflammation	40%–75%
Strawberry cervix	2%

FIGURE 6-8 Physical findings in women with vaginal trichomoniasis. Physical findings in women with vaginal trichomoniasis, like symptoms, are highly variable. Only a minority manifest the complete classic picture of a yellowish, frothy, foul-smelling discharge accompanied by inflammatory changes of the vulva, vaginal walls, and cervix. (Rein MF: *Trichomonas vaginalis. In* Mandell GL, Bennett JE, Dolin R (eds.): *Principles and Practice of Infectious Diseases*, 4th ed. New York: Churchill Livingstone; 1995:2497. Wolner-Hanssen P, Krieger JN, Stevens CE, *et al.*: Clinical manifestations of vaginal trichomoniasis. *JAMA* 1989, 261:571–576.)

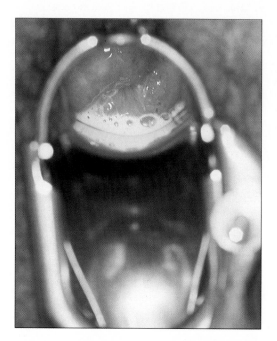

FIGURE 6-9 Frothy vaginal discharge in trichomoniasis. Speculum examination of woman with trichomoniasis reveals a profuse, foul-smelling discharge containing bubbles. The discharge is loose and pools in the posterior fornix. Redness of the exocervix is also appreciated. Some workers claim that the bubbles in trichomoniasis appear larger than those frequently accompanying bacterial vaginosis. The cervical discharge is seen to be mucoid; *Trichomonas vaginalis* causes vaginitis and exocervicitis but not endocervicitis; thus, a mucopurulent cervical discharge should raise suspicion of coincident gonococcal or chlamydial infection. (*From* Rein MF: *In* Holmes KK, *et al.* (eds.): *Sexually Transmitted Diseases.* New York: McGraw-Hill; 1984; with permission.)

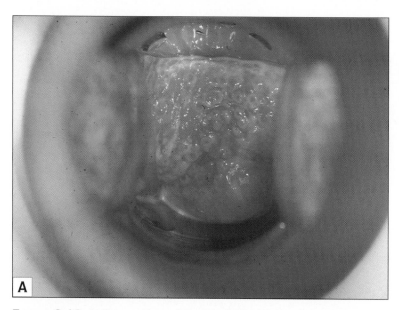

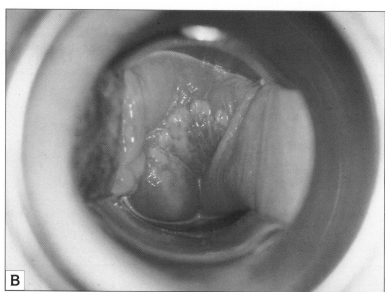

FIGURE 6-10 Inflammation of the vaginal walls in trichomoniasis. Inflammation in trichomoniasis may be pronounced. Accompanying edema may result in apparent hypertrophy of the vaginal rugae, which may be seen during speculum examination or felt on bimanual examination. **A,** The vaginal walls are highly inflamed and hypertrophied. **B,** Severe inflammation of the vaginal wall with desquamation giving the appearance of a pseudomembrane. (*Courtesy of* H.L. Gardner, MD.)

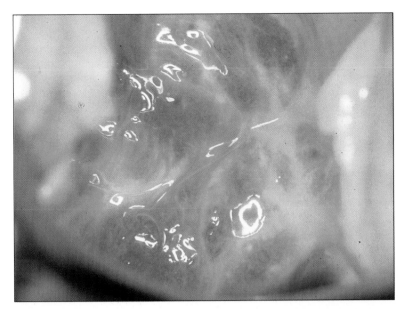

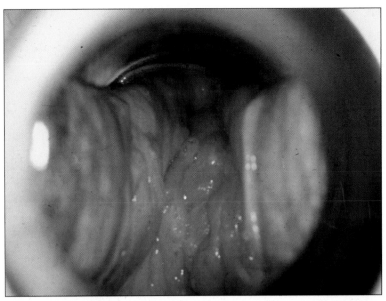

FIGURE 6-11 Speculum examination demonstrating florid granular vaginitis in a woman with chronic trichomoniasis. With the naked eye, the vaginal walls are recognized as erythematous in one to two thirds of women with trichomoniasis. In severe infection, the vaginal walls are characterized by dilation of blood vessels and capillary proliferation, yielding the granular appearance. When viewed through the colposcope, such inflamed vaginal walls reveal a characteristic double cresting of capillaries. (Kolstad P: The colposcopic picture of *Trichomonas vaginalis. Acta Obstet Gynecol Scand* 1965, 43:388–398.) (*From* Rein MF: Clinical manifestations of urogenital trichomoniasis in women. *In* Honigberg BM (ed.): *Trichomonads Parasitic in Humans.* New York: Springer-Verlag; 1989:228; with permission.)

FIGURE 6-12 Vaginitis emphysematosa. Vaginitis emphysematosa, in which gas-filled blebs appear in the vaginal walls, is an uncommon complication of vaginal trichomoniasis, although it develops in other settings as well. If associated with trichomoniasis, as in this case, it will resolve when the underlying infection is cured. (Josey WE, Campbell WG Jr: Vaginitis emphysematosa: A report of four cases. *J Reprod Med* 1990, 35:974–977.) (*Courtesy of* H.L. Gardner, MD.)

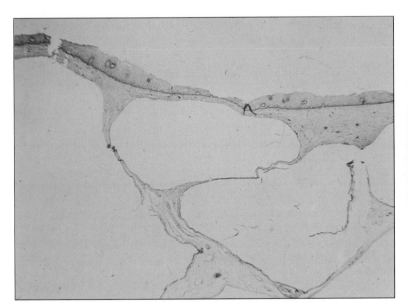

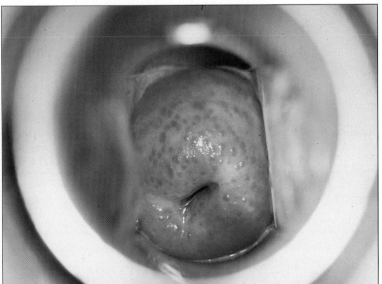

FIGURE 6-13 Historic appearance of vaginitis emphysematosa. Thin-walled blebs are apparent, with the characteristic absence of an inflammatory response. The nature of the gas in the blebs has been disputed, but current opinion favors carbon dioxide.

FIGURE 6-14 Speculum examination showing colpitis macularis (strawberry cervix) in trichomoniasis. Colpitis macularis, the strawberry cervix, is the most specific clinical finding for the diagnosis of trichomoniasis. It is observed in only 2% of infected women by visual inspection, but colposcopy reveals the diagnosis in 45%. Women with colpitis macularis have a higher parasite burden than those without the finding, but the organisms isolated from cases with and without the finding do not vary in experimental virulence. (Krieger JN, Wolner-Hanssen P, Stevens C, Holmes KK: Characteristics of *Trichomonas vaginalis* isolates from women with and without colpitis macularis. *J Infect Dis* 1990; 161:307–312.) (*Courtesy of* H.L. Gardner, MD.)

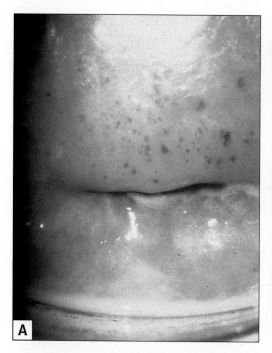
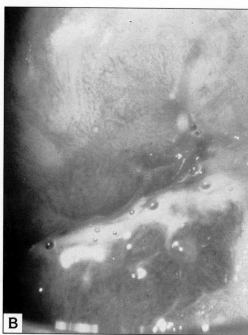

FIGURE 6-15 Colposcopic views of colpitis macularis in trichomoniasis. **A,** Small hemorrhages. **B,** Purulent vaginal discharge characteristic of trichomoniasis. Such hemorrhages are quite specific for trichomoniasis. Microscopic examination of biopsy specimens reveals superficial ulcerations and infiltration with polymorphonuclear neutrophils. (Gupta PK, Frost JK: Cytopathology and histopathology of the female genital tract in *Trichomonas vaginalis* infection. *In* Honigberg BM (ed.): *Trichomonads Parasitic in Humans.* New York: Springer-Verlag; 1989:274–290.)

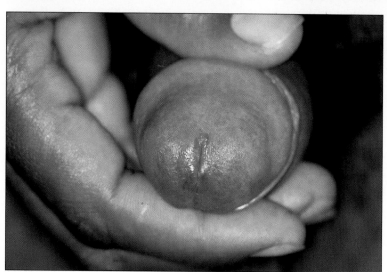

FIGURE 6-16 Urethral trichomoniasis in a man. Urethral trichomoniasis in men is often asymptomatic, but trichomoniasis may produce symptoms or signs of nongonococcal urethritis. The discharge is heavy and purulent, resembling that seen with gonococcal urethritis, in about 5% of infected men; more commonly, it is thin and scanty, crusting around the meatus. This man has nongonococcal urethritis of undetermined etiology but manifests a small amount of discharge, which would be typical of men with symptomatic trichomonal urethritis. Men with milder symptoms may be aware of discharge only upon arising from sleep. (Krieger JN, Jenny C, Verdon M, *et al.*: Clinical manifestations of trichomoniasis in men. *Ann Intern Med* 1993, 118:844–849. Krieger JN: Trichomoniasis in men: Old issues and new data. *Sex Transm Dis* 1995, 22:83–96.)

LABORATORY DIAGNOSIS

Laboratory diagnosis of vaginal trichomoniasis

Test	Sensitivity
pH > 4.5	66%–91%
Positive whiff test	75%
Wet mount	
Excess PMNs	75%
Trichomonads	66%–80%
Fluorescent antibody	90%
Gram stain	< 1%
Acridine orange stain	60%
Giemsa stain	50%
Papanicolaou smear	70%

PMNs—polymorphonuclear neutrophils.

FIGURE 6-17 Laboratory diagnosis of vaginal trichomoniasis. The diagnosis of vaginal trichomoniasis is supported by the finding of a vaginal pH elevated above the normal value of 4.5, although this finding also occurs in more common bacterial vaginosis. Likewise, the whiff test, an aminelike, fishy odor generated by the addition of potassium hydroxide to vaginal discharge, is positive in about 75% of cases but is more commonly associated with bacterial vaginosis. Trichomoniasis is definitively diagnosed by demonstrating *Trichomonas vaginalis* in the vaginal discharge. (Rein MF: *Trichomonas vaginalis. In* Mandell GL, Bennett JE, Dolin R (eds.): *Principles and Practice of Infectious Diseases,* 4th ed. New York: Churchill Livingstone; 1995:2493–2497.)

Diagnosis of trichomoniasis in men

Relative sensitivity of culture	
Urethra	40/50 (80%)
First-void urine	34/50 (68%)
External genitalia	6/50 (12%)
Semen	11/15 (73%)

FIGURE 6-18 Diagnosis of trichomoniasis in men. The diagnosis of trichomoniasis in men is difficult, and culture is the only technique with acceptable sensitivity. Direct culture of a urethral swab into Diamond's medium is the most sensitive technique. (Krieger JN, Jenny C, Verdon M, *et al.*: Clinical manifestations of trichomoniasis in men. *Ann Intern Med* 1993, 118:844–849. Krieger JN: Trichomoniasis in men: Old issues and new data. *Sex Transm Dis* 1995, 22:83–96.)

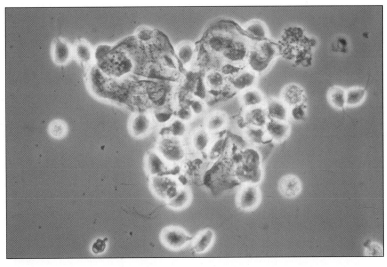

FIGURE 6-19 Phase photomicrograph of cultured vaginal discharge in trichomoniasis. Discharge reveals normal squamous epithelial cells and very large numbers of *Trichomonas vaginalis*, which are recognized by their flagella. *T. vaginalis* are recognized easily in live preparations by their characteristic twitching motility. (Original magnification, × 400.) (*Courtesy of* the Centers for Disease Control and Prevention.)

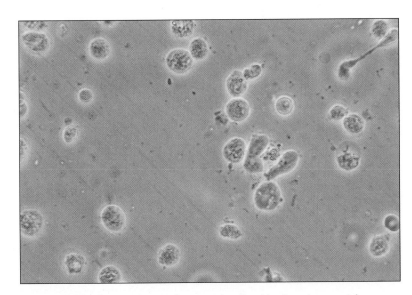

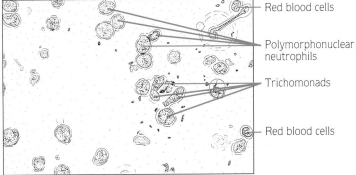

FIGURE 6-20 Phase photomicrograph of vaginal wet mount in trichomoniasis. Wet mount shows four trichomonads, numerous, polymorphonuclear neutrophils (which are close in size to trichomonads), and occasional red blood cells. The vaginal discharge from women with trichomoniasis usually contains large numbers of poly- morphonuclear neutrophils, which apparently can kill *Trichomonas vaginalis*. (Original magnification, × 400.) (Rein MF, Sullivan JA, Mandell GL: Trichomonacidal activity of human polymorphonuclear neutrophils: Killing by disruption and fragmentation. *J Infect Dis* 1980, 142:575–585.)

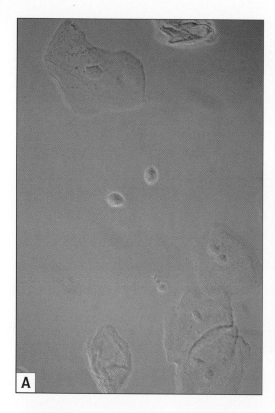
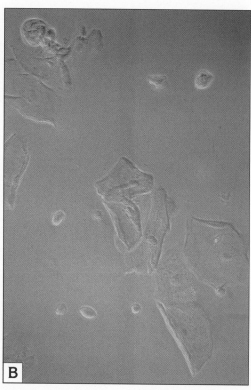

FIGURE 6-21 Light micrograph of vaginal wet mount in trichomoniasis. **A** and **B**, *Trichomonas vaginalis* can be visualized in the wet mount using conventional light microscopy. The substage condenser should be racked down and the substage diaphragm closed to increase contrast, as one would look at a urine sediment. The protozoa must be differentiated from polymorphonuclear neutrophils, which they resemble in size. *T. vaginalis* are usually ovoid or pear-shaped and should be actively motile. The sensitivity of the wet mount for *T. vaginalis* is only about 66% under optimal conditions.

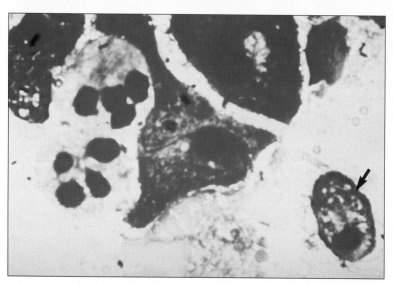

FIGURE 6-22 Gram stain of vaginal discharge revealing *Trichomonas vaginalis*. *T. vaginalis* (*arrow*) can be identified only with great difficulty on Gram stain. This stain should not be used for diagnosis of trichomoniasis. (*Courtesy of* the Centers for Disease Control and Prevention.)

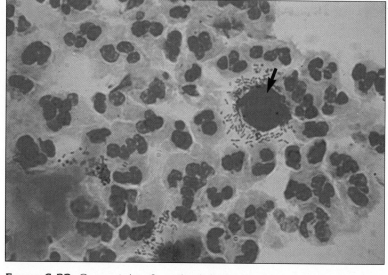

FIGURE 6-23 Gram stain of urethral discharge from a man with trichomoniasis. The patient had proven trichomonal urethritis. *Trichomonas vaginalis* is the large organism in the upper right (*arrow*). The surrounding gram-negative rods are unexplained. Urethral trichomoniasis is difficult to diagnose, and culture remains the most effective technique.

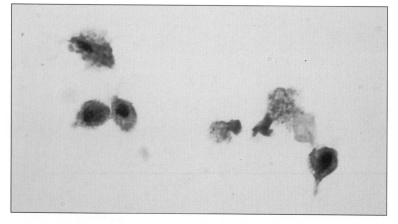

FIGURE 6-24 Cultured *Trichomonas vaginalis* stained with the Giemsa technique revealing characteristic dense nuclei. Although more sensitive than the Gram stain in clinical specimens, the Giemsa technique is less sensitive than the wet mount for diagnosis of trichomoniasis in women.

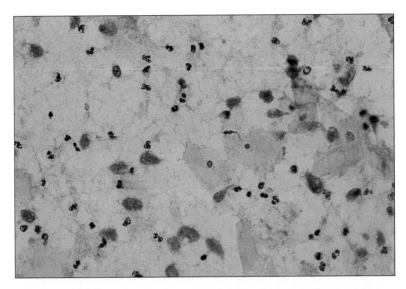

FIGURE 6-25 Papanicolaou-stained specimen containing *Trichomonas vaginalis*. The Papanicolaou smear, which stains the trichomonads green, has a sensitivity of about 60%. False-positive smears are also reported, even by experienced cytologists. Thus, cytologic diagnosis should be confirmed using another method. (Krieger JN, Tam MR, Stevens CE, *et al.*: Diagnosis of trichomoniasis: Comparison of conventional wet-mount examination with cytologic studies, cultures and monoclonal antibody staining of direct specimens. *JAMA* 1988, 259:1223–1227.)

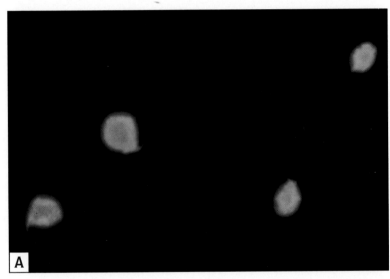

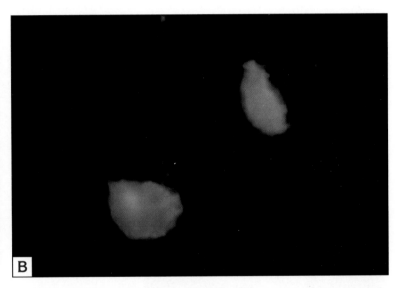

FIGURE 6-26 A and **B**, Cultured *Trichomonas vaginalis* stained with different monoclonal antibodies conjugated with fluorescent dyes. Four recent clinical isolates of *T. vaginalis* were used to prepare a panel of nine murine monoclonal antibodies, which were examined by indirect immunofluorescence against strains of *T. vaginalis* from several geographic sites. Wells containing fixed *T. vaginalis* were covered with one of the antibodies. After rinsing, each well was flooded with a fluorescein-isothiocyanate–conjugated goat anti- murine IgG. After subsequent washing, slides were counterstained with Evans blue dye and examined on a fluorescence microscope. Organisms with typical morphology are readily apparent. (Original magnification, × 400.) (Krieger JN, Holmes KK, Spence MR, *et al.*: Geographic variation among *Trichomonas vaginalis*: Demonstration of antigenic heterogeniety using monoclonal antibodies and the indirect immunofluorescence technique. *J Infect Dis* 1985, 152:979–984.)

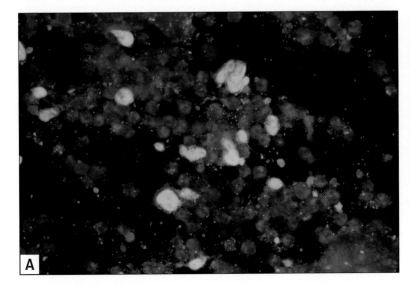

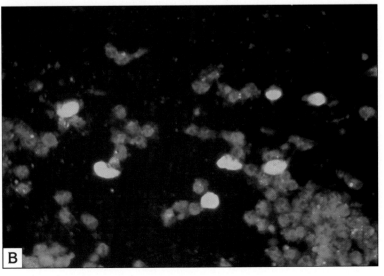

FIGURE 6-27 *Trichomonas vaginalis* identified by monoclonal antibody staining. **A** and **B**, Staining reveals a marked inflammatory response consisting principally of polymorphonuclear neutrophils (PMNs). (*contiened*)

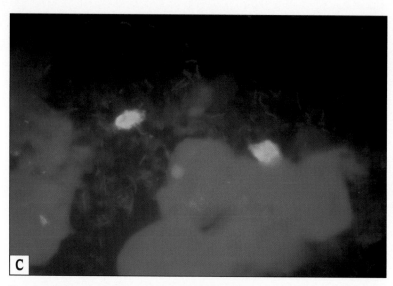

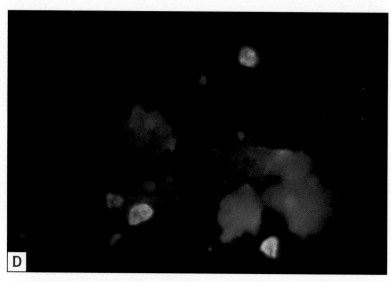

FIGURE 6-27 (*continued*) **C** and **D.** Whereas it might be difficult to differentiate *Trichomonas vaginalis* from polymorphonuclear neutrophils on fixed preparations by conventional staining, fluo- rescent monoclonal antibody staining permits rapid diagnosis, even in settings where few organisms are present.

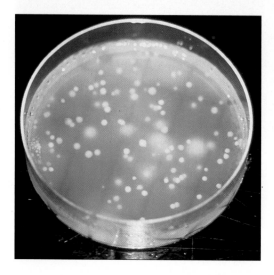

FIGURE 6-28 *Trichomonas vaginalis* culture in pour plates. *T. vaginalis* is usually cultured in liquid media but can be quantitated in pour plates. After 4 to 5 days of incubation, individ- ual colonies of *T. vaginalis* are apparent and can be counted with a dissecting microscope. Quantitative cultures suggest that most infected women carry between 10 and 100,000 organisms per milliliter of vaginal fluid (Philip A, *et al.*: An agar culture technique to quantitate *Trichomonas vaginalis* from women. *J Infect Dis* 1987, 155:304–308.)

THERAPY

Sites of colonization with *Trichomonas vaginalis* from 387 symptomatic women

								Totals
Urethra	+			+		+	+	82.5%
Paraurethral glands		+			+	+	+	97.8%
Vagina			+	+	+	+	+	98.4%
Cervix							+	13.1%
Totals	1.7%	3.2%	3.2%	0.6%	12.7%	68.8%	13.1%	

FIGURE 6-29 Site of colonization with *Trichomonas vaginalis*. Trichomoniasis is more than a simple vaginitis because organisms are frequently isolated from the urethra as well as the vagina. Thus, systemic therapy with one of the 5'-nitroimidazoles has proven more successful than strictly topical therapy. Obviously, topical therapy has no role in the treatment of infected men. The percent- ages indicate the proportion of patients having that finding exclu- sively. (Grys E: Topography of trichomoniasis in the reproductive organ of the woman. *Wiad Parazytol* 1964, 10:122–124.)

Recommended therapy for trichomoniasis*

Metronidazole 2 g orally immediately
or
Metronidazole 250 mg orally three times a day × 7 days

---

*Treat sex partners simultaneously.

FIGURE 6-30 Recommended therapy for trichomoniasis. Metronidazole is the only 5′-nitroimidazole available in the United States. In other countries, treatment with single doses of tinidazole, ornidazole, or nimorazole have proven equally effective. Advantages of the single-dose regimens include lower cost, avoidance of noncompliance, and smaller total exposure to the drug. Treatment of male sexual partners, even if they are asymptomatic, significantly improves the cure rate in women treated with the single-dose regimen.

Prevalence of *Trichomonas vaginalis* in sexual partners of infected women

Days since last exposure	Patients examined, *n*	Positive
2	23	70%
4	29	55%
6	27	26%
8	25	37%
10	21	37%
12	5	20%
14	25	33%

FIGURE 6-31 Prevalence of *Trichomonas vaginalis* in sexual partners of infected women. Trichomoniasis appears to be self-limited in many men. It becomes harder to isolate *T. vaginalis* from the urethras of men as the time from their last sexual exposure increases. If women are treated with the 1-week regimen, they may be less susceptible to reinfection from untreated sexual partners.

SELECTED BIBLIOGRAPHY

Honigberg BM (ed.): *Trichomonads Parasitic in Humans*. New York: Springer-Verlag; 1990.

Krieger JN: Trichomoniasis in men: Old issues and new data. *Sex Transm Dis* 1995, 22:83–96.

Krieger JN, Jenny C, Verdon M, *et al.*: Clinical manifestations of trichomoniasis in men. *Ann Intern Med* 1993, 118:844–849.

Rein MF: *Trichomonas vaginalis*. *In* Mandell GL, Bennett JE, Dolin R (eds.): *Principles and Practice of Infectious Diseases*, 4th ed. New York: Churchill Livingstone, 1995:2493–2497.

Wolner-Hanssen P, Krieger JN, Stevens CE, *et al.*: Clinical manifestations of vaginal trichomoniasis. *JAMA* 1989, 261:571–576.

CHAPTER 7

Vulvovaginal Candidiasis

Jack D. Sobel

EPIDEMIOLOGY

Classification of vulvovaginal candidiasis

Sporadic vaginitis	Recurrent vaginitis (≥ 3 episodes/yr)
Primary	Primary/idiopathic
Secondary	Secondary
Antibiotic therapy	Uncontrolled diabetes mellitus
Pregnancy	AIDS
	Estrogen replacement therapy
	Immunosuppressive therapy

FIGURE 7-1 Classification of vulvovaginal candidiasis. Most women suffer from sporadic, occasional attacks of vulvovaginal candidiasis, the most common precipitating factor being antibiotic use. Recurrent vulvovaginitis affects only a small percentage and, apart from in uncontrolled diabetics and immunocompromised hosts, is usually idiopathic.

Epidemiology of vulvovaginal candidiasis

Second only on anaerobic bacterial vaginosis (*Gardnerella*)

Approx. 75% of adults have at least one attack of vulvovaginal candidiasis

Three subpopulations:
  No attacks
  Infrequent episodes
  Recurrent/chronic vulvovaginal candidiasis

45% have more than one episode

FIGURE 7-2 Epidemiology of vulvovaginal candidiasis. Vulvovaginal candidiasis is second only to bacterial vaginosis in prevalence, and because of its hormonal dependence, the infection is rare before puberty and after menopause.

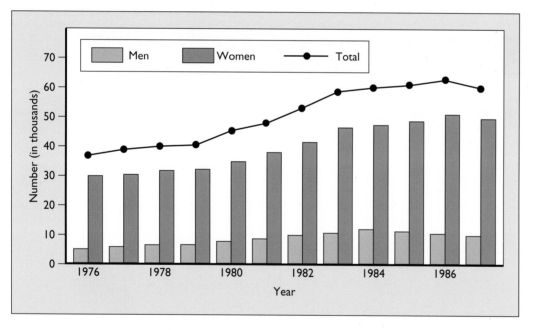

FIGURE 7-3 Incidence of genital candidiasis in the United Kingdom. Although vulvovaginal candidiasis is not a reportable disease in the United States, data from the United Kingdom show a continued increase in its prevalence. (*Data from* the Annual Reports of the Chief Medical Officer, Department of Health and Social Security, 1976–1984, England and Wales.)

ETIOLOGY

Microbiology of vulvovaginal candidiasis

> 80% due to *Candida albicans*
3%–15% due to *Candida glabrata*
Incubation period: 24–96 hrs
Inoculum: 10^2 microorganisms

FIGURE 7-4 Microbiology of vulvovaginal candidiasis. By far, the commonest pathogen in vulvovaginal candidiasis is *Candida albicans*; however, 5% to 15% of cases are due to non–*albicans Candida* species, the commonest of which is *Candida (Torulopsis) glabrata*. The minimal inoculum causing disease has been experimentally defined as 100 microorganisms.

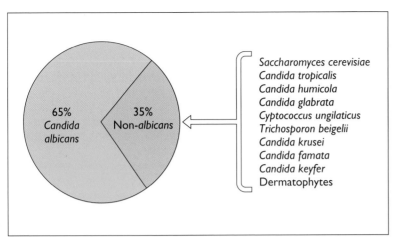

FIGURE 7-5 Subspeciation of yeast causing vulvovaginal candidiasis. Some authors have claimed a markedly increased prevalence of both *Candida glabrata* and *Candida tropicalis* in vulvovaginal candidiasis, although the data to support these recent claims have not been substantiated. Possibly women with HIV infection are more prone to infection with *C. glabrata*. (Horowitz BJ, Giaqunta D, Ito S: Evolving pathogens in vulvovaginal candidiasis: Implications for patient care. *J Clin Pharmacol* 1992, 32:248–255.)

Saccharomyces cerevisiae
Candida tropicalis
Candida humicola
Candida glabrata
Cyptococcus ungilaticus
Trichosporon beigelii
Candida krusei
Candida famata
Candida keyfer
Dermatophytes

65% Candida albicans

35% Non-albicans

Chronologic speciation of vaginal isolates from women with acute *Candida* vaginitis, 1983–1992

	1983	1986	1987	1988	1989	1990	1991	1992
Candida albicans	85%	85.2%	82.5%	87.2%	86.3%	87.7%	93%	87.8%
Non-*albicans*	15%	14.8%	17.5%	12.8%	13.7%	12.3%	7%	12.2%
C. glabrata	12%	4.9%	8.8%	7.4%	7.6%	6.6%	2.6%	6.1%
C. parapsilosis	1%	6.2%	6.1%	1.1%	2.3%	1.6%	0.9%	1.2%
C. tropicalis	1%	—	1.7%	2.1%	2.3%	1.6%	0.9%	1.2%
C. lusitaniae	1%	—	0.9%	—	0.8%	—	—	—
Saccharomyces cerevisiae	—	1.2%	—	1.1%	0.8%	0.8%	1.7%	1.2%
C. krusei	—	—	—	—	—	0.8%	—	1.2%
C. kefyr	—	—	—	1.1%	—	0.8%	—	—
Trichosporon beigelii	—	2.5%	—	—	—	—	0.9%	1.2%

FIGURE 7-6 Chronologic speciation of vaginal isolates from women with acute *Candida* vaginitis between 1983 and 1992. Isolates were obtained from women with recurrent and chronic vaginitis referred to the Vaginitis Clinic at the Detroit Medical Center over a 10-year period. Given the intractability of vulvovaginal candidiasis in most patients and their previous long-term, intensive, highly diversified therapy, if there were to be a major or minor change in prevalence of pathogenic yeast species and susceptibility, it would be readily apparent in this series. No such change has been documented by these data, which do not show any increase in vaginitis due to non-*albicans* species.

PATHOGENESIS

Transformation From Asymptomatic to Symptomatic Infection

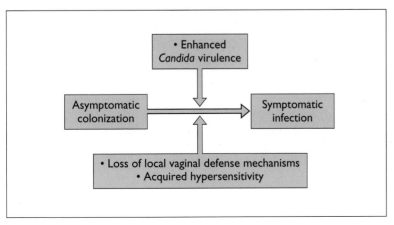

• Enhanced
Candida virulence

Asymptomatic colonization

Symptomatic infection

• Loss of local vaginal defense mechanisms
• Acquired hypersensitivity

FIGURE 7-7 Transformation from asymptomatic colonization to symptomatic vaginitis. Low numbers of *Candida* colonize the vagina as commensals but are capable of causing symptomatic vaginitis in the presence of local factors that enhance yeast virulence (*eg*, uncontrolled diabetes) or reduce local vaginal defense mechanisms (*eg*, antibiotics).

Factors influencing transformation from asymptomatic colonization to symptomatic vaginitis

Factors enhancing *Candida* virulence	Factors associated with loss of local defense mechanisms
Pregnancy	Local/systemic antimicrobials
Uncontrolled diabetes	AIDS
Exogenous hormones (estrogen, corticosteroids)	Sexual intercourse (?)
Use of tight-fitting noncotton underclothing	Hypersensitivity reactions (?)
"Candy binge"	
Switching colonies(?)	

FIGURE 7-8 Factors influencing the transformation from asymptomatic colonization to symptomatic vaginitis. Transformation to symptomatic vaginitis may occur as a result of enhanced virulence expression or loss of local defense mechanisms. In most episodes of acute *Candida* vaginitis, no exogenous precipitating factors are usually evident. Factors involving sexual behavior, such as frequency of vaginal intercourse, receptive oral sex, and use of spermicides and oral contraceptives, may contribute to exacerbation of symptoms. In the absence of precipitating events, attention has focused on spontaneous "switch" in yeast phenotype.

Comparison of asymptomatic vaginal colonization and symptomatic vaginitis

	Asymptomatic colonization	Symptomatic vaginitis
Candida strain type	Identical	Identical
Predominant phenotype	Blastospore and budding	Germ tube and mycelia
Concentration	$\leq 10^3$/mL	$\geq 10^4$/mL
Proteolytic activity	+ to + +	+ + to + + +
White/opaque colonies	Fewer opaque	More opaque

FIGURE 7-9 Comparison of *Candida* characteristics in asymptomatic vaginal colonization versus symptomatic vaginitis. The mechanism by which asymptomatic colonization of the vagina is transformed to symptomatic vaginitis remains unclear. During asymptomatic carriage, *Candida* organisms exist predominantly in the nonfilamentous form and in low numbers. Symptomatic vaginitis develops in the presence of factors that enhance *Candida* virulence or as a result of loss of local defense mechanisms. (*From* Sobel JD: Genital candidiasis. *In* Bodey GP (ed.): *Candidiasis: Pathogenesis, Diagnosis, and Treatments*, 2nd ed. New York: Raven Press; 1993:230; with permission.)

Natural anti-*Candida* vaginal defense mechanisms

Vaginal microbial flora dominated by *Lactobacillus*
Intact vaginal (compartmentalized) cell-mediated immunity
Cervicovaginal immunoglobulins
   Candida-specific sIgA and IgG
Minor protective factors (?)
   Complement
   Phagocytic cells
Hormonal influence (anti-estrogen)

FIGURE 7-10 Natural anti-*Candida* defense mechanisms of the vagina. In contrast to oral thrush, vaginal candidiasis is not an opportunistic infection, as it occurs in otherwise healthy women. The normal *Lactobacillus*-dominant flora provides an essential defense mechanism, together with local vaginal cell-mediated immunity that involves *Candida*-specific T-lymphocyte clones expressing Th1 activity. Vaginal secretions contain antibodies that appear to have a minor protective role.

Risk factors for vulvovaginal candidiasis

Pregnancy
Uncontrolled diabetes mellitus
Corticosteroid therapy
Tight-fitting synthetic underclothing
Antimicrobial therapy (oral, parental, topical)
Estrogen therapy
Contraceptive use
  IUD
  Sponge
  Nonoxynol-9 (?)
  Diaphragm (?)
  High-dose estrogen contraceptives
Increased frequency of coitus
"Candy binge"
Women frequenting STD clinics
HIV infection

IUD—intrauterine device; STD—sexually transmitted diseases.

FIGURE 7-11 Risk factors for vulvovaginal candidiasis. The list of known exogenous and endogenous risk factors is large, but most episodes of vulvovaginal candidiasis occur in the absence of a recognizable precipitating factor. Although vulvovaginal candidiasis is not a sexually transmitted disease, sexual behavior, and possibly coital frequency, may contribute to symptomatic infection.

Microbial Virulence Factors

Candida virulence factors

Adherence to epithelial cells
Protease elaboration
Germination (hyphae, pseudohyphae)
Phospholipase production
Switching colonies/phenotype variation
Immunosuppression
Hemolysin production
Iron utilization
Complement-binding receptors
Mycotoxins

FIGURE 7-12 Microbial virulence factors expressed in *Candida*. In order to colonize, yeast blastospores adhere to epithelial cells and persist despite relatively antagonistic bacterial flora. Elaboration by *Candida* of phospholipase and proteases facilitates tissue invasion. Hemolysins lyse erythrocytes, releasing iron needed by *Candida*. The ability of *Candida* blastospores to bind activated complement components interferes with complement binding to immunoglobulins and may prevent efficient phagocytosis of *Candida* in invasive candidiasis. The hyphal form of *Candida* is more virulent and invasive and is the morphotype associated with symptomatic vaginitis. (*See also* Fig. 7-20.)

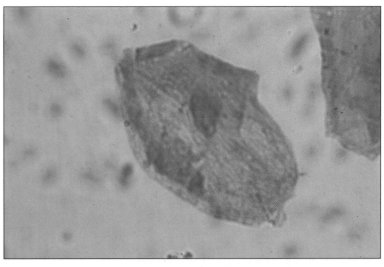

FIGURE 7-13 Normal vaginal squamous epithelial cells. A Gram stain shows normal squamous epithelial cells of the vagina without adherent bacteria or yeast.

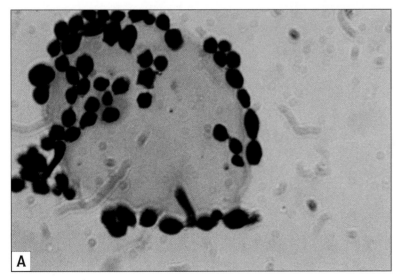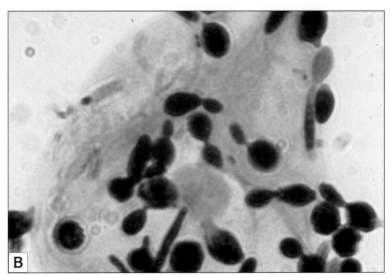

FIGURE 7-14 Gram stain of vaginal squamous epithelial cell with adherent blastospores in budding phase. Yeasts are densely Gram-positive. **A.** Low-power view. **B.** High-power view.

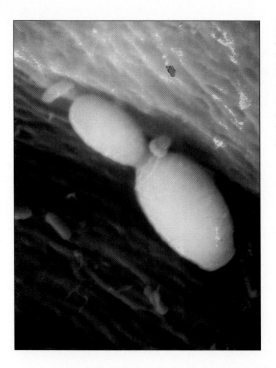

FIGURE 7-15
Scanning electron micrograph of budding yeast (blastospore) of *Candida albicans* adherent to a vaginal squamous cell.

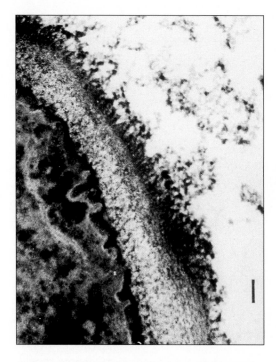

FIGURE 7-16
Transmission electron micrograph of *Candida albicans* cell wall. The micrograph shows the mannan surface layer containing mannoprotein (binding) ligands or adhesins. These mucopolysaccharide components adhere to fucose-containing receptors expressed on epithelial cells.

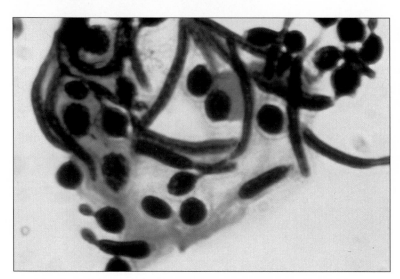

FIGURE 7-17 Gram stain of vaginal squamous epithelial cell with adherent blastospores, budding yeast, and pseudohyphae. The pseudohyphae often have a beaded appearance on Gram stain.

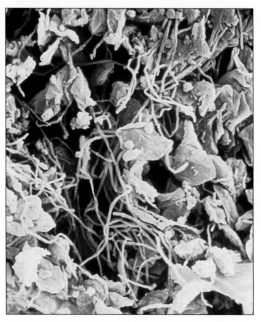

FIGURE 7-18 Scanning electron micrograph of a a mass of interwoven hyphae of *Candida albicans* and desquamated vaginal epithelial cells. The specimen was obtained by vaginal biopsy from a patient with vaginitis. (*Courtesy of* M. Borgers, PhD.)

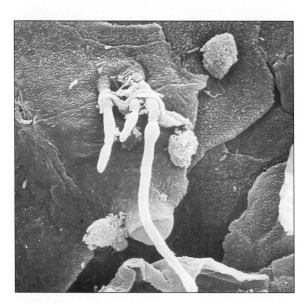

FIGURE 7-19 Scanning electron micrograph of mycelia of *Candida albicans* invading the intact surface of vaginal epithelial cells. (*Courtesy of* M. Borgers, PhD.)

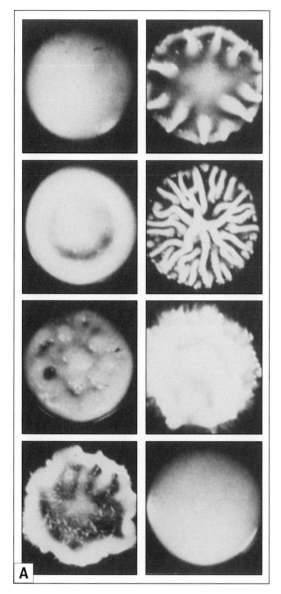

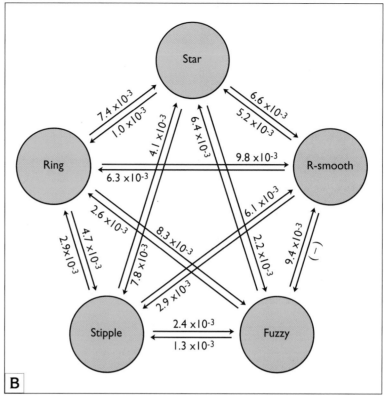

FIGURE 7-20 Switch colony phenotypes of *Candida albicans*. **A**, Switch colony phenotypes of *C. albicans* develop *in vitro* when plated on Lee's medium at 25° C. Switching of colony phenotypes may represent an *in vivo* virulence factor responsible for selection of more virulent vaginopathic strains of identical species. Spontaneous switching of phenotype may be responsible for episodes of vaginitis that occur in the absence of identifiable precipitating events or risk factors. **B**, Switching of colony phenotypes is thought to represent a heritable change in physical characteristics of yeast blastospores occurring at a relatively high frequency and may represent an adaptation to a changing, often adverse microenvironment.

Pathogenesis of Recurrent Vulvovaginal Candidiasis

Pathogenesis of recurrent vulvovaginal candidiasis

Absence of recognized predisposing factors in women with recurrent vulvovaginal candidiasis

FIGURE 7-21 Pathogenesis of idiopathic recurrent vulvovaginitis. In the vast majority of patients, episodes of vulvovaginal candidiasis recur in the absence of recognizable risk factors. In some women, recurrent vulvovaginal candidiasis is due to uncontrolled diabetes, hormone replacement therapy, or use of immunosuppressive agents.

Pathogenesis of recurrent vulvovaginal candidiasis

Source	Mechanism
1. More frequent vaginal inoculation/reinfection	1. Enhanced *Candida* virulence
Intestinal reservoir theory	2. Host
Sexual transmission	Depressed mucosal immunity (CMI)
2. Vaginal relapse	Immediate hypersensitivity reactivity (IgE)
	Loss of bacterial "colonization resistance"

CMI—cell-mediated immunity.

FIGURE 7-22 Pathogenesis of idiopathic recurrent vulvovaginal candidiasis. For many years, recurrent vulvovaginal candidiasis was thought to be due to repeated reinfection from a gastrointestinal reservoir or possibly from sexual transmission. New evidence suggests that frequent reinfection is less likely to be responsible, and evidence instead points to frequent vaginal relapses resulting from subclinical persistence of yeasts in the vagina. Relapses occur because of the use of fungistatic antifungal agents and impaired local host defense mechanisms. Enhanced *Candida* virulence may rarely be due to antimycotic drug resistance. (*From* Sobel JD: Genital candidiasis. *In* Bodey GP (ed.): *Candidiasis: Pathogenesis, Diagnosis, and Treatment*, 2nd ed. New York: Raven Press; 1953:232; with permission.)

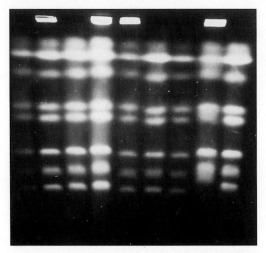

FIGURE 7-23 Contour clamped homogeneous field (CHEF) karotyping of vaginal isolates of *Candida albicans*. CHEF electrophoretic analysis involves mounting yeasts in a gel, extracting the DNA, and subjecting it sequentially to electrical pulses of varying voltage at several different angles. The pulses cause the chromosomes to migrate through the gel matrix with a velocity dependent on their charge and molecular weight. The resulting bands are stained with ethidium bromide. Yeasts may be subspeciated on the basis of the resulting banding pattern. This figures shows CHEF karyotyping of vaginal isolates of *Candida albicans* obtained longitudinally from a single patient with recurrent bouts of *Candida* vaginitis. All isolates obtained over 2 years had identical karyotypes, supporting the hypothesis of relapsing vaginitis.

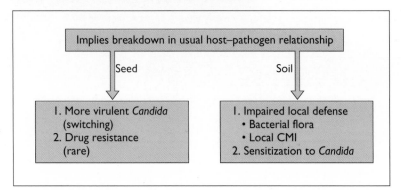

FIGURE 7-24 Pathogenesis of vaginal relapse recurrent *Candida* vulvovaginitis. Vaginal relapse implies that most successful courses of treatment of vaginitis result in persistence of small numbers of organisms in the vagina, which later proliferate to cause recurrent vaginitis. (CMI—cell-mediated immunity.)

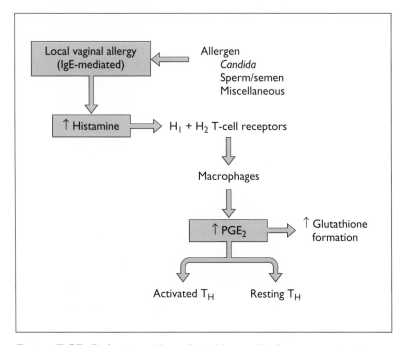

FIGURE 7-25 Defective cell-mediated immunity in recurrent vulvovaginal candidiasis (VVC). Among the theories directed at explaining recurrent VVC is impaired local cell-mediated immunity of the vaginal mucosal. Some investigators attribute impaired T-cell (CD4) function to the presence of suppressor cells or to prostaglandin E_2 (PGE_2) excess produced by local macrophages. (Witkin SS, Hirsch J, Ledger WJ: A macrophage defect in women with recurrent *Candida* vaginitis and its reversal *in vitro* by prostaglandin inhibitors. *Am J Obstet Gynecol* 1986, 155:790–795.)

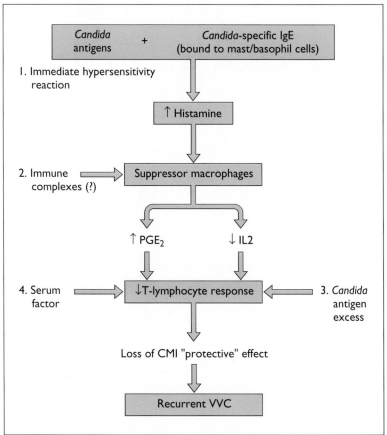

FIGURE 7-26 Immunopathogenesis of recurrent vulvovaginal candidiasis (VVC). It is postulated that after acquisition of *Candida*-specific local IgE antibodies, repeat reintroduction of *Candida* into the vagina results in an antigen–antibody reaction. Following binding to mast cells, histamine is released, which causes local symptoms and also serves to suppress the protective vaginal cell-mediated immunity (CMI). (IL2—interleukin-2; PGE_2—prostaglandin E_2.)

Vulvovaginal Candidiasis in HIV Infection

Vulvovaginal candidiasis in HIV-infected women

First sign of HIV infection
Tends to precede oral thrush
Vaginitis more severe and persistent
Tendency to recur

FIGURE 7-27 Characteristics of vulvovaginal candidiasis in HIV-infected women. Preliminary studies suggested that vulvovaginal candidiasis in HIV-positive women was more likely to recur, resulting in a pattern of relapsing *Candida* vaginitis. However, clinical episodes are identical to those in HIV-negative women and respond to conventional therapy. (Rhoads JL, Wright DC, Redfield RR, Burke DS: Chronic vaginal candidiasis in women with HIV infection. *JAMA* 1987, 257:3105–3197.)

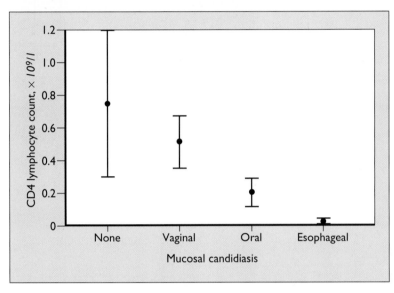

FIGURE 7-28 Occurrence of mucosal candidiasis correlating with CD4 cell counts in HIV-positive women. Esophageal candidiasis invariably occurs at CD4 counts < 100/mm^3, whereas oral candidiasis frequently manifests at CD4 counts of 200 to 400/mm^3. Women reporting only vulvovaginal candidiasis (VVC) had CD4 counts within the normal range. The authors interpreted these findings as indicating that only a minimal immunosuppressive effect of HIV will result in chronic and recurrent VVC. This view has not been substantiated. (*From* Imam N, Carpenter CC, Mayer KH, *et al.*: Hierarchical pattern of mucosal candida infections in HIV-seropositive women. *Am J Med* 1990, 89:142–146; with permission.)

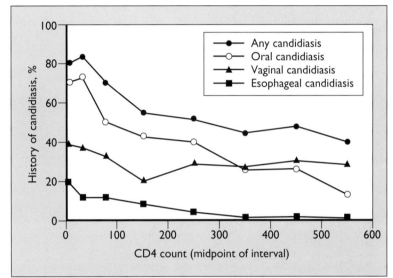

FIGURE 7-29 History of candidiasis by CD4 count. With a decline in CD4 cell counts in HIV-positive women, an increased susceptibility to oral and esophageal candidiasis is evident. However, no increased frequency of vulvovaginal candidiasis accompanies a decline in CD4 count.

CLINICAL MANIFESTATIONS

Symptoms of acute vulvovaginal candidiasis

Pruritus
Discharge
Soreness, irritation, burning
Dysuria
Dyspareunia
Minimal nonoffensive odor
Penile rash (men)

FIGURE 7-30 Symptoms of acute *Candida* vulvovaginitis. The symptoms of vulvovaginal candidiasis are nonspecific, not allowing diagnosis by history alone. Symptoms typically increase premenstrually and improve with onset of menstrual flow. A small portion of the male partners of women with vulvovaginal candidiasis will develop superficial genital candidiasis.

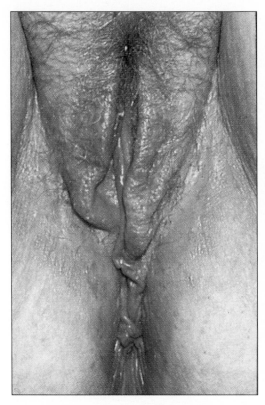

FIGURE 7-31 Vulvar edema and erythema. Characteristic findings in vulvovaginal candidiasis include edema, erythema, and fissures, with prominent vulvar manifestations.

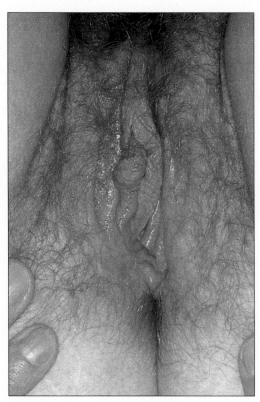

FIGURE 7-32 Vulvar erythema and pruritus extending into perianal area. Signs of vulvovaginal candidiasis are also nonspecific and preclude diagnosis without laboratory confirmation.

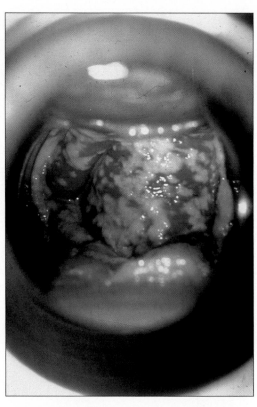

FIGURE 7-33 Typical cottage cheese–like discharges in vulvovaginitis candidiasis. The typical "cottage cheese," white discharge seen on speculum examination is found in only a minority of patients with *Candida* vaginitis.

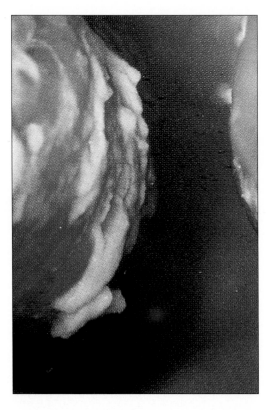

FIGURE 7-34 Curd-like, white, floccular discharge adherent to vaginal surface in a patient with *Candida* vaginitis. This discharge is easily removed by wiping.

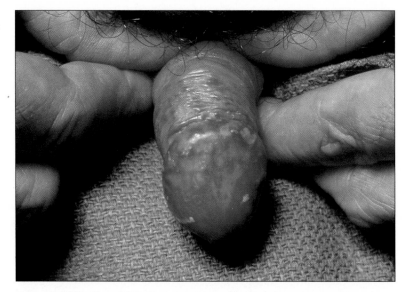

FIGURE 7-35 *Candida* balanoposthitis. Candida balanoposthitis presents with penile itching, irritation, and soreness, accompanied by edema, erythema, and excoriation. It is seen in the male partners of women with a vaginal culture positive for *Candida albicans*. Only a small fraction of the male partners of women with vulvovaginal candidiasis will develop superficial genital candidiasis.

DIFFERENTIAL DIAGNOSIS

↑pH	Normal pH
Bacterial vaginosis	Physiologic leukorrhea
Trichomoniasis	Allergic/hypersensitivity vaginitis
Atrophic vaginitis	Chemical/irritant (*eg,* nonoxynol-9)
Desquamative inflammatory vaginitis	Cytolytic vaginosis
Mixed (above + vulvovaginal candidiasis)	Vestibular adenitis/vulvovdynia
Erosive planus (vagina)	Erosive planus (vulva)
	Lichen simplex
	Lichen sclerosus
	Squamous papulomatosis
	Genital herpes

Differential diagnosis of vulvovaginal candidiasis

FIGURE 7-36 Differential diagnoses in vulvovaginal candidiasis. Considerations in the differential diagnosis of vulvovaginal candidiasis differ depending on measurement of the vaginal pH.

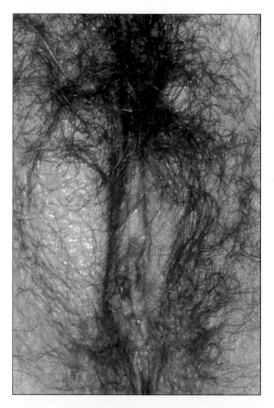

FIGURE 7-37 Chronic lichen simplex. Chronic lichen simplex is seen in a patient presenting with pruritus vulvae but with negative vaginal and vulvar yeast cultures. Lichen simplex chronicus, manifesting as erythematous lichenified plaques, appears in response to a cycle of protracted itching and scratching. The itching is often perceived as being worse at night, and the patient may scratch without being aware that she is doing so. The condition is also referred to as *squamous cell hyperplasia* in the classification prepared by the International Society for the Study of Vulvovaginal Disease. (Ridley CM, *et al*.: ISSVD: New nomenclature for vulvar disease. *Am J Obstet Gynecol* 1989, 160:769.)

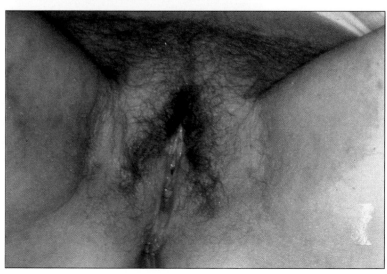

FIGURE 7-38 Tinea cruris. The borders of the lesions of tinea cruris are usually sharper than those of candidiasis, tend to have a brownish color, and are less likely to be accompanied by weeping or fissures. In men, genital candidiasis often involves the scrotum, whereas tinea cruris characteristically spares the scrotum.

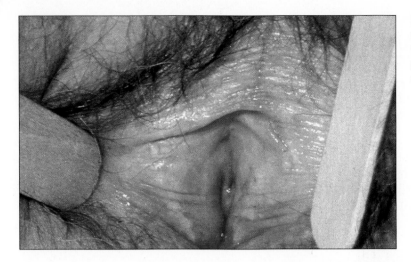

FIGURE 7-39 Lichen sclerosus (et atrophicus). Lichen sclerosus may also present with chronic irritation, discomfort, and pruritus vulvae. The involved skin is pale and fragile and may display superficial ulceration. The lesions sometimes present a finely crinkled appearance.

DIAGNOSIS

Diagnostic tests in vulvovaginitis	
pH estimation	Nonspecific but extremely useful in suggesting bacterial and protozoal infection (*see* Fig. 7-7)
Amine test (whiff test, sniff test)	Low sensitivity and specificity; useful in suggestion bacterial vaginosis or trichomoniasis
Saline microscopy	Essential study in evaluating patients with vulvovaginitis; sensitivity in diagnosis of VVC only 30%–40%
10% KOH microscopy	↑ sensitivity in diagnosing VVC (60%–80%)
Vaginal yeast culture	Gold standard for diagnosing presence of yeast, but a positive culture does not indicate vaginitis; culture uncommonly needed

KOH—potassium hydroxide; VVC—vulvovaginal candidiasis.

FIGURE 7-40 Diagnostic tests in vulvovaginitis. Diagnosis of *Candida* vulvovaginitis typically includes measurement of vaginal pH, saline microscopy, and 10% potassium hydroxide microscopic examination. For each test, a swab is obtained from the middle third of the vagina.

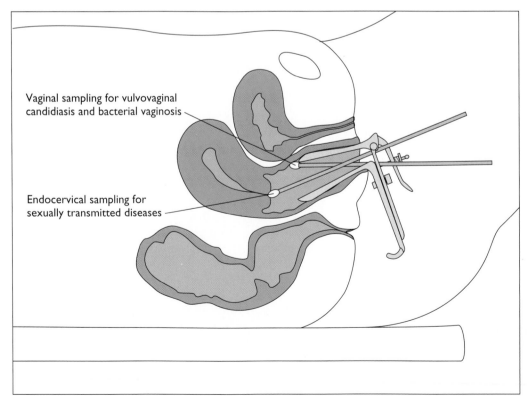

Vaginal sampling for vulvovaginal candidiasis and bacterial vaginosis

Endocervical sampling for sexually transmitted diseases

FIGURE 7-41 Vaginal sampling sites for diagnosis of vulvovaginal candidiasis. A cross-sectional diagram shows that for a diagnosis of vulvovaginal candidiasis (or bacterial vaginosis), a swab sample should be obtained from the middle third of the vagina.

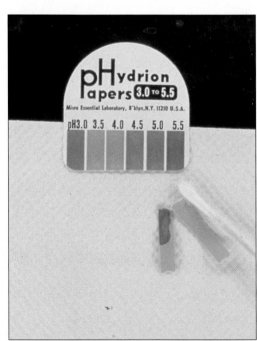

FIGURE 7-42 Vaginal pH testing. An elevated vaginal pH (normal, 4.5) suggests a major disruption in vaginal flora that is not seen in *Candida* vulvovaginitis (*see* Fig. 7-43). Other causes of an elevated pH include the sampling of cervical mucosa and presence of semen.

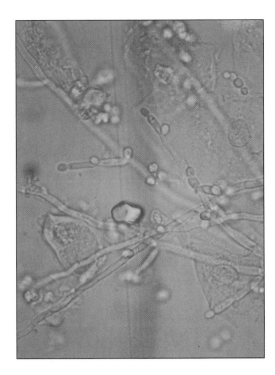

FIGURE 7-43 Saline microscopy. Although a number of techniques are used, most frequently a swab obtained from the middle third of the vagina is immediately placed in 0.5 mL of saline in a test tube. Then, a single drop of the resultant solution is placed on a clean dry slide and a coverslip applied. Initially under low power, the presence of motile trichomonads, polymorphonuclear neutrophils (PMNs), and hyphae can be detected. Under high-power magnification, a search is made for clue cells, trichomonads, PMNs, yeast blastospores and pseudohyphae, and epithelial cell maturation (squamous versus basal and parabasal cells). Finally, the bacterial flora is assessed (rods versus cocci).

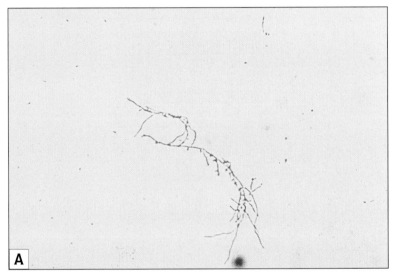

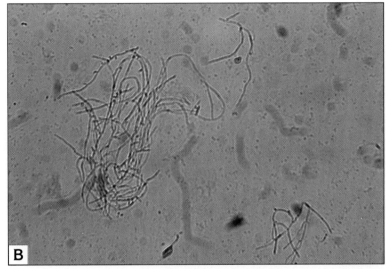

FIGURE 7-44 Potassium hydroxide (KOH) microscopy showing hyphae and blastospores. **A** and **B**, Ten percent potassium hydroxide (KOH) microscopy facilitates the diagnosis of *Candida* vulvovaginitis. KOH, by destroying epithelial cells, allows easier recognition of yeast and hyphae, improving on the sensitivity of the saline microscopy (30%–40%) to reach levels of 60% to 80%. With the exception of *Candida glabrata* and *Saccharomyces cerevisiae*, KOH examination allows recognition of pseudohyphae and hyphae as well as blastospores.

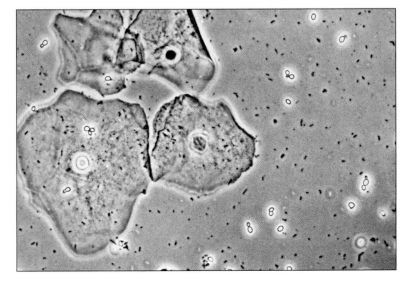

FIGURE 7-45 Phase contrast microscopy showing yeast cells without hyphae. Large numbers of yeast cells are seen as singlets or as budding yeast, but there is a complete absence of pseudohyphae and hyphae. This appearance is almost pathognomonic of *Candida glabrata* or *Saccharomyces cerevisiae*, two species of yeast that may resemble typical *Candida albicans* vaginitis but tend to be difficult to cure with conventional therapy.

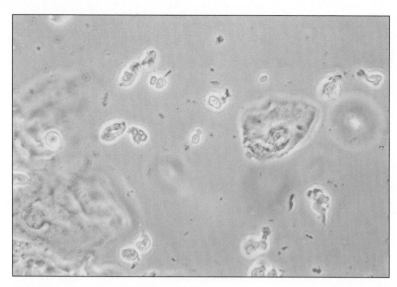

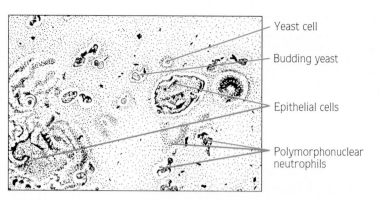

FIGURE 7-46 Phase microscopic examination (wet mount) of vaginal discharge in vulvovaginal candidiasis (VVC). Many patients with symptomatic VVC have small numbers of yeasts in the vaginal pool. The overall sensitivity of wet mount in the diagnosis of VVC may be as low as 50%, and thus, a negative wet mount does not rule out the diagnosis. This figure shows a single budding yeast and, above it and to the right, a single yeast cell. There are several epithelial cells, alone or in clumps. Polymorphonuclear neutrophils are present, as are bacilli, which presumably represent normal lactobacillary flora. (*Courtesy of* M.F. Rein, MD.)

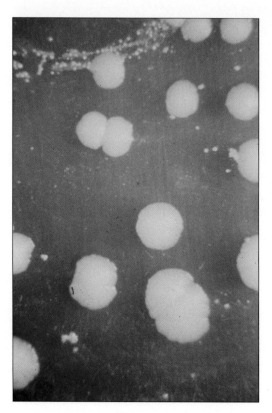

FIGURE 7-47 Vaginal yeast culture. Creamy white colonies of *Candida albicans* can be visualized on a Sabouraud's agar in a Petri dish. Tiny white bacterial colonies are also seen.

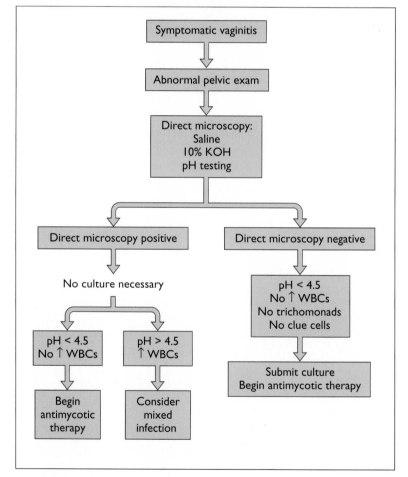

FIGURE 7-48 Diagnostic steps in vulvovaginitis candidiasis. All patients with symptomatic vaginitis require physical examination, pelvic examination, and vaginal swabs for laboratory diagnosis. If direct microscopy is positive for yeast, confirmatory culture for *Candida* is unnecessary; however, if saline microscopy and potassium hydroxide (KOH) preparation are negative for yeast, culture is essential. A low pH in this situation would be a useful indication for a latex agglutination slide test. (WBCs—white blood cells.)

TREATMENT

Treatment of Primary Vulvovaginal Candidiasis

Antimycotic agents

Local	Systemic
Creams	Oral
Lotions	
Aerosol sprays	
Vaginal tablets	
Suppositories	
Coated tampons	

FIGURE 7-49 Available formulations of imidazole antimycotic agents for treatment of acute *Candida* vaginitis. Given the available broad armamentarium of effective topical and oral antifungal regimens, every effort should be made to individualize therapy. Patients should participate in selecting method of therapy. No evidence exists that formulation influences therapeutic efficacy.

Topical azole antimycotics for acute *Candida* vaginitis

Single day	
Clotrimazole (Mycelex)	500-mg vaginal tablets
Tioconazole (Vagistat)	6.5% cream
3 days	
Butoconazole (Femstat)	2% cream (5 g)
Clotrimazole (Mycelex, Gynelotrim)	200-mg vaginal tablet
Miconazole (Monistat)	200-mg vaginal suppository
Tioconazole	2% cream
Terconazole (Terazol)	0.8% cream (5 g)
	80-mg vaginal suppository
7 days	
Clotrimazole	1% cream
	100-mg vaginal tablet
Miconazole	2% cream
	100-mg vaginal suppository
Terconazole	0.4% cream (5 g)

FIGURE 7-50 Topical azole preparations antimycotics for treatment of acute *Candida* vaginitis, stratified by duration of therapy. All the agents achieve 75% to 85% cure rates. The choice of formulation should be determined by patient preference and distribution of inflammation. Severity of inflammation also influences duration of therapy.

Nonazole topical agents for acute *Candida* vaginitis

14 days	
Nystatin (Mycostatin)	100,000-U vaginal tablet or suppository daily
Boric acid	600-mg vaginal suppository daily
Gentian violet	7–14 days

FIGURE 7-51 Nonazole topical agents for acute *Candida* vaginitis. Nonazole agents are also effective in treating *Candida* vulvovaginitis. Cure rates are slightly lower, 70% to 75%, and treatment requires more prolonged administration because of slower "killing rates" (*ie*, relatively more fungistatic). These agents may be particularly useful in therapy of non-*albicans* vaginitis and are also inexpensive despite protracted therapy.

Factors determining outcome of therapy in acute *Candida* vulvovaginitis

Host	Yeast	Drug
History of recurrent VVC	*Candida albicans* vs	Fungicidal
Severity (of signs and symptoms)	non-*albicans*	Fungistatic
Duration (of symptoms)		Half-life in tissues
Diabetes mellitus		
Pregnancy		
Immunocompromised host		

VVC—vulvovaginal candidiasis.

FIGURE 7-52 Factors determining outcome of therapy in acute *Candida* vulvovaginitis. Clinicians need to individualize therapy depending on host considerations, the yeast pathogen, and drug selected. Mild episodes respond to all formulations and to short courses. In contrast, moderate-to-severe and severe, often-neglected attacks, especially in women with a history of recurrent infection, need more prolonged therapy.

Oral/systemic therapy for vulvovaginal candidiasis	
Ketoconazole	400 mg/d × 5 days
Itraconazole	200 mg/d × 3 days
	200 mg 2 times a day × 1 day
Fluconazole	150 mg/d × 1 day

FIGURE 7-53 Oral/systemic therapy for vulvovaginal candidiasis (VVC). Three agents—ketoconazole, itraconazole, and fluconazole—are all highly effective in achieving therapeutic cure in VVC. Ketoconazole is associated with significant toxicity, notably hepatotoxicity, and like the triazole itraconazole, is not approved for use for this indication in the United States. Single-dose fluconazole is approved and is now widely used for VVC.

Short-course azole therapy	
Clotrimazole	100 mg/d × 7 days
	200 mg/d × 3 days
	500 mg single dose

FIGURE 7-54 Short-course azole therapy. Short courses of both topical and systemic azole agents have become established as effective and more convenient than conventional 5- to 14-day regimens. Most azoles are now marketed as single-dose regimens, which are effective for mild to moderate disease but may be insufficient for severe vaginitis. Three short-course regimens of clotrimazole are shown as examples, although similar regimens are possible with miconazole and with the oral triazoles, itraconazole and fluconazole.

Treatment of Recurrent Vulvovaginal Candidiasis

Therapy of recurrent vulvovaginal candidiasis
Confirm diagnosis
Eliminate predisposing factors
Treatment of sexual partner (?)
Reassure
Induction and maintenance regimen

FIGURE 7-55 Principles of therapy of recurrent vulvovaginal candidiasis. Because many women have been mislabeled as having chronic and recurrent vulvovaginal candidiasis, before any prolonged maintenance regimen is initiated, the role of *Candida* species as the cause of the chronic syndrome must be established by culture. Predisposing factors are usually absent, but when they are present (*eg*, uncontrolled diabetes), efforts to control precipitating factors should be attempted. No evidence exists that treatment of male partners is beneficial. After a more intensive initial induction regimen, patients should be placed on a maintenance regimen for about 6 months.

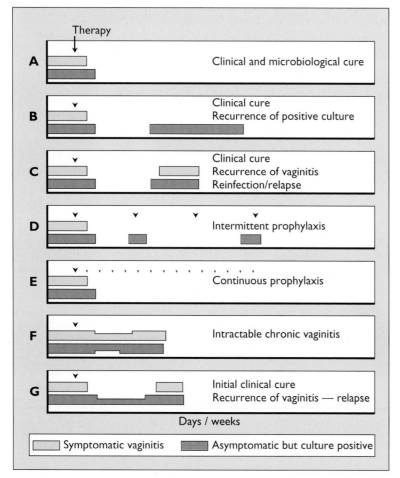

FIGURE 7-56 Clinical and microbiologic patterns following antimycotic therapy. *Green bars* indicate the duration of signs and symptoms of vulvovaginal candidiasis, and *purple bars* reflect the patient's culture-positive status. Invariably following antimycotic therapy, symptoms disappear and a culture-negative status follows (*A*). In normal healthy women, vaginal recolonization with the same strain occurs in 20% to 25% of cases within 4 to 6 weeks, but is not associated with recurrence of symptoms (*B*). Women with recurrent vulvovaginal candidiasis do predictably develop recurrence of symptoms within 3 months of previous "successful" therapy (*C*). Because of these frequent recurrences following "successful" therapy, there is a need for maintenance therapy that can be prescribed on a weekly (*D*) or even daily basis (*E*). Infrequently, partial or incomplete symptomatic relief (*F*) or partial mycologic response only (*G*) follows appropriate intensive therapy. This is due to partial or complete resistance of yeast and requires that vaginal cultures and, rarely, fungal susceptibility tests be performed.

Maintenance regimens for recurrent vulvovaginal candidiasis	
Ketoconazole	100 mg daily
Clotrimazole	500 mg weekly
Miconazole	(undetermined)
Fluconazole	100–200 mg weekly

FIGURE 7-57 Maintenance regimens for recurrent vulvovaginal candidiasis (VVC). Two oral regimens (ketoconazole and fluconazole) and one topical regimen (weekly clotrimazole) are highly effective in providing > 90% protection against recurrence of VVC while prophylaxis is taken. Maintenance suppressive prophylaxis is prescribed for 6 months and then discontinued. Slightly more than half of women with recurrent VVC will remain in long-term remission. The remainder rapidly return to the same pattern of recurrent VVC and should be placed on maintenance suppressive therapy for 1 year and then reassessed.

SELECTED BIBLIOGRAPHY

Sobel JD: Genital candidiasis. *In* Bodey GP (ed.): *Candidiasis: Pathogenesis, Diagnosis, and Treatment*, 2nd ed. New York: Raven Press; 1993.

Sobel JD: Genital candidiasis. *In* Holmes KK, *et al.* (eds.): *Sexually Transmitted Diseases*, 2nd ed. New York: McGraw-Hill; 1990.

CHAPTER 8

Syphilis: Epidemiology and Laboratory Testing

Sandra A. Larsen

ETIOLOGY AND PATHOGENESIS

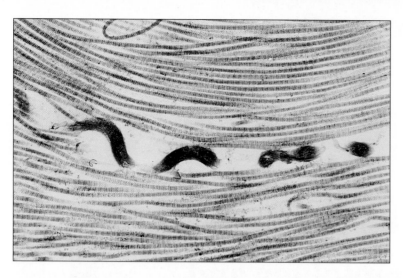

FIGURE 8-1 Electron micrograph of *Treponema pallidum* in scar tissue. *T. pallidum* is a member of the order Spirochaetales and family Spirochaetaceae.

Pathogenic subspecies of *Treponema pallidum*

	ssp *pallidum*	ssp *pertenue*	ssp *endemicum*
Disease	Syphilis	Yaws	Bejel
Infection	Systemic, cutaneous	Nonsystemic, cutaneous	Nonsystemic, cutaneous
Transmission	Sexually, congenital	Nonvenereal	Nonvenereal
Distribution	Worldwide	Tropics	Desert
Patient age	Adolescent–adult (sexually active)	All ages	All ages
	Newborns (congenital)		

FIGURE 8-2 Pathogenic subspecies of *Treponema pallidum*. The three pathogenic subspecies of *T. pallidum* are *pallidum* (syphilis), *pertenue* (yaws), and *endemicum* (bejel or nonvenereal syphilis). *Treponema carateum*, the etiologic agent of pinta, which is rarely seen, exists as a separate species. The three subspecies and *T. carateum* cannot be distinguished from each other serologically, morphologically, biochemically, or genetically. These treponemes are distinguished on the basis of geography, means of transmission, age of the individuals infected, and appearance of the lesion.

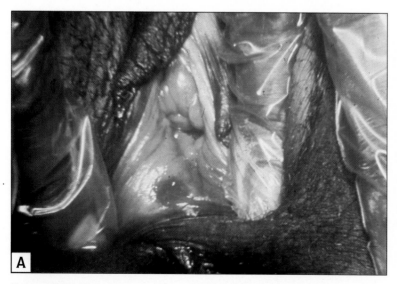

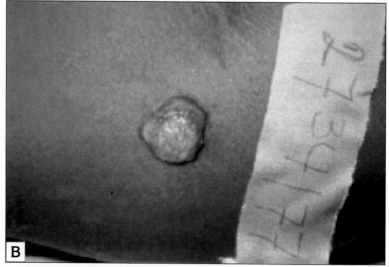

FIGURE 8-3 Primary lesions in *Treponema* infections. **A,** The primary lesion of infection with *Treponema pallidum* ssp *pallidum* is typically a small, discrete ulcer (chancre) occurring at the site of infection, which may be genital, oral, or anal. **B,** A papilloma is the typical primary lesion of *T. pallidum* ssp *pertenue* infection (yaws). The lesion is usually nontender but often may be pruritic, crusted, or ulcerated; it occurs most frequently on exposed skin. (*continued*)

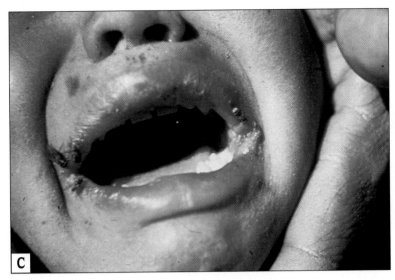
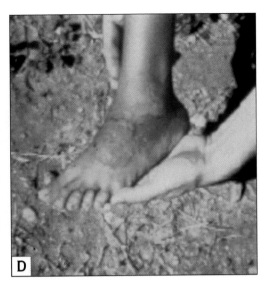

Figure 8-3 (*continued*) **C**, The most common early manifestation of endemic syphilis (bejel) is a mucocutaneous lesion occurring on the lips, tongue, pillars of the fauces, tonsils, and buccal mucosa. **D**, Erythematosquamous plaque of early *Treponema carateum* infection (pinta). The primary lesion of pinta is a papule, usually occurring on the legs or dorsum of the foot. The lesion enlarges with time to become a pruritic plaque resembling psoriasis that progressively changes in color from copper, to lead gray, to slate blue, and eventually to the achromic scars of late pinta. (Perine PL, Hopkins DR, Niemel PLA, *et al.*: *Handbook of Endemic Treponematoses*. Geneva: World Health Organization; 1984.) (Panels 3B, 3C, and 3D *courtesy of* P.L. Perine, MD.)

Stages of syphilitic infection

Stage	Time of appearance (days postinfection)	Symptoms
Primary	10–90 days (avg. 21 days)	Chancre, single or multiple, on skin or mucous membranes Regional lymphadenopathy
Secondary	6 wks–6 mos	Multiple secondary lesions (skin or mucous membrane) Lymphadenopathy, fever, malaise Condylomata lata Alopecia Asymptomatic or symptomatic central nervous system involvement (meningitis)
Latent	≤ 1-yr duration (early) > 1-yr duration (late)	Asymptomatic
Late	Months to years	Gummatous (monocytic infiltrates, tissue destruction of any organ) Cardiovascular (aortic aneurysm) Neurosyphilis (paresis, tabes dorsalis, meningovascular syphilis)

Figure 8-4 Stages of syphilitic infection. Syphilis can be a chronic disease that advances through a series of stages. Although disseminated infection occurs in virtually all infected individuals, multiple secondary lesions arise in only 25% of the infected persons. Longitudinal observations of patients with untreated syphilis at the beginning of the 20th century indicated that approximately one third of infected individuals remain latently infected for life, one third have biologic cure, and the remaining one third develop late manifestations.

Unique features of *Treponema pallidum*

Periplasmic flagella
Lipid-rich outer membrane
Protein-deficient outer membrane
Fluid outer membrane
Host dependent
Inability to synthesize lipids
Limited DNA repair capacity
Binds fibronectin reversibly

FIGURE 8-5 Unique features of *Treponema pallidum*. The unique features of the pathogenic treponemes account for both the organism's inability to be maintained outside an animal host and the organism's survival within the host without the production of a strong cellular immune response. The flagella of the treponemes are enclosed within an outer limiting membrane. The rotation of the flagella apparently causes the treponemes to rotate, enabling their penetration of materials of high viscosity. The outer membrane is apparently very rich in lipids and is extremely fluid. Despite the lipid nature of the outer membrane, treponemes appear to be unable to synthesize their own lipids and acquire them exclusively from the host. *T. pallidum* has an extremely long generation time of 33 hours and is defective in DNA repair in comparison to most bacteria. As a result, the treponeme depends on the host for protection against DNA-damaging chemicals, such as oxygen radicals. Degraded fragments of fibronectin are found in immune complexes with treponemal antigens, and this binding to treponemal proteins may be related to the autoimmune-like clinical symptoms observed in late syphilis.

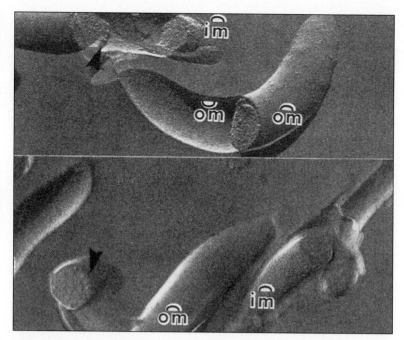

FIGURE 8-6 Freeze fracture electron micrograph of *Treponema pallidum*. There is a lack of immunodeterminants (transmembrane proteins) visualized as intramembranous particles on both the inner (*im*) and outer membranes (*om*). The lack of exposed proteins enables the organism to avoid the host's immune surveillance. *Arrowheads* indicate periplasmic flagella. (Chiu MJ, Radolf JD: Syphilis. *In* Hoeprich PD, Jordan MC, Ronald AR (eds.): *Infectious Diseases*, 5th ed. Philadelphia: J.B. Lippincott; 1994.) (*Courtesy of* J. Radolf, MD.)

EPIDEMIOLOGY

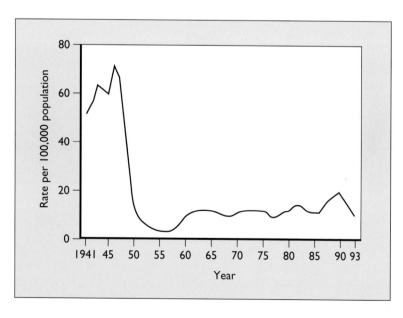

FIGURE 8-7 Annual rates of primary and secondary syphilis in the United States between 1941 and 1993. The annual incidence of syphilis decreased dramatically with the introduction of penicillin treatment. However, levels of syphilis periodically have increased, then decreased. Frequently, the increases have correlated with behavioral changes, such as the introduction of birth control pills in the 1960s, proliferation of gay bath houses in the 1970s and 1980s, and use of crack cocaine in the 1990s. In 1990, the rate of primary and secondary cases per 100,000 population was 20.3, the highest rate since 1952. The rate for 1993 declined to approximately 12 cases per 100,000 population. (Division of STD/HIV Prevention: *Sexually Transmitted Diseases Surveillance, 1993*. Atlanta: Centers for Disease Control and Prevention; 1994.)

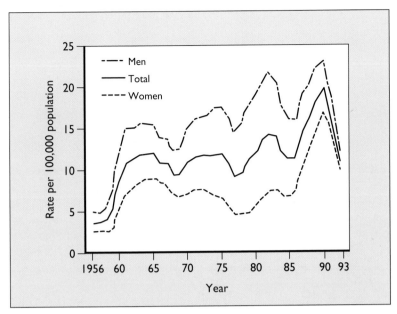

FIGURE 8-8 Annual rates of primary and secondary syphilis by gender in the United States between 1956 and 1993. In the 1980s, with the recognition of HIV infection in the homosexual population, the rate of syphilis in men decreased. In contrast, the proportion of adolescent women aged 15 to 19 years who reported having sexual intercourse increased from 29% in 1970 to 52% in 1988. The male-to-female ratio of cases has approached 1 since 1991, suggesting that much of the transmission of syphilis is primarily heterosexual. Because of acquired syphilis in the heterosexual population, the number of infants born with congenital syphilis increased to 107.2 per 100,000 live births in 1991. The rate began to decline in 1992 and continued to decline in 1993. (Division of STD/HIV Prevention: *Sexually Transmitted Diseases Surveillance, 1993.* Atlanta: Centers for Disease Control and Prevention; 1994.)

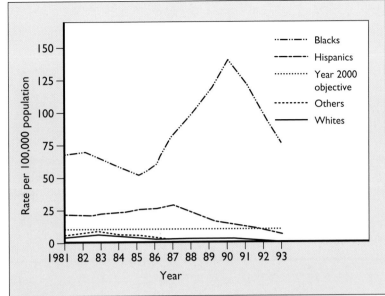

FIGURE 8-9 Annual rates of primary and secondary syphilis by race and ethnicity in the United States between 1981 and 1993. Although rates of syphilis have declined among all racial and ethnic groups since 1990, the risk for syphilis appears to be much higher in blacks and Hispanics than in whites. For blacks, rates of primary and secondary syphilis are approximately 60-fold higher than for whites, and rates for Hispanics are fivefold higher than for whites. In 1993, black men aged 10 to 29 years had the highest rates of syphilis for any age group, nearly 200 cases per 100,000 population. (Division of STD/HIV Prevention: *Sexually Transmitted Diseases Surveillance, 1993.* Atlanta: Centers for Disease Control and Prevention; 1994.)

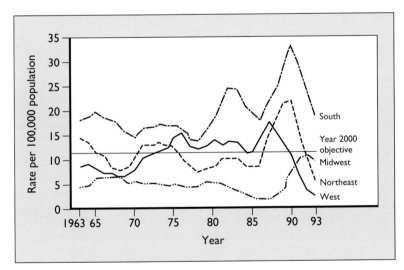

FIGURE 8-10 Annual rates of syphilis by region in the United States between 1963 and 1993. Rates for syphilis remain the highest in the southern United States. Rates increased in the midwest in 1987 because of the shift in populations from the south to Minnesota, Wisconsin, and Kansas. As with the remainder of the nation, the rates of syphilis began to decrease in the midwest in 1992. Risk factors for syphilis appear to be poverty, chronic unemployment, illicit drug use, low education, and racial isolation. (Division of STD/HIV Prevention: *Sexually Transmitted Diseases Surveillance, 1993.* Atlanta: Centers for Disease Control and Prevention; 1994.)

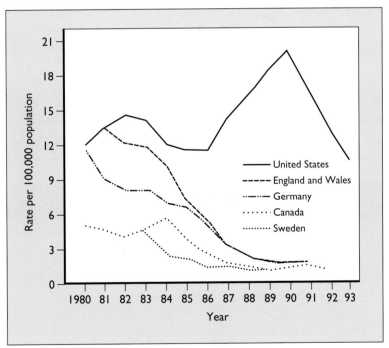

FIGURE 8-11 International rates of syphilis. Among the industrialized world, the United States has the highest rate of syphilis. In 1993, only 312 cases of syphilis were reported for England and Wales. In the nonindustrialized nations, syphilis remains a significant health problem, especially because there is a strong association between genital ulcer disease and HIV infection. (Division of STD/HIV Prevention: *Sexually Transmitted Diseases Surveillance, 1993.* Atlanta: Centers for Disease Control and Prevention; 1994.)

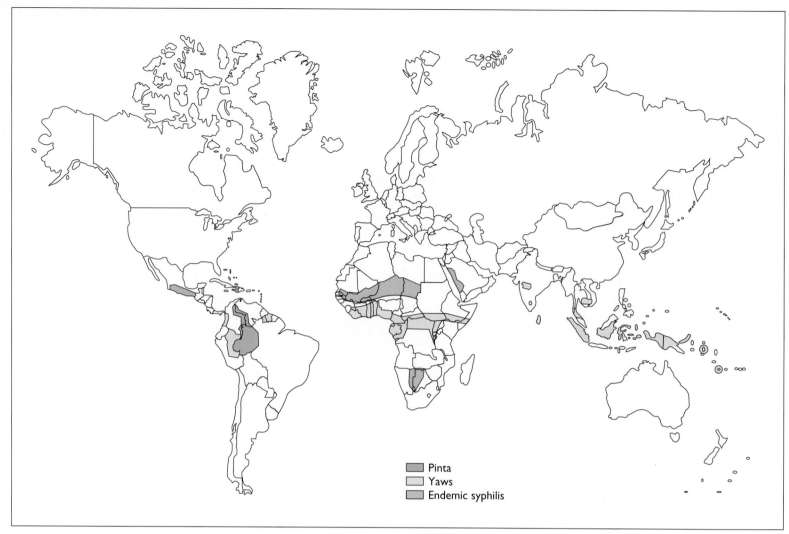

Pinta
Yaws
Endemic syphilis

FIGURE 8-12 Geographic distribution of endemic nonvenereal treponematoses in the early 1990s. Yaws, endemic syphilis, and pinta were common infections prior to the World Health Organization's eradication program that began in 1948. In the early 1950s, more than 200 million people were estimated to have been exposed to yaws at some time during their life. Areas where the nonvenereal treponematoses are endemic are now more restricted, but decreased surveillance has led to a return of disease in many areas. (*Adapted from* Meheus A, Antel GM: The endemic treponematoses: Not yet eradicated. *World Health Stat Q* 1992, 45:228–231; with permission.)

LABORATORY EXAMINATIONS

Current tests for syphilis

Direct microscopic examination
Nontreponemal tests—screening tests
Treponemal tests—confirmatory tests

FIGURE 8-13 Current tests for syphilis. The tests for syphilis comprise direct microscopic examination of lesion material or tissue and serologic tests for antibody response to either cardiolipin-like material (nontreponemal tests) or treponemal antigens (treponemal tests). The nontreponemal tests are used for screening because they are sensitive, inexpensive, and easily performed, and reactivity in these tests disappears following treatment of the patient. In contrast, the treponemal tests, used to confirm reactivity in the nontreponemal tests, are specific but more costly and complicated to perform, and reactivity in these tests does not usually disappear after the patient has been treated.

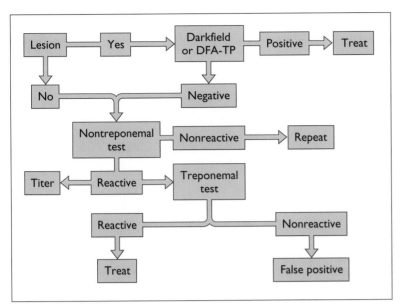

FIGURE 8-14 Routine testing scheme for syphilis. If lesions are present, routine testing consists of direct microscopic examination, either by darkfield microscopy or direct fluorescent antibody for *Treponema pallidum* (DFA-TP). If lesions are not present or are healing, then first a nontreponemal test is used to screen for syphilis, with a reactive result confirmed by a treponemal test. The nontreponemal tests can be quantitated to determine an endpoint titer. A fourfold decrease in titer after treatment indicates a successful response to treatment, whereas a fourfold increase in titer usually indicates relapse or reinfection. The routine testing scheme does not need to be altered for HIV-positive individuals, but direct microscopic examination is even more important in these individuals because a delay in antibody response may occur in immunosuppressed individuals. (Larsen SA, Steiner BM, Rudolph AH: Laboratory diagnosis and interpretation of tests for syphilis. *Clin Microbiol Rev* 1995, 8:1–21.)

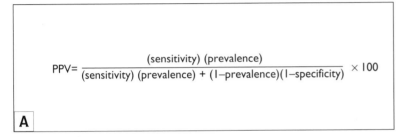

$$PPV = \frac{(\text{sensitivity})\,(\text{prevalence})}{(\text{sensitivity})\,(\text{prevalence}) + (1-\text{prevalence})(1-\text{specificity})} \times 100$$

A

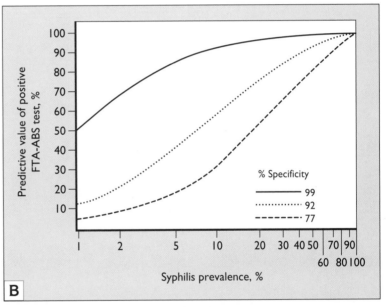

B

FIGURE 8-15 Positive predictive value in sequential tests. In most instances in which tests are used as screening procedures, the disease status of the individual is unknown. **A,** Calculation of positive predictive value (PPV). When a PPV is determined on the basis of either the prevalence of the disease in a population or a clinical estimate of the probability of the disease in a given patient, the risk of disease is known as the pretest or *a priori* probability. **B,** PPV in relation to syphilis prevalence. Although the specificities of the Venereal Disease Research Laboratory (VDRL) and fluorescent treponemal antibody absorption (FTA-ABS) tests are similar, screening with the VDRL to increase the prevalence of the disease in the samples to be confirmed with the FTA-ABS test improves the PPV value of the FTA-ABS test. Assuming that the PPV of the VDRL is 70%, then by screening with the VDRL before confirming with the FTA-ABS, the prevalence of the disease in the population is increased to 70% and the PPV of the FTA-ABS approaches 100% (if the sensitivity and specificity of the FTA-ABS test are assumed to be 99%). In contrast, if the FTA-ABS test is used as a screening test in a low-prevalence population, then the PPV of the FTA-ABS test could be less than 50%.

Direct Microscopic Examination

Direct microscopic examination: Techniques
Darkfield examination Direct fluorescent antibody for *Treponema pallidum* (DFA-TP)

FIGURE 8-16 Types of direct microscopic examination.

Darkfield Microscopy

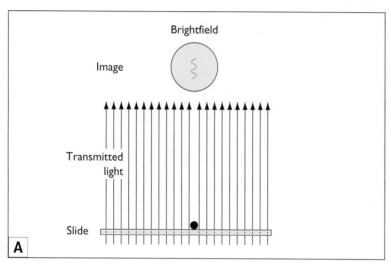

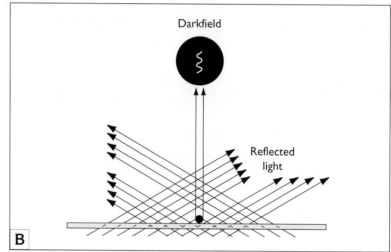

FIGURE 8-17 Optics of darkfield microscopy. **A**, Brightfield examination. In the compound microscope, light rays are concentrated and directed straight upward through the microscope slide and objective lens into the barrel of the microscope. Because of their narrow width, treponemes cannot be observed with the ordinary light microscope. In addition, treponemes cannot be stained with ordinary laboratory stains, such as Gram stain, and instead require silver stains such as the Steiner stain.

Use of silver stains does not permit the identification of *Treponema pallidum* but only identifies the presence of a spiral organism. **B**, Darkfield microscopy. For identification of *T. pallidum* in lesion material, a microscope equipped with a darkfield condenser must be used. On darkfield examination, the background is dark, and objects, visualized by reflected light, are bright against the background. Brownian movement of very small objects can be seen on darkfield examination.

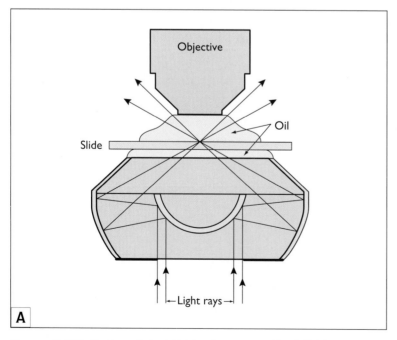

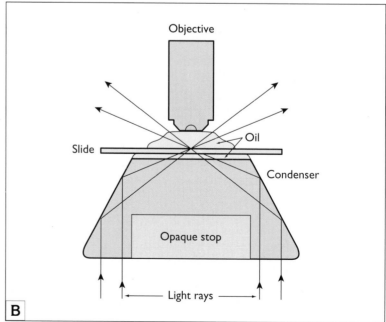

FIGURE 8-18 Optics of darkfield microscopy. Darkfield condensers may be either double or single reflecting. **A**, In the double-reflecting darkfield condenser, two reflecting surfaces produce an intense illumination; however, this type of condenser requires precise focusing and accurate centering. **B**, The single-reflecting condenser contains one reflecting surface that does not produce a sharp focusing of the hollow cone of rays. However, the single-reflecting condenser is easier to manipulate, but less intense illumination is produced. Thus, the single-reflecting condenser is less desirable.

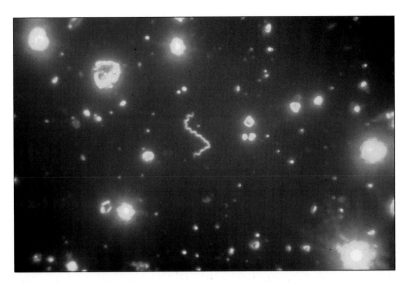

FIGURE 8-19 Darkfield examination. Illumination for darkfield microscopy is obtained when light rays strike the object in the field at an oblique angle so that no light rays pass directly from the condensor to the objective of the microscope, but only the light rays that are reflected from the object will enter. A treponema is seen in the center of the field, distinguished by its corkscrew, spiral shape.

Sources of specimens for direct microscopic examination
Chancres
Condyloma latum
Regional lymph nodes
Cerebrospinal fluid
Amniotic fluid
Mucous patches
Oral and rectal lesions (direct fluorescent antibody only)

FIGURE 8-20 Sources of specimens for darkfield examination for syphilis. Samples for direct microscopic examination are obtained under any scab or crust covering a lesion. A dry gauze sponge is used to remove any secondary infectious exudate, and then the lesion is squeezed to deliver tissue fluid. A glass slide should be applied to the oozing lesion, or a sterile loop can be used to transfer fluid from the lesion to the slide. Exudates from anal or oral lesions are inappropriate for darkfield examination but may be examined by direct fluorescent antibody for *Treponema pallidum*.

	Treponema pallidum ssp *pallidum*	*Treponema refringens*	*Treponema phagedenis (reiteri)*	*Treponema denticola*
Number of coils (range)	10–13 (6–20)	2–3	10–12 (10–30)	6–8
Length, µm (range)	Medium 10 (6–20)	Short 5–8 (5–16)	Medium-long 10–12 (10–30)	Medium 8 (6–16)
Width, µm	Very thin 0.13–0.15	Thick 0.20–0.30	Thick 0.20–0.25	Very thin 0.15–0.20
Spiral wave length, µm (range)	Tight 1.1 (1.0–1.5)	Loose ≈ 1.8	Loose 1.4–1.6	Tight ≈ 0.9
Spiral depth, µm	Deep 0.5–0.7	Shallow 0.2–0.3	Shallow 0.2–0.3	Shallow 0.1–0.4

FIGURE 8-21 Morphologic characteristics of *Treponema* species on darkfield examination. In the darkfield examination, *Treponema pallidum* is distinguished on the basis of morphology from other nonpathogenic treponemes that may be part of the normal bacterial flora. *T. pallidum* is a delicate, corkscrew-shaped organism with rigid, uniform, tightly wound, deep spirals. The length of the organism is 6 to 20 µm, and the width is 0.13 to 0.15 µm. The length of the spiral wave is 1.0 to 1.5 µm, and the spiral depth is 0.5 to 0.7 µm. The source of the specimen may suggest which organisms will be present, as *Treponema refringens* and *Treponema phagedenis* are part of the normal genital flora and *Treponema denticola* is part of the normal oral flora. Because *T. pallidum* and *T. denticola* have very similar appearances, it is advisable that specimens not be collected from the mouth; if the mouth is the only possible collection site, a fluorescent antibody test should be used, as *T. pallidum* will fluoresce but *T. denticola* will not.

	Treponema pallidum ssp *pallidum*	*Treponema refringens*	*Treponema phagedenis*	*Treponema denticola*
Translation (forward/backward)	Slow, deliberate	Rapid	Slow, jerky, deliberate	Slow, deliberate
Rotation (turns through longitudinal axis)	Slow to rapid Like a corkscrew; may rotate in place	Very rapid, looks straight Active serpentine-like; may rotate so rapidly that it looks straight	Slow to rapid Rotates in place	Slow to rapid, often jerky
Flexion (bending)	Soft bending in middle Pops back into place like a spring	Marked bending, relaxed coils	Jerky Twisting or undulating side to side	Soft bending Bending, twisting, or undulating
Distortion (twists out of original shape)	Circular	Straight	Straight middle, rotating ends	Normally not seen

FIGURE 8-22 Motility characteristics of *Treponema* species on darkfield examination. Motility of *Treponema pallidum* is an important characteristic for identification, but its evaluation requires that the samples be examined within a few minutes after collection. The characteristic motion of *T. pallidum* is a deliberate forward-and-backward movement with rotation about the longitudinal axis. Rotation may be accompanied by a soft bending, twisting, or undulation of the organism from side to side. When attached to or obstructed by heavier particles, the organism may contort, convolute, or bend and thereby distort the coils, but the organism will snap back to its original coillike form. Organisms easily confused with *T. pallidum* are *Treponema refringens* and *Treponema denticola*.

Outcomes of darkfield examination

Positive findings
  Specific and immediate diagnosis of syphilis
  Diagnosis of primary syphilis before the appearance of reactive
    serologic tests
Negative findings
  Exclude diagnosis of syphilis, when collection is not a problem
  Do not exclude the diagnosis of syphilis, if:
    Too few organisms are present to be demonstrated
    The spirochete has been altered by systemic or topical treatment

FIGURE 8-23 Outcomes of darkfield examination. The identification of *Treponema pallidum* by direct microscopic examination is definitive for syphilis, if infection with the other pathogenic treponemes can be excluded. A negative result or darkfield examination does not always rule out the possibility of syphilis, because the condition of the lesion and systemic or topical antimicrobial therapy can alter the organism's motility or reduce the numbers of organisms in the lesion.

Direct Fluorescent Antibody Test

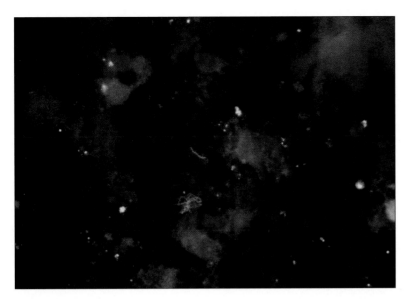

FIGURE 8-24 Direct fluorescent antibody for *Treponema pallidum* (DFA-TP). A tissue impression smear from a brain biopsy specimen shows fluorescent treponemes. In the DFA-TP test, a monoclonal antibody labeled with fluorescein isothiocyanate specific for *T. pallidum* binds to the treponemes in either smears or tissue sections prepared from paraffin-embedded tissue blocks. Because a monoclonal antibody is used in the DFA-TP test, motility of the organism is not required for identification.

Nontreponemal Tests

Standard nontreponemal tests for syphilis
Venereal Disease Research Laboratory (VDRL) slide
Unheated serum reagin (USR)
Rapid plasma reagin (RPR) 18-mm circle card
Reagin screen test (RST)
Toluidine red unheated serum test (TRUST)

FIGURE 8-25 Standard nontreponemal tests for syphilis. The antigen for all of the standard nontreponemal tests is composed of cardiolipin, cholesterol, and lecithin with or without various stabilizers, and particles to enhance the visualization of the test. All the nontreponemal tests measure IgG and IgM antibodies to lipoidal material released from damaged host cells as well as to lipoprotein-like material released from the treponemes. The nontreponemal tests can be used as qualitative tests for initial screening or as the quantitative tests to follow treatment.

Specimens for the nontreponemal tests

Test	Specimen
VDRL	Unheated serum, unheated CSF
USR	Heated or unheated serum
RPR, TRUST, RST	Heated or unheated serum, unheated plasma

CSF—cerebrospinal fluid; RPR—rapid plasma reagin; RST—reagin screen test; TRUST—toluidine red unheated serum; USR—unheated serum reagin; VDRL—Venereal Disease Research Laboratory.

FIGURE 8-26 Specimens for nontreponemal tests. Serum is the specimen of choice for all nontreponemal tests. The macroscopic card tests may also be performed with plasma samples. Plasma cannot be used in the Venereal Disease Research Laboratory (VDRL) test because the sample must be heated before testing, and plasma cannot be used in confirmatory tests for syphilis. The VDRL slide test is the only test that can be modified for testing cerebrospinal fluid. When using unheated plasma with the rapid plasma reagin, toluidine red unheated serum, and reagin screen tests, the manufacturer's recommendations must be followed to ensure accuracy.

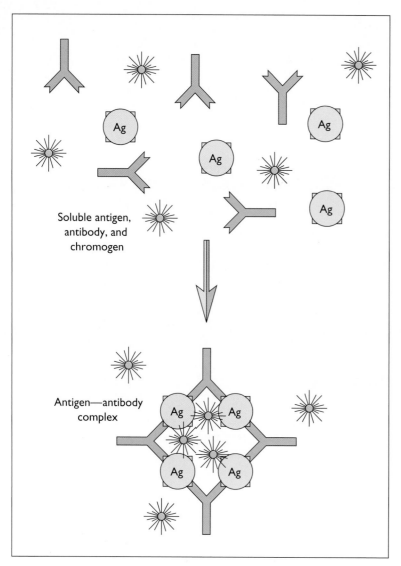

Soluble antigen, antibody, and chromogen

Antigen—antibody complex

FIGURE 8-27 Antigen–antibody complexing in nontreponemal tests. For all nontreponemal tests, the patient's serum is mixed with antigen (Ag) on a solid matrix. If antibodies are present, the antigen and antibody combine to form a flocculent that is read microscopically (if no visualization particles are added). If appropriately sized particles have been added by the reagent manufacturer to the antigen, the results may be read macroscopically.

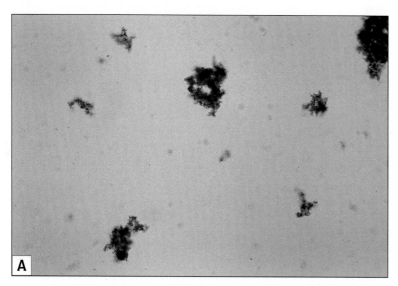

A

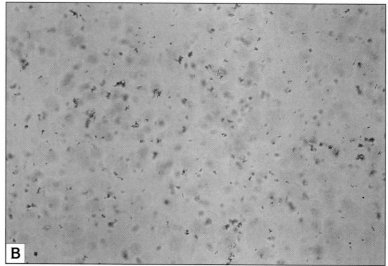

B

FIGURE 8-28 Venereal Disease Research Laboratory (VDRL) test results. **A**, In a reactive VDRL test result, large clumps are formed. **B**, With a weakly reactive serum, small defined clumps are formed. (*continued*)

FIGURE 8-28 (*continued*) **C.** With nonreactive serum, smooth antigen dispersion or slight roughness is observed in the VDRL test. (Magnification, × 100.)

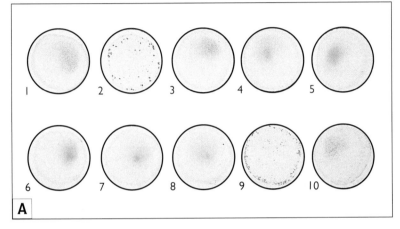

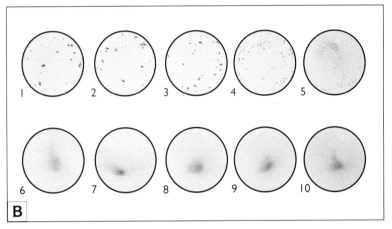

FIGURE 8-29 Macroscopic card tests. **A,** Rapid plasma reagin test. The macroscopic card tests are read as reactive (*circles* 2 and 9), reactive minimal (*circles* 1 and 10), or nonreactive (remaining *circles*) based on the amount of flocculation observed. However, results are reported only as reactive or nonreactive, with minimally reactive results reported as reactive. **B,** Toluidine red unheated serum test (TRUST). A quantitative TRUST result with a titer of 32. The reading of the result in *circle* 6 (1:32) is reactive minimal. (Portnoy J, Brewer JH, Harris A: Rapid plasma reagin card test for syphilis and other treponematoses. *Public Health Rep* 1962, 77:645. Pettit DE, Larsen SA, Harbec PS: Toluidine red unheated serum test, a nontreponemal test for syphilis. *J Clin Microbiol* 1983, 18:1141.)

Sensitivity and specificity of standard nontreponemal tests

	Sensitivity, %				Specificity, %
	Primary	Secondary	Latent	Late	Nonsyphilis
VDRL	78 (74–87)*	100	96 (88–100)	71 (34–34)	98 (96–99)
RPR	86 (77–99)	100	98 (95–100)	73	98 (36–99)
USR	80 (72–88)	100	95 (88–100)	—	99
RST	82 (77–86)	100	95 (88–100)	—	97
TRUST	85 (77–86)	100	95 (95–100)	—	93 (98–99)

*Numbers in parentheses are ranges.
RPR—rapid plasma reagin; RST—reagin screen test; TRUST—toluidine red unheated serum test; USR—unheated serum reagin; VDRL—Venereal Disease Research Laboratory.

FIGURE 8-30 Sensitivity and specificity of standard nontreponemal tests. The sensitivities of the nontreponemal tests vary according to the stage of syphilis. In early primary and untreated syphilis of > 1 year's duration, the nontreponemal tests are < 100% sensitive. The specificities of the tests in individuals without syphilis are similar. The tests are less specific in individuals who are intra-venous drug users or who have autoimmune diseases. (Larsen SA, Hunter EF, Kraus SJ (eds.): *A Manual of Tests for Syphilis*. Washington, DC: American Public Health Association, 1990. Schroeter AL, Lucas JB, Price EV, Falcone VH: Treatment of early syphilis and reactivity of serologic tests. *JAMA* 1972, 221:471.)

A. Advantages of the nontreponemal tests
Widely available Inexpensive Easily performed Applicable to mass screening Useful for monitoring treatment

B. Limitations of the nontreponemal tests
Lack of sensitivity in early darkfield positive primary cases The prozone phenomenon Failure of the tests to distinguish between the infections with 　other pathogenic treponemes Failure of the titers to decline in some patients False-positive results

FIGURE 8-31 Advantages and disadvantages of nontreponemal tests for syphilis. **A.** The nontreponemal tests have several advantages that make them useful in screening and in monitoring treatment. **B.** There are also several limitations to the tests. Antibodies are detectable in serologic tests for syphilis usually 1 week after lesion formation in early primary syphilis. Serum samples containing large amounts of nontreponemal antibody occasionally demonstrate a prozone reaction in the nontreponemal tests in which no flocculation can be observed. In the prozone, flocculation is inhibited as a result of poor lattice formation and steric hindrance caused by this extreme antibody excess. In addition to intravenous drug use, any disease or condition that results in tissue damage may cause a false-positive nontreponemal test result.

Treponemal Tests

Standard treponemal tests for syphilis	
FTA-ABS	Fluorescent treponemal antibody absorption
FTA-ABS-DS	FTA-ABS double staining
MHA-TP	Microhemagglutination assay for antibodies to 　*Treponema pallidum*

Uses of the treponemal tests
Confirmation of reactive nontreponemal tests Confirmation of a clinical impression Resolution of problem cases

FIGURE 8-32 Standard treponemal tests for syphilis. Three tests are currently considered as standard treponemal tests. Several treponemal tests using the enzyme-linked immunosorbent assay (ELISA) and one using Western blot are being evaluated. All tests are based on the detection of antibodies directed against treponemal cellular components. The treponemal tests are qualitative procedures and cannot be used to monitor the efficacy of treatment.

FIGURE 8-33 Uses of the treponemal tests for syphilis. The major use of the treponemal test is for confirmation of reactive nontreponemal test results.

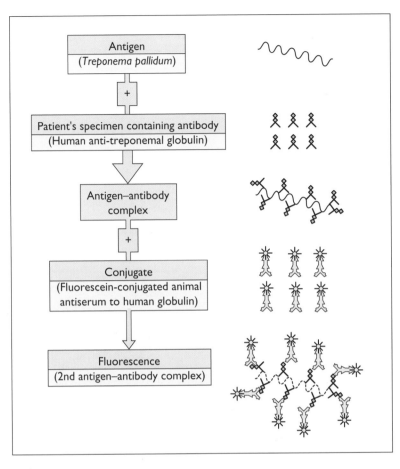

FIGURE 8-34 Mechanisms of reactivity in the fluorescent treponemal antibody absorption (FTA-ABS) test. In the FTA-ABS test, the patient's serum (diluted 1:5 in sorbent) is reacted with the whole treponeme (antigen). If antibodies are present in the patient's serum, the antigen and antibody react to form complexes. A fluorescein isothiocyanate–labeled antihuman conjugate is then added that allows the antigen–antibody complexes to be visualized. Unstained treponemes in a nonreactive test must be located with a darkfield condenser to ensure that treponemes are actually present in the field being read. (Hunter EF, Deacon WE, Meyer PE: An improved FTA test for syphilis, the absorption procedure (FTA-ABS). *Public Health Rep* 1964, 79:410.)

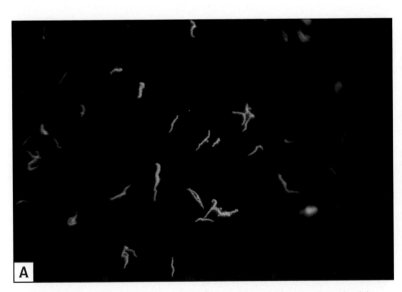

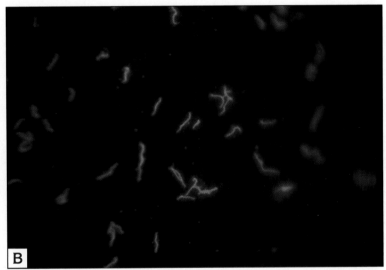

FIGURE 8-35 Fluorescent treponemal antibody absorption double-staining (FTA-ABS-DS) test. The FTA-ABS-DS test was developed for use with incident light fluorescent microscopes that are not equipped with a darkfield condenser. **A,** An antitreponemal conjugate labeled with fluorescein isothiocyanate is used as the counterstain to facilitate location of the treponemes in a nonreactive test.

B, A tetramethyl-rhodamine isothiocyanate–labeled antihuman conjugate recognizing heavy-chain IgG only is used as the indicator of the antigen–antibody reaction in a reactive test. (Hunter EF, McKinney RM, Maddison SE, Cruce DD: Double-staining procedure for the fluorescent treponemal antibody absorption (FTA-ABS) test. *Br J Vener Dis* 1979, 55:105.)

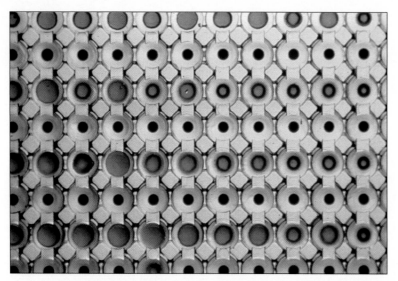

Figure 8-36 Microhemagglutination assay for antibodies to *Treponema pallidum*. In the hemagglutination test, the patient's serum is reacted with sonicated fragments of the treponemes attached to a red blood cell carrier (*rows* 1, 3, 5, and 7). Antibodies are detected by the formation of typical mat patterns of agglutination. The patient's serum is also reacted with red blood cells without treponemal antigen (*rows* 2, 4, 6, and 8) to detect the presence of nonspecific agglutination, as seen in row 8, well 5 (*bottom row*). (Rathlev T: Hemagglutination tests utilizing antigens from pathogenic and a pathogenic *Treponema pallidum*. *Br J Vener Dis* 1967, 43:181.)

Sensitivity and specificity of treponemal tests

	Sensitivity, %				Specificity, %
	Primary	Secondary	Latent	Late	Nonsyphilis
FTA-ABS	84 (70–100)	100	100	96	97 (94–100)
FTA-ABS-DS	80 (70–100)	100	100	—	98 (97–100)
MHA-TP	76 (69–90)	100	97 (97–100)	94	99 (98–100)

FTA-ABS—fluorescent treponemal antibody absorption; FTA-ABS-DS—FTA-ABS double-staining; MHA-TP—microhemagglutination assay for antibodies to *Treponema pallidum*.

Figure 8-37 Sensitivity and specificity of treponemal tests. The sensitivities of the treponemal tests vary with the stage of syphilis. Most notably, the microhemagglutination assay for antibodies to *Treponema pallidum* is less sensitive than the fluorescent treponemal antibody absorption tests in primary syphilis. The specificities of the tests are similar. (Larsen SA, Hunter EF, Kraus SJ (eds.): *A Manual of Tests for Syphilis*. Washington, DC: American Public Health Association, 1990.)

Limitations of the treponemal tests

Remain reactive after treatment in 85% of the cases
False-positive results
Nonspecific agglutination in the MHA-TP
Failure of the tests to distinguish between the infections with other pathogenic treponemes
Cost and complexity
Decreased sensitivity of the MHA-TP in primary syphilis

MHA-TP—microhemagglutination assay for antibodies to *Treponema pallidum*.

Figure 8-38 Limitations of the treponemal tests. The treponemal tests have few limitations, but these emphasize the reasons that these tests are used as confirmatory tests rather than as screening tests for the detection of recent infections.

Selected Bibliography

Chiu MJ, Radolf JD: Syphilis. *In* Hoeprich PD, Jordan MC, Ronald AR (eds.): *Infectious Diseases*, 5th ed. Philadelphia: J.B. Lippincott; 1994.

Jaffe HW, Musher DM: Management of the reactive syphilis serology. *In* Holmes KK, Mårdh P-A, Sparling PF, *et al.* (eds.): *Sexually Transmitted Diseases*, 2nd ed. New York: McGraw-Hill, 1990.

Larsen SA, Hunter EF, Kraus J (eds.): *A Manual of Tests for Syphilis*. Washington, DC: American Public Health Association, 1990.

Larsen SA, Steiner BM, Rudolph AH: Laboratory diagnosis and interpretation of tests for syphilis. *Clin Microbiol Rev* 1995, 8:1–21.

Norgard MV: Clinical and diagnostic issues of acquired and congenital syphilis encompassed in the current syphilis epidemic. *Curr Opin Infect Dis* 1993, 6:9–16.

CHAPTER 9

Primary and Secondary Syphilis

Nicholas J. Fiumara

EPIDEMIOLOGY

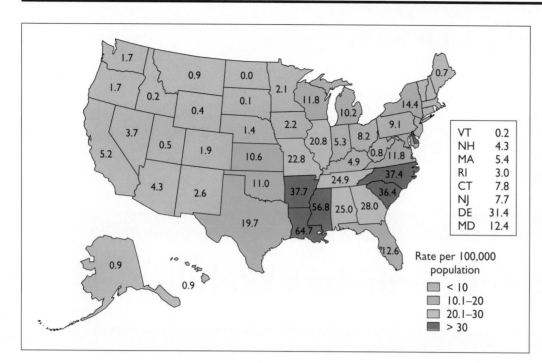

VT	0.2
NH	4.3
MA	5.4
RI	3.0
CT	7.8
NJ	7.7
DE	31.4
MD	12.4

Rate per 100,000 population

- < 10
- 10.1–20
- 20.1–30
- > 30

FIGURE 9-1 Incidence of primary and secondary syphilis by state in the United States in 1992. Since 1990, the rates of primary and secondary syphilis have declined among all ethnic groups. In the early 1980s, a disproportionate incidence occurred among homosexual men. In the 1990s, the overall rate of primary and secondary syphilis in cities with a population exceeding 200,000 declined from 33.4 cases per 100,000 in 1991 to 25.1 in 1992. The total rate for the United States in 1992 was 13.7 cases per 100,000 population. New cases tend to be concentrated in the southeast. (*From* Division of STD/HIV Prevention: *Sexually Transmitted Disease Surveillance, 1992.* Atlanta: Centers for Disease Control and Prevention; 1993:7.)

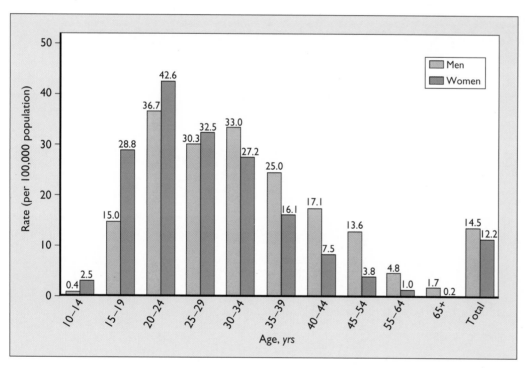

FIGURE 9-2 Age- and gender-specific rates for primary and secondary syphilis in the United States in 1992. Compared with gonorrhea, syphilis is more likely to be acquired by slightly older individuals, particularly men. The male-to-female ratio is nearly one, suggesting that the current transmission of syphilis is primarily heterosexual. The high incidence of early syphilis among women of childbearing age has given rise to an alarming recent increase in congenital syphilis (*see* Chapter 11). (*From* Division of STD/HIV Prevention: *Sexually Transmitted Disease Surveillance, 1992.* Atlanta: Centers for Disease Control and Prevention; 1993:10.)

PRIMARY SYPHILIS

Penile Chancres

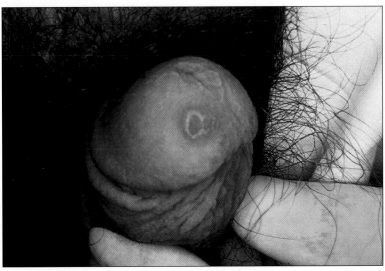

FIGURE 9-3 Typical chancre of primary syphilis on glans penis. The typical appearance of the chancre of primary syphilis on the glans penis is shown. Such lesions are usually indurated, indolent, and nontender. The ulcerations may be large or small but are always indurated and sharply demarcated. The chancre appears after an average of 3 weeks after infection, but the incubation period can range from 9 to 90 days. Intercurrent antibiotics can delay or dramatically modify the appearance of the chancre. Regional lymphadenopathy accompanies the chancre. Classically referred to as satellite bubo, involved nodes are moderately enlarged, discrete, and nontender. The inguinal nodes regularly enlarge because syphilis first spreads throughout the lymphatic vessels. The chancre heals spontaneously within about 3 to 6 weeks but may persist for up to 3 months and overlap the manifestations of secondary syphilis.

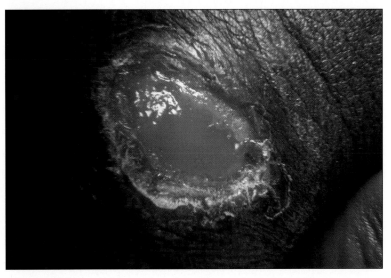

FIGURE 9-4 Chancre of primary syphilis on penile shaft. A large, indurated, nontender ulceration is seen on the distal penile shaft. The borders of the lesion are sharply circumscribed. Induration is characteristic of syphilis, in contrast to the lesions of chancroid (historically referred to as *soft chancre*), donovanosis, or herpes genitalis.

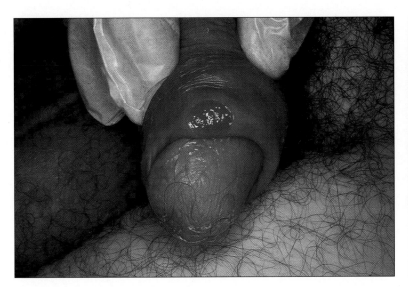

FIGURE 9-5 Chancre on the prepuce in primary syphilis. Chancres of the prepuce, like those of the glans, are indurated and nontender. Several studies have suggested an increased incidence of sexually transmitted diseases among uncircumcised men; the mechanism is unknown, but theories include delays in diagnosis of hidden lesions, increased proliferation of organisms beneath the foreskin, or even increased susceptibility of the foreskin itself.

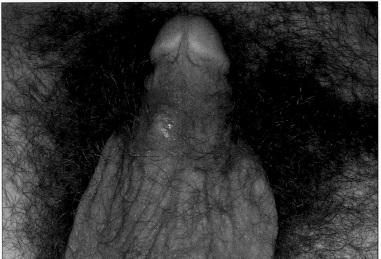

FIGURE 9-6 Chancre of primary syphilis at base of penis. A typical chancre is seen at the base of the penis. Chancres of the penis occur, in descending order of frequency, on the corona, prepuce, shaft, and base. Such lesions at the base of the penis or in the pubic hair sometimes occur in patients who have worn condoms but become infected in areas that remain uncovered.

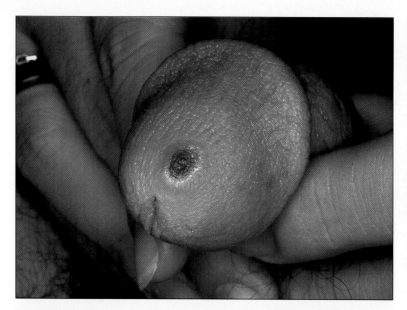

FIGURE 9-7 Chancre of the glans in primary syphilis. Although inguinofemoral adenopathy is often seen with a chancre on the shaft of the penis, the glans drains preferentially to the deep iliac nodes, causing the palpable inguinofemoral adenopathy to be minimal or delayed in appearance when the chancre is at this site. Lymphatic drainage is similar for the cervix and proximal third of the vagina.

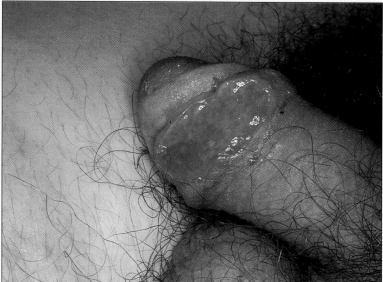

FIGURE 9-8 Multiple penile chancres in primary syphilis. Multiple chancres have merged together, forming a large ulceration at the corona of the penis, which is the most common site for penile chancres. Multiple chancres are seen in approximately 40% of cases. The rapid plasma reagin blood test is universally reactive when the chancre is 7 days old.

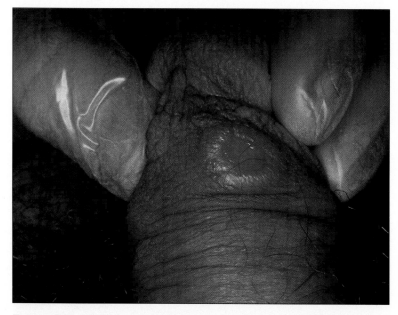

FIGURE 9-9 Multiple penile chancres in primary syphilis. Multiple chancres occur more frequently in patients who have a chronic dermatosis, such as eczema or psoriasis, or a penis traumatized by oral sex or by biting during sexual foreplay followed by genital intromission.

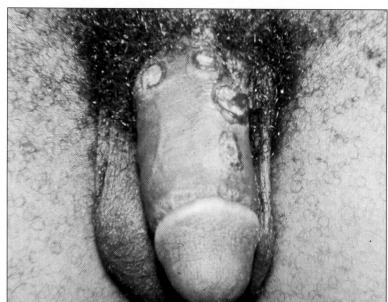

FIGURE 9-10 Multiple chancres of primary syphilis on the penile shaft. The ulcerated lesions are raised above the surface of the surrounding skin, a feature frequently seen in syphilis. (*Courtesy of* the Centers for Disease Control and Prevention.)

Oral and Facial Chancres

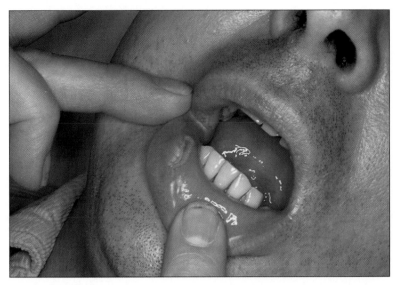

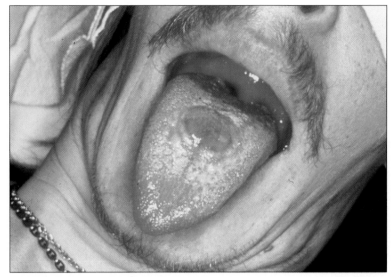

FIGURE 9-11 Oral chancres in primary syphilis. A chancre developed on the lower lip of a man, caused by performing fellatio. Most chancres of the lip result from open-mouth or "wet" kisses and tend to occur on the upper lip in the man and the lower lip in the woman (due to the mechanics of kissing in our culture). The infecting partner is usually in the secondary stage of syphilis, with mucous patches in the mouth. Chancres resulting from fellatio are usually on the lower lip or at the commissure of the mouth. During preliminary sex play, whether kissing or fellatio, microscopic tears occur that become the portal of entry for the spirochete of syphilis. (*From* Fiumara NJ: *Pictorial Guide to Sexually Transmitted Diseases.* New York: Cahners Publ.; 1989:42; with permission.)

FIGURE 9-12 Oral chancres of primary syphilis on the tongue. An indurated, nontender ulceration occurred on the tongue, along with bilateral anterior cervical lymphadenopathy, in this married, bisexual patient. The chancre was caused by performing fellatio on a partner with secondary syphilis. The ulcerations of primary syphilis are deep, in contrast to the shallow ulcers of herpes and staphylococcal or streptococcal infections. The chancres have a punched-out appearance with sharp margins, unlike the irregular ulcerations seen in herpes and other infections. (*From* Fiumara NJ: *Pictorial Guide to Sexually Transmitted Diseases.* New York: Cahners Publ.; 1989:42; with permission.)

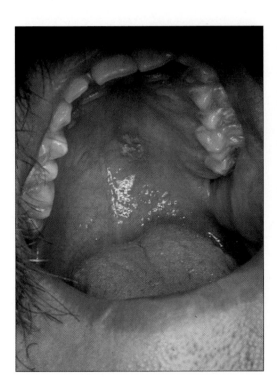

FIGURE 9-13
Oral chancres of primary syphilis on the hard palate. A chancre is seen on the hard palate, contracted by performing fellatio. The lesion must be distinguished from mucous patches, which may also involve the tongue. Intraoral lesions of syphilis contain large numbers of organisms. Previously, when dentists practiced bare-handed, a chancre of the finger (dentist's finger) was occasionally seen in health-care workers.

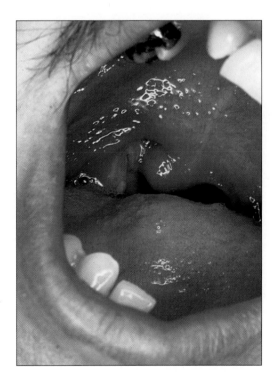

FIGURE 9-14
Oral chancre on the tonsil in primary syphilis. A chancre on the left tonsil was caused by performing deep-throat fellatio. All chancres of the tonsil are reported to occur on the left tonsil (with only one known exception), but the reason for this anatomic predisposition is unknown.

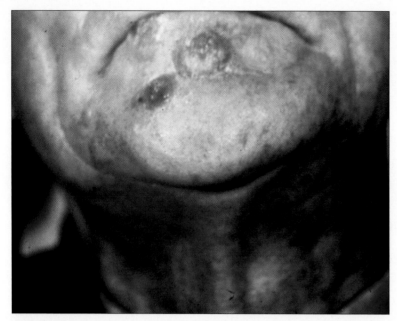

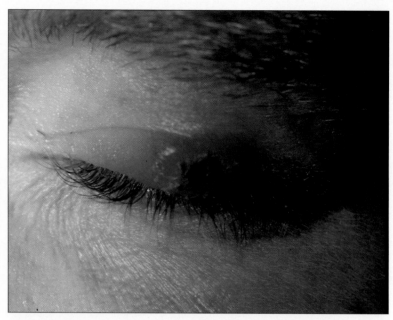

FIGURE 9-15 Facial chancres in primary syphilis. Multiple chancres occurred on the chin of this patient due to open-mouth kissing with a partner who had secondary syphilis with mucous patches of the tongue. Chancres form at the site of primary inoculation and initial multiplication of *Treponema pallidum*. The spirochetes can infect through intact mucous membranes or through microscopic defects in grossly intact skin. Thus, one must consider the possibility of syphilis when evaluating lesions that appear even at some distance from the genitalia.

FIGURE 9-16 Facial chancre of primary syphilis on the eyelid. A chancre on the left upper eyelid resulted from open-mouth kissing with a partner who had secondary syphilis.

Perianal Chancres

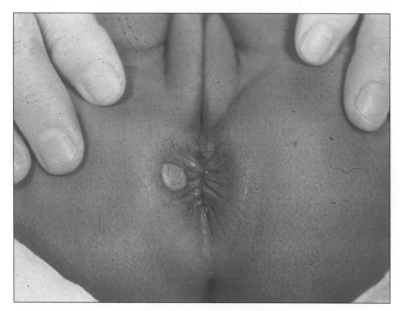

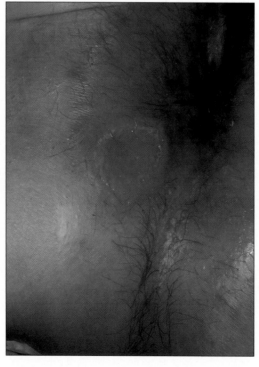

FIGURE 9-18 Large perianal chancre in primary syphilis. Chancres of the anus are not painful, unless they occur on the sphincter or a hemorrhoid. Chancres of the skin, including the anus, are not painful because they result from ischemic necrosis histologically, whereas those on the sphincter involve muscles, and on a hemorrhoid, a phlebitis.

FIGURE 9-17 Perianal chancre in an infant. This lesion has the classic morphologic appearance and induration and resulted from sexual abuse. Such lesions must be differentiated from those of secondary syphilis, which might result from *in utero* infection.

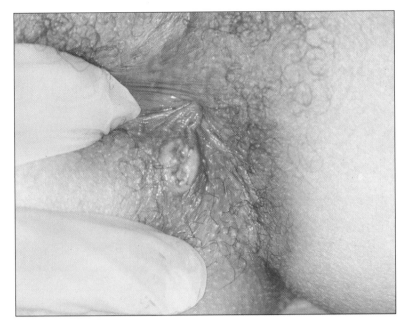

FIGURE 9-19 Perianal chancre of primary syphilis in a woman who practiced receptive anal intercourse. The lesion was not painful, although the patient was aware of its presence. The lesion was firm and, characteristically, elevated above the surface of the surrounding skin. (*Courtesy of* M.F. Rein, MD.) (*From* Tramont EC: *Treponema pallidum* (syphilis). *In* Mandell GL, Bennett JE, Dolin R (eds.): *Principles and Practice of Infectious Disease*, 4th ed. New York: Churchill Livingstone; 1995:2121; with permission.)

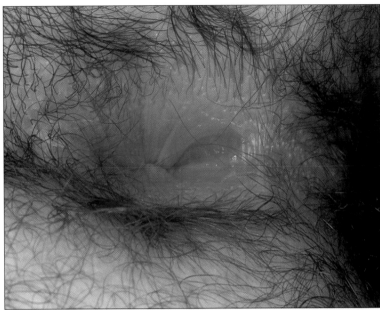

FIGURE 9-20 Large, nontender chancre in the perianal region. Because the chancre develops at the site of initial inoculation and multiplication of the spirochete, the presence of a perianal chancre, particularly in a man, suggests the possibility of receptive anal intercourse. The anus should be carefully examined for evidence of other sexually transmitted disease, and the patient should be strongly encouraged to undergo testing for HIV.

Vaginal Chancres

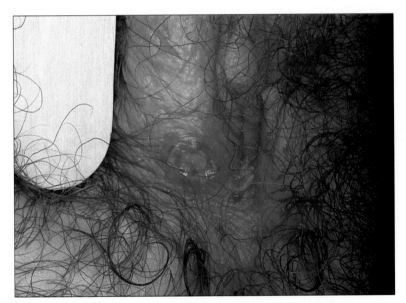

FIGURE 9-21 Vaginal chancre in primary syphilis. A typical indurated, nontender chancre is seen on the lower pole of the right labium. The right inguinal node is discretely enlarged and also nontender. Most chancres in women appear in the lower portions of the labia. Whereas the external genitalia and distal two thirds of the vagina drain to the inguinofemoral nodes, the cervix and proximal third of the vagina drain to the deep iliac nodes. Thus, chancres at these latter locations may not be accompanied by palpable lymphadenopathy.

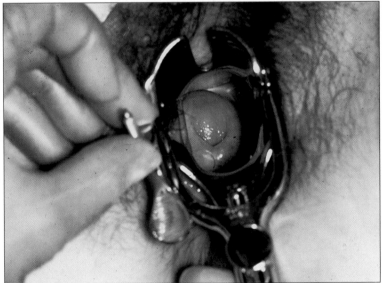

FIGURE 9-22 Cervical chancre in primary syphilis. A sharply circumscribed ulceration is seen on the cervix. Chancres are often not noticed in women, and primary syphilis is usually not detected unless the woman is identified as a contact of an individual with infectious syphilis.

Diagnostic Evaluations

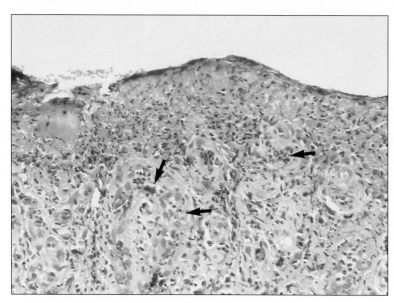

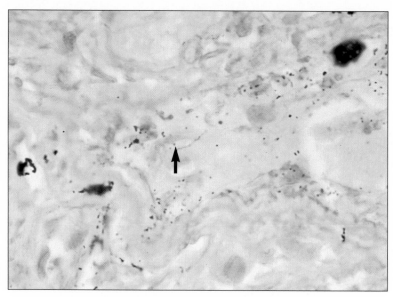

FIGURE 9-23 Histologic appearance of the syphilitic chancre. The patient noted a penile papule, which subsequently eroded into a painless ulcer with raised, firm, indurated borders and a clean base. The biopsy specimen, stained with hematoxylin-eosin, reveals superficial ulceration, plasma cell infiltration, and endarteritis with endothelial proliferation (*arrows*). Not shown but classically described is capillary proliferation and a hyperplastic surrounding epithelium with tongues of epidermis projecting into the dermis (so-called pseudoepitheliomatous hyperplasia). (*From* Wong T-Y, Mihm MC Jr: Primary syphilis [images]. *N Engl J Med* 1994, 331:1492; with permission.)

FIGURE 9-24 Histologic examination of the syphilitic chancre on high-power microscopy. The generation time of *Treponema pallidum* in the human host is quite long, about 30 hours. By the time the chancre is clinically manifest, however, large numbers of spirochetes are present. These are usually demonstrable on dark-field examination of expressed tissue fluid (*see* Chapter 8). The organisms within tissue are harder to reveal. Here, silver staining demonstrates a spirochete about 6 to 15 µm long with regularly spaced spirals (*arrow*). (*From* Wong T-Y, Mihm MC Jr: Primary syphilis [images]. *N Engl J Med* 1994, 331:1492; with permission.)

Differential diagnosis of genital ulcers

Sexually transmitted diseases
  Syphilis
  Herpes
  Chancroid
  Donovanosis
  Lymphogranuloma venereum
  Gonorrhea (rarely)
  Trichomoniasis (rarely)
Nonsexually transmitted diseases
  Trauma
  Fixed drug eruption
  Tularemia
  Behçet's syndrome
  Malignancy
  Candidiasis
  Histoplasmosis
  Mycobacterial infection
  Amebiasis

FIGURE 9-25 Differential diagnosis of genital ulcers. The differential diagnosis of genital ulcer disease can be challenging because the relative frequency of etiologies differs with the population being examined. For example, chancroid was diagnosed in 40% to 90% of some Indian series, and donovanosis is endemic in India, New Guinea, the West Indies, and parts of Africa and South America. In the United States, genital herpes still accounts for most genital ulcers, but chancroid is becoming more common in inner cities. Features of differential diagnostic significance include the morphology of the ulcer base and edge, number of ulcers, degree of tenderness, and accompanying regional lymphadenopathy. Serpiginous lesions heal in one area while progressing in another. (Dangor Y, Ballard RC, Exposito FDL, *et al.*: Accuracy of clinical diagnosis of genital ulcer disease. *Sex Transm Dis* 1990, 17:184-189. Rein MF: Skin and mucous membrane lesions. *In* Mandell GL, Bennett JE, Dolin R (eds.): *Principles and Practice of Infectious Diseases*, 4th ed. New York: Churchill Livingstone; 1995:1055-1063.)

Differential features of sexually transmitted genital ulcers

	Lesions	Tenderness	Edge	Base	Adenopathy
Syphilis	Usually single	None or mild	Indurated	Clean	Indolent
Chancroid	Usually multiple	Marked	Soft	Dirty	Tender, fluctuant
Herpes	Multiple	Marked	Soft	Clean	Tender
Donovanosis	Multiple	None	Serpiginous, may be white	Beefy red, granulation tissue	Erosive lesions overlying nodes
LGV	Single	None	Soft	Eroded papule	Prominent, tender

LGV—lymphogranuloma venereum.

Figure 9-26 Differential features of sexually transmitted genital ulcers. The differential diagnosis of genital ulcers may be difficult, and the "classic" descriptions of these lesions for individual conditions are often misleading. For example, the syphilitic chancre is described as a single, painless, indurated lesion, but in some series, almost half of men with chancres had multiple lesions; in contrast, some 40% to 70% of men presenting with chancroid manifest only a single lesion. Lesional tenderness is described by up to 30% of patients with chancres. Multiple infections of lesions are common in some parts of the world. Thus, differential diagnosis requires attention to all clinical details. Genital ulcers have assumed a particularly ominous role because they can apparently serve as portals of entry or exit for HIV. (Chapel TA: The variability of syphilitic chancres. *Sex Transm Dis* 1978, 5:68–70. Rein MF: Skin and mucous membrane lesions. *In* Mandell GL, Bennett JE, Dolin R (eds.): *Principles and Practice of Infectious Diseases*, 4th ed. New York: Churchill Livingstone; 1995:1055–1063.) (*Courtesy of* M.F. Rein, MD.)

SECONDARY SYPHILIS

Early systemic manifestations of secondary syphilis

Sore throat	53%
Malaise	42%
Headache	24%
Weight loss	18%
Fever	14%
Meningismus	8%
Abdominal discomfort	7%
Arthralgias	7%
Vaginal discharge	3%
Deafness	2%
Hoarseness	2%
Myalgias	2%

Figure 9-27 Early systemic manifestations of secondary syphilis. Secondary syphilis appears 2 to 12 weeks after the development of chancre, but the interval is highly variable. Constitutional symptoms are common but nonspecific. (*Adapted from* Stokes JH, Beerman H, Ingraham NR: *Modern Clinical Syphilology*, 3rd ed. Philadelphia: W.B. Saunders; 1944:599; with permission.)

Dermatologic manifestations of secondary syphilis

Rash	
Macular	90%
Maculopapular	54%
Large macular	28%
Follicular	16%
Papulopustular	11%
Mucous membrane lesions	
Mucous patches	2%
Genital mucosa	58%

Figure 9-28 Dermatologic lesions in secondary syphilis. Rash is a hallmark of secondary syphilis. Papulosquamous eruptions may resemble pityriasis rosea. Vesicles and bullae are distinctly rare in secondary syphilis in adults, although they may be manifest in congenital syphilis. The generalized rash of secondary syphilis almost always involves the mouth or genitals, and classic teaching suggests that a generalized eruption sparing these sites is unlikely to be secondary syphilis. Involvement of the palms and soles is by no means diagnostic of syphilis but should suggest that possibility to the clinician. (Stokes JH, Beerman H, Ingraham NR: *Modern Clinical Syphilology*, 3rd ed. Philadelphia: W.B. Saunders; 1944:526–527.) (*Courtesy of* M.F. Rein, MD.)

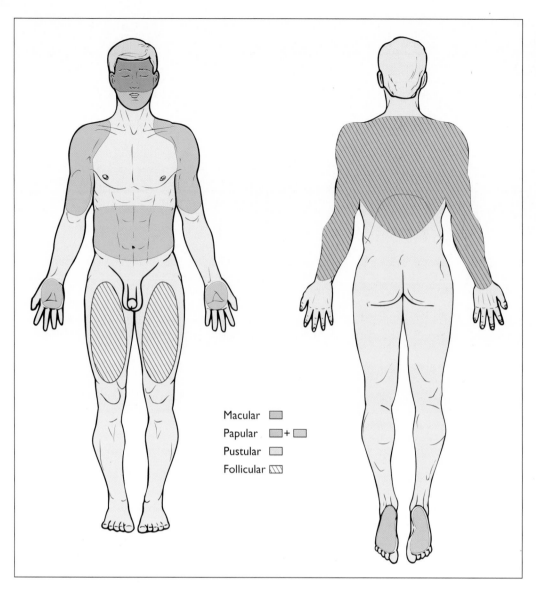

FIGURE 9-29 Distribution of skin lesions in secondary syphilis. Clinicians in the 1930s and 1940s observed that various types of syphilitic lesions had a predilection for certain anatomic sites. The reason for this specific distribution is unknown but may relate to skin temperature, vascularity, and distribution of skin appendages, such as hair follicles. Thus, one is most likely to see macules over the flanks and abdomen, shoulders, upper arms, back, and chin; papules in the same distribution but with an increased predilection for the face, palms, and soles; pustules over the face and scalp; and follicular lesions over the back and extensor surfaces. (Stokes JH, Beerman H, Ingraham NR: *Modern Clinical Syphilology*, 3rd ed. Philadelphia: W.B. Saunders; 1944:7.) (*Courtesy of* M.F. Rein, MD.)

Macular
Papular
Pustular
Follicular

Maculopapular Rash

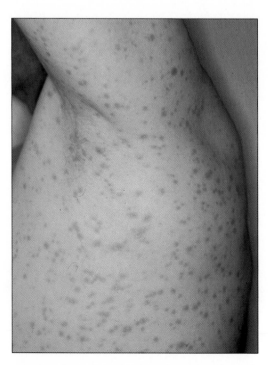

FIGURE 9-30 Maculopapular rash of secondary syphilis on the trunk. The symptoms of secondary syphilis appear about a month after the onset of primary syphilis or about 8 weeks after the infectious exposure. This patient had flulike symptoms, rash, and generalized adenopathy. The rash may be macular, maculopapular, papular, or pustular. In this patient, the maculopapular rash also involved the midface, with mucous patches in the mouth, oval lesions in the lines of cleavage of the skin, which superficially resembled pityriasis rosea, and lesions on the palms and soles.

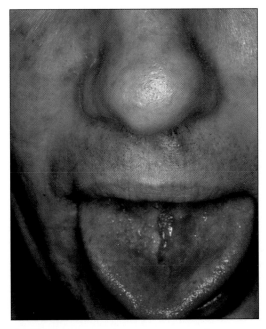

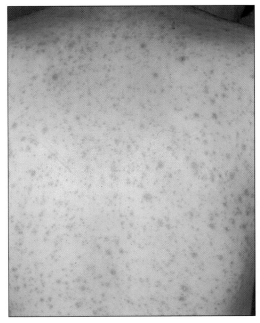

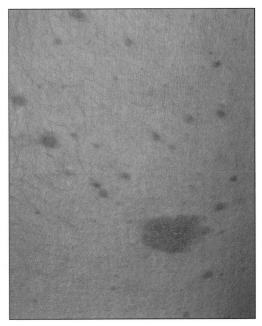

FIGURE 9-31 Maculopapular rash of secondary syphilis on the midface. A coppery-red rash is seen on the midface and nose, and mucous patches also are evident on the tongue and buccal mucous membrane. Rash is the most common manifestation of secondary syphilis and often begins as a macular rash on the trunk, shoulders, and arms, progressing to a maculopapular eruption involving the face, chest, back, abdomen, arms, and sometimes, legs. The rash is classically minimally pruritic and is often described as having a "sinister" coppery color. The rash has a symmetrical distribution, and lesions are usually 3 to 10 mm in diameter. Although the rash is highly variable in adults, vesicular or bullous lesions are not seen.

FIGURE 9-32 Maculopapular rash of secondary syphilis involving the back. Maculopapular rashes are observed in about one quarter of patients with secondary syphilis. They are classically described as nonpruritic, but some 40% of patients describe mild itching. (Chapel TA: The signs and symptoms of secondary syphilis. *Sex Transm Dis* 1980, 7:161–164.)

FIGURE 9-33 Pityriasis rosea-like lesions of secondary syphilis involving the chest. The differential diagnosis of secondary syphilis can be challenging. One condition that invites confusion is pityriasis rosea, a disease of unknown etiology. Both diseases produce symmetrical, minimally pruritic, papulosquamous lesions, and both frequently involve the mouth. The rash of pityriasis rosea is often preceded by a single large lesion, termed the *herald patch*, which is suggested by the large lesion seen in this syphilitic patient. The differential diagnosis is most easily made by a serologic test for syphilis, which should be reactive in all patients with secondary syphilis.

Papular Lesions

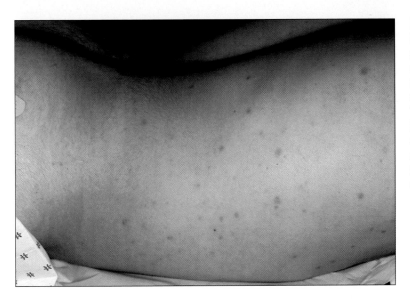

FIGURE 9-34 Papular lesions on the chest in secondary syphilis. Reddish-brown papular lesions are seen on the chest, along with generalized adenopathy. The quantitative rapid plasma reagin (RPR) and Venereal Disease Research Laboratory tests are always reactive in secondary syphilis. The quantitative RPR is used to detect the prozone reaction and to follow the titer posttreatment. The prozone phenomenon occurs when antibody production is so high that antibody excess renders the nontreponemal tests nonreactive on undiluted or very low dilutions of serum. If secondary syphilis is suspected, one should order a *quantitative* nontreponemal test, so that the patient's serum is tested at sufficiently high dilutions to prevent the prozone phenomenon (*see* Chapter 8).

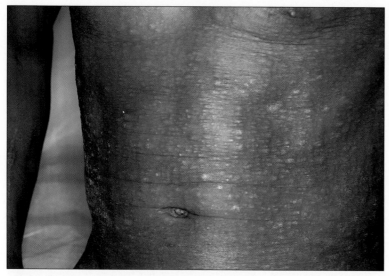

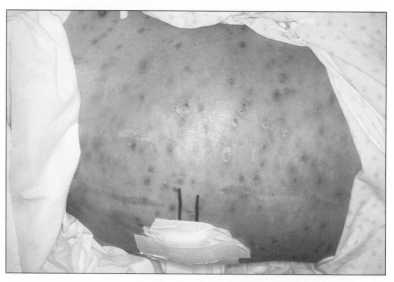

FIGURE 9-35 Papular lesions of secondary syphilis on the abdomen of a black man. In secondary syphilis, the treponemal tests, such as the microhemagglutinin antibody assay to *Treponema pallidum* or fluorescent treponemal antibody absorption assays, are always reactive (positive). Whenever a reagin test, such as the rapid plasma reagin (RPR) or Venereal Disease Research Laboratory (VDRL) test, is reactive, a treponemal test should be performed. If the RPR or VDRL test is positive but the treponemal tests are negative, then the patient has a biologic false-positive reaction, which may be due to an autoimmune disease or another infectious disease.

FIGURE 9-36 Papular lesions of the chest and abdomen in secondary syphilis. The lesions are reddish-brown to dark red in color and nonpuritic. Papular lesions traditionally develop after the maculopapular eruption, and lesions are larger and fewer in number.

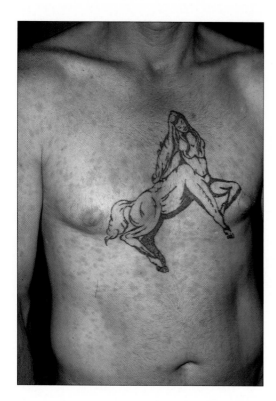

FIGURE 9-37 Papular lesions of secondary syphilis on the chest in a patient with an exotic tattoo, a centaur. Oval lesions, following lines of skin cleavage, may invite confusion with pityriasis rosea.

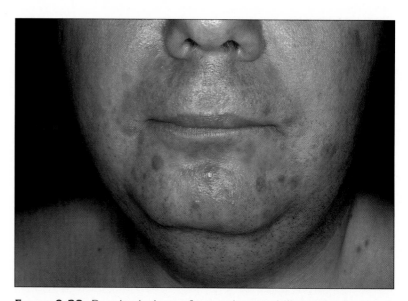

FIGURE 9-38 Papular lesions of secondary syphilis on the face and chin. Papular lesions are seen on the middle of the face and the chin in this patient who also has AIDS. A few case reports suggest an increased frequency of malignant syphilis, with rapidly progressive and destructive lesions, in patients with advanced HIV disease. These lesions may also occur on the upper trunk.

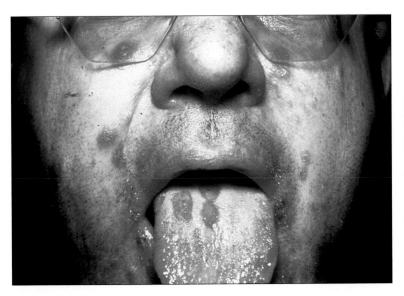

FIGURE 9-39 Papular lesions of secondary syphilis involving the face and tongue. Papular lesions are present on the forehead, face, chin, and tongue. Lesions were also present on the body, palms, and soles of this patient who also has AIDS.

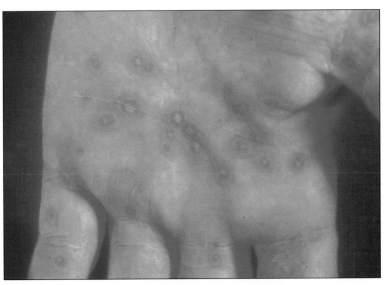

FIGURE 9-40 Palmar lesions of secondary syphilis. Papular lesions of the palms are seen crossing the creases. If lesions of secondary syphilis are present on the palms, they should also be looked for elsewhere on the skin and mucous membranes.

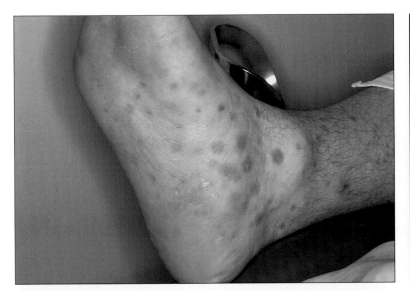

FIGURE 9-41 Papular lesions of secondary syphilis on the soles and ankles. These lesions are hard, nontender, and nonpruritic. One half to two thirds of patients will have lesions on the palms and soles.

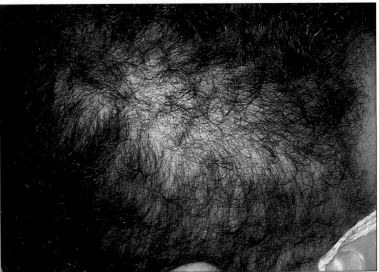

FIGURE 9-42 Papular lesions of the scalp in secondary syphilis. Involvement of hair follicles will produce papular lesions of the scalp, leading to patchy, moth-eaten, nonerythematous, nonscarring alopecia. The hair regrows after treatment. The differential diagnosis may initially include superficial fungal infection, but in syphilis, broken hair shafts are not observed.

FIGURE 9-43 Papular lesions of secondary syphilis. Papular lesions of the face, with patchy alopecia of the beard and eyebrows.

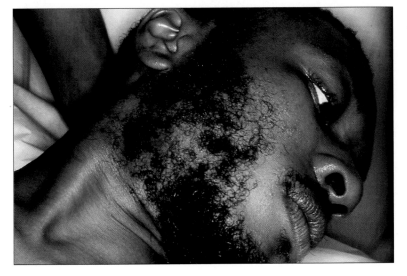

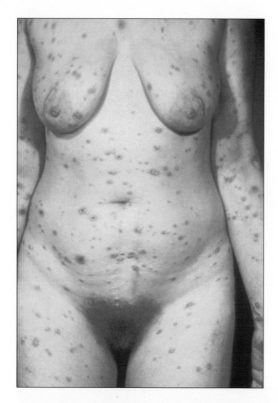

FIGURE 9-44 Generalized pustular rash of secondary syphilis. Generalized pustular lesions resembling a chickenpox eruption are seen. This patient also had lesions on the face, mucous patches, and pustules on the palms and soles. Pustular lesions are less common than either macular or papular rashes and form when papules have ulcerated and then crusted. They may be related to diminished host resistance. (*From* Fiumara NJ: *Pictorial Guide to Sexually Transmitted Diseases.* New York: Cahners Publ.; 1989:43; with permission.)

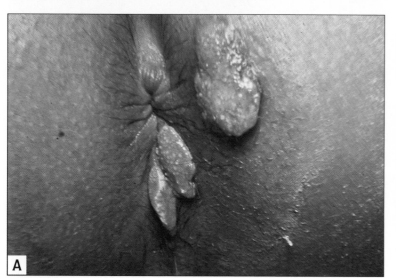

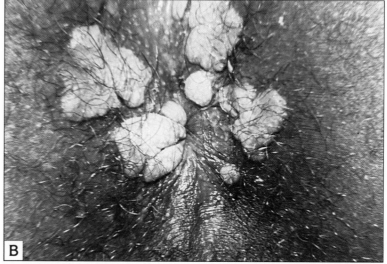

FIGURE 9-45 Condyloma lata in the perianal region. **A** and **B**, Papular lesions on moist, intertriginous areas may coalesce to form broad, moist, highly infectious plaques called *condyloma lata*. These flat, wartlike lesions develop at sites to which *Treponema pallidum* has disseminated and are frequently seen around the anus, as in these two images. They may also occur on the vulva or scrotum and are less commonly found in the axillae, under the breasts, or between the toes. Condyloma lata must be differentiated from condyloma acuminata, caused by human papillomavirus (*see* Chapter 12), which are generally more verrucous and exuberant.

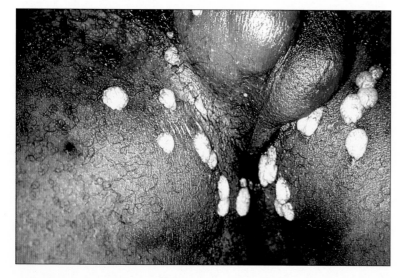

FIGURE 9-46 Condyloma lata in the scrotal region. Condyloma lata develop in a small percentage of patients in anatomic locations where skin is oppressed to skin. These lesions contain many spirochetes, which makes them highly contagious but also makes them a prime site for sampling for darkfield microscopy. (*Courtesy of* M.J. Chiu, MD.)

Mucous Membrane Lesions

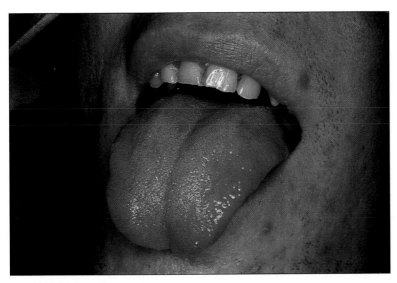

FIGURE 9-47 Mucous patches on the tongue in secondary syphilis. Secondary syphilis results from systemic dissemination of the spirochetes. Lesions on the skin contain small numbers of organisms and are not contagious. Mucous membrane lesions, on the other hand, contain large numbers of organisms and can easily result in disease transmission. Mucous patches are painless ulcerations, often displaying a dirty, yellowish base.

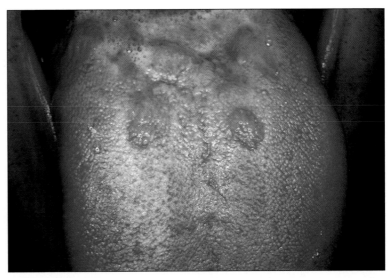

FIGURE 9-48 Papular lesions of the tongue in secondary syphilis. Very early in syphilis, spirochetes disseminate widely. Organisms arriving at the mouth can cause mucous patches, which are shallow ulcerations (*see* Figs. 9-12, 9-13, and 9-14). Such dissemination may also result in papular lesions.

TREATMENT

Recommended treatment of early syphilis
Adults
Benzathine penicillin G, 2.4 MU intramuscularly × single dose
Children
Benzathine penicillin G, 50,000 U/kg intramuscularly, up to the adult dose of 2.4 MU × single dose
Penicillin allergy (nonpregnant)
Doxycycline, 100 mg orally 2 times a day × 2 wks
or
Tetracycline, 500 mg orally 4 times a day × 2 wks

FIGURE 9-49 Recommended treatment of early syphilis. For purposes of therapy, early syphilis is defined as primary, secondary, or early latent syphilis. Early latent disease refers to syphilis without signs or symptoms but which is known to have been present for < 1 year (*eg*, because of a recent previous nonreactive serologic test or a well-defined history of specific recent exposure). These regimens are recommended by the Centers for Disease Control and Prevention but remain somewhat controversial, with some experts (including the author) recommending two doses of benzathine penicillin, 2.4 MU given intramuscularly, separated by 1 week. Other tetracyclines can be used in equivalent dosages. Pregnant patients allergic to penicillin should be desensitized. Use of erythromycin in this setting is associated with treatment failures. (Centers for Disease Control and Prevention: 1993 Sexually transmitted disease treatment guidelines. *MMWR* 1993, 42(RR-14):30–32.)

Clinical features of the Jarisch-Herxheimer reaction
Fever, chills
Myalgias
Headache
Palpitations
Flushing
Hypotension
Intensification of skin lesions
Edema around lesions
Appearance of a faint rash resembling secondary syphilis
Increased size of involved lymph nodes
Tenderness of involved lymph nodes
Fetal distress, early labor

FIGURE 9-50 Clinical features of the Jarisch-Herxheimer reaction. Treatment of secondary syphilis with penicillin or other antibiotics frequently elicits the Jarisch-Herxheimer reaction. This reaction is observed in about 70% of patients treated for secondary syphilis and perhaps 30% of patients treated for primary syphilis. It usually begins within 1 or 2 hours of initiating treatment, is usually managed with aspirin, and resolves within 24 to 48 hours. Occasionally, it is more severe and may cause end-organ damage if the central nervous system is involved. The reaction is referred to historically as *therapeutic shock*, but the exact mechanism remains unclear. Material released from rapidly lysing organisms triggers the inflammatory response.

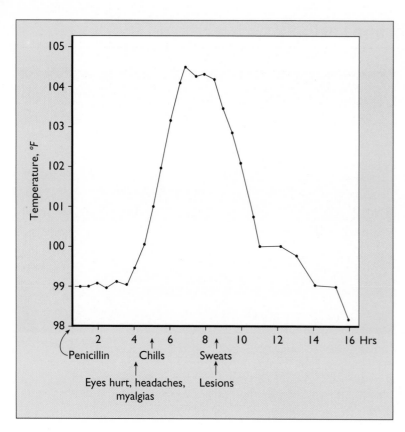

FIGURE 9-51 Clinical course of the Jarisch-Herxheimer reaction. A characteristic feature of syphilis' response to therapy is the appearance of a Jarisch-Herxheimer reaction. The illustrated example occurred in a patient with secondary syphilis who was given 1.2 MU of procaine penicillin. The onset of the reaction occurred 4 hours later with the characteristic headache, myalgias, and chills, followed by lesions and sweats at 8 hours and resolution by 16 hours. One study in a medical observation unit found that most patients treated for secondary syphilis developed such a reaction. (Young EJ, Weingarten NM, Baughn RE, Duncan WC: Studies on the pathogenesis of the Jarisch-Herxheimer reaction: Development of an animal model and evidence against a role for classical endotoxin. *J Infect Dis* 1982, 146:606–615.) (*Courtesy of* D.M. Musher, MD.)

SELECTED BIBLIOGRAPHY

Engelkens HJ, Stolz E: Genital ulcer disease. *Int J Dermatol* 1993, 32:169–181.

Fiumara NJ: Infectious syphilis. *Dermatol Clin North Am* 1983, 1:3–21.

Fiumara NJ: Treatment of primary and secondary syphilis: The serologic response. *J Am Acad Dermatol* 1986, 14:487–491.

Musher DM, Hamill RJ, Baughn RE: Effect of human immunodeficiency virus (HIV) infection on the course of syphilis and on the response to treatment. *Ann Intern Med* 1990, 113:872–881.

Rolfs RT: Treatment of syphilis, 1993. *Clin Infect Dis* 1995, 20(supp 1):S23–S38.

CHAPTER 10

Late Syphilis

Michael F. Rein
Daniel M. Musher

Natural History of Untreated Syphilis

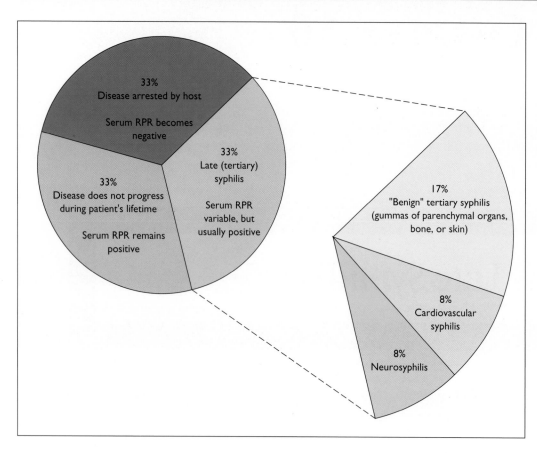

Figure 10-1 Natural history of untreated syphilis. Studies conducted in Oslo at the beginning of the 20th century, based on follow-up observations throughout the life-time of infected persons, showed that in the absence of treatment for syphilis, one third of infected persons appeared to resolve the infection, as inferred from the absence of recurrent syphilitic disease and the disappearance of the reactive nontreponemal serologic test (*see* Chapter 8). One third retained a reactive serologic test but did not, during their lifetimes, have further syphilitic disease. One third developed late (tertiary) syphilis. Tertiary syphilis is categorized into benign, cardiovascular, and neurologic syphilis. Benign tertiary syphilis receives its name because nonvital structures, such as the skin, soft tissues, and bones, are involved, or because the condition affects parenchymal organs, such as liver or testes, but without risk to patient survival. (RPR—reactive plasma reagin.) (Gjestland T: The Oslo study of untreated syphilis. *Acta Derm Venereol (Stockh)* 1955, 35(suppl 34): 1–368.)

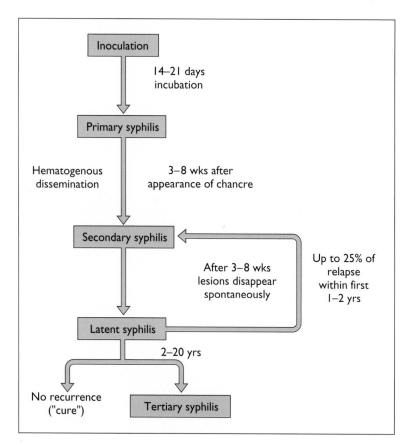

Figure 10-2 Time course of untreated syphilis. Soon after initial infection by *Treponema pallidum*, a primary lesion or chancre usually appears at the site of inoculation, followed in about 6 weeks by disseminated secondary disease. After the secondary phase subsides, the patient enters a latent phase, during the first 1 to 2 years of which ("early" latency) relapses to the secondary stage may occur. During the "late" latency phase, patients remain reactive on serologic tests for syphilis but have no apparent signs of disease, although progression of disease continues. One third of untreated patients go on to develop tertiary syphilis after a highly variable period ranging from 2 to 20 years or more. Treatment at any stage with accepted doses of penicillin nearly always eliminates disease (except in late tertiary syphilis and HIV infection). (*Adapted from* Musher DM: Syphilis. *In* Gorbach SL, Bartlett JG, Blacklow NR (eds.): *Infectious Diseases.* Philadelphia: W.B. Saunders; 1992:826; with permission.)

BENIGN LATE SYPHILIS

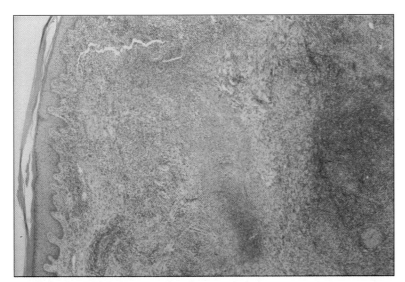

FIGURE 10-3 Histologic appearance of syphilitic gumma. The classic lesion of benign syphilis is the gumma. A specimen from a lesion, stained with hematoxylin-eosin, shows an accumulation of lymphocytes at its center and macrophages at the periphery. *Treponema pallidum* is generally not demonstrated within such lesions, even by use of special stains, and the gumma is regarded as an immunologically mediated response to an undetermined antigenic stimulus. One modern study, however, has used fluorescent antibody assays to demonstrate treponemes in a gumma, albeit in an unusual case. (Handsfield HH, Lukehart SA, Sell A, *et al*.: Demonstration of *Treponema pallidum* in a cutaneous gumma by indirect immunofluorescence. *Arch Dermatol* 1983, 719:677.)

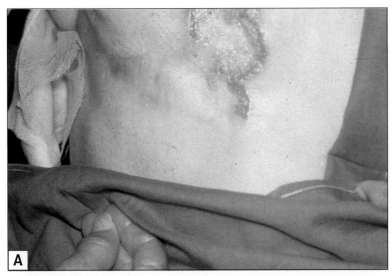

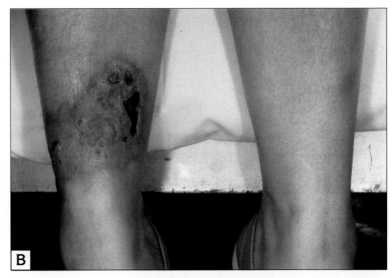

FIGURE 10-4 Cutaneous gummas in late syphilis. Gummas may affect virtually any part of the body and range from small nodules to deep, necrotizing, ulcerative lesions. They are typically indolent and painless and develop from 2 to 35 years after initial infection. **A.** Cutaneous gumma on the lower back. **B.** Cutaneous gumma on the lower leg. These two lesions show nearly all of the typical characteristics of late cutaneous syphilis, as described by Stokes: 1) solitary character; 2) asymmetry; 3) induration; 4) indolence; 5) arciform (circinate) configuration; 6) sharp margination of the lesion, with a punched-out appearance of ulcers; 7) tissue destruction and replacement; 8) tendency to one-sided healing with extension; 9) scar formation that is atrophic and noncontractile, retaining the arciform configuration of the original lesion; 10) peripheral hyperpigmentation that persists. (Stokes JH: *Modern Clinical Syphilology: Diagnosis–Treatment–Case Study*. Philadelphia: W.B. Saunders; 1934.) (*Courtesy of* J.F. Mullins, MD.)

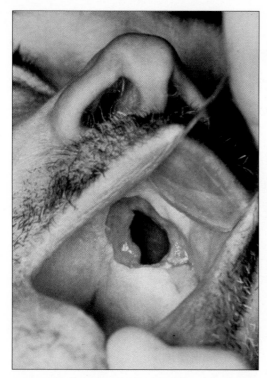

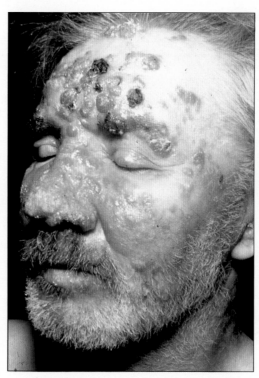

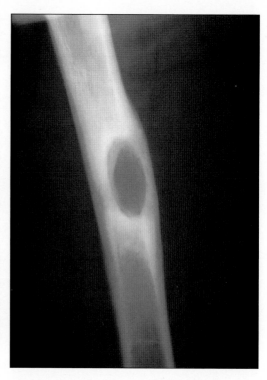

FIGURE 10-5 Perforation of the hard palate due to late syphilis. Cases of perforated palate were relatively common in the pre-penicillin era but are now exceedingly rare. The differential diagnosis would include squamous cell carcinoma and midline granuloma. (*Courtesy of* J.F. Mullins, MD.)

FIGURE 10-6 Nodular gummatous syphilis involving the forehead. Nodules in this form of syphilis may range in size from microscopic to large nodules measuring many centimeters. The nodules are pink or purplish red and tend to appear on the face, upper body, and extremities. The nodules may break down into an ulcerative form. If untreated, the lesion may heal over many weeks or months with significant scarring. (*Courtesy of* M.J. Chiu, MD.)

FIGURE 10-7 Syphilitic osteomyelitis (gumma) of the femur. Anteroposterior radiograph of the femur of a 62-year-old man with late syphilis reveals a punched-out lesion in the midshaft occupied by a gumma. Deep granulomatous lesions may break down to form punched-out lesions. Gummas of the bone may result in a pathologic fracture or joint destruction. (*Courtesy of* J.T. Mader, MD.)

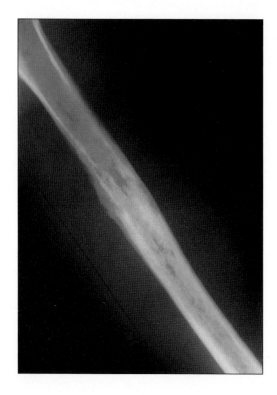

FIGURE 10-8 Syphilitic osteomyelitis (gumma) of the femur. Anteroposterior radiograph of a femur from a 70-year-old man with late syphilis shows diffuse lytic and sclerotic changes in the shaft consistent with chronic osteomyelitis. (*Courtesy of* J.T. Mader, MD.)

NEUROSYPHILIS

Clinical comparison of early and late neurosyphilis

Late neurosyphilis	Early neurosyphilis
Predominant form	Perhaps 2% of all neurosyphilis in the prepenicillin era
Onset 5–40 yrs after infection, usually 17–25 yrs	Onset in first year after infection, usually after incomplete course of therapy
Ectodermal structures, specifically neuronal tissue	Mesodermal structures—meninges, vessels
Tabes dorsalis, paresis, dementia, death	Meningitis, cranial nerve abnormalities, cerebrovascular accidents

FIGURE 10-9 Clinical comparison of early and late neurosyphilis. Treponemes invade the central nervous system in the early stages of syphilis in at least 40% of cases and can be found in the cerebrospinal fluid of one quarter of patients with secondary syphilis. In the absence of treatment, neurologic disease usually appears an average of 20 years (usual range, 12–40 yrs) after initial infection with *Treponema pallidum*. This form of late neurosyphilis involves neuronal tissue (ectodermal structures) and causes a range of syndromes, including tabes dorsalis, paresis, dementia, and death. Cerebrovascular accidents may also occur. In a tiny proportion of cases (80/4500 in one series), an early form of neurosyphilis occurs. The onset is in the first year of infection, usually following an adequate course of treatment for early syphilis. Mesodermal structures, such as the meninges and blood vessels, are involved, and the principal findings are meningitis, cranial nerve abnormalities, and cerebrovascular accidents. (Chesney AM, Kemp JE: Incidence of *Spirochaeta pallida* in cerebrospinal fluid during early stage of syphilis. *JAMA* 1924, 83:1725–1728. Lukehart SA, Hook EW III, Baker-Zander SA, *et al.*: Invasion of the central nervous system by *Treponema pallidum*: Implications for diagnosis and treatment. *Ann Intern Med* 1988, 109:855–862. Stokes JH: *Modern Clinical Syphilology: Diagnosis–Treatment–Case Study.* Philadelphia: W.B. Saunders; 1934. Adams RD, Solomon HC: *Neurosyphilis.* Oxford, UK: Oxford University Press; 1946.)

Clinical manifestations of late neurosyphilis

Meningovascular
  Hemiplegia or hemiparesis
  Seizures
    Generalized
    Focal
  Aphasia
Parenchymatous
  General paresis
    Changes in personality, affect, sensorium, intellect, insight, judgment
    Hyperactive reflexes
    Speech disturbances (slurring)
    Pupillary disturbances (Argyll Robertson pupils)
    Optic atrophy tremors (face, tongue, hands, legs)
  Tabes dorsalis
    Shooting or lightning pains
    Ataxia
    Pupillary disturbances (Argyll Robertson pupils)
    Impotence
    Bladder disturbances
    Fecal incontinence
    Peripheral neuropathy
    Romberg sign
    Cranial nerve involvement (II–VII)

FIGURE 10-10 Clinical manifestations of late neurosyphilis. Late symptomatic neurosyphilis is divided into two major clinical categories that have been correlated with pathologic findings, although a great deal of overlap occurs between these groups in individual patients. Meningovascular neurosyphilis, which is an inflammatory process, refers to the development of typical endarteritis obliterans affecting the small blood vessels of the meninges, brain, and spinal cord and leading to multiple small areas of infarction; resultant disorders range from hemiplegia to progressive neurologic deficits due to gradual destruction of nerve tissue by small-vessel endarteritis. Parenchymatous neurosyphilis, which includes tabes dorsalis and general paresis, is a degenerative condition that involves the actual destruction of nerve cells, principally in the cerebral cortex, and results in a combination of psychiatric and neurologic manifestations. (*From* Tramont EC: *Treponema pallidum* (syphilis). *In* Mandell GL, Bennett JE, Dolin R (eds.). *Principles and Practice of Infectious Diseases*, 4th ed. New York: Churchill Livingstone; 1995:2124; with permission.)

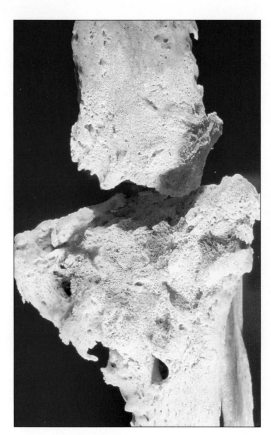

FIGURE 10-11 Damaged knee joint in tabes dorsalis. In tabes dorsalis, the posterior columns of the spinal cord are involved, and the major sensory loss affects proprioception. During walking, the loss of appropriate neurologic feedback that would modify the placement of the feet results in extensive trauma to the joints of the legs and feet, as seen in this damaged knee joint at autopsy. (*Courtesy of* J.A. Tschen, MD.)

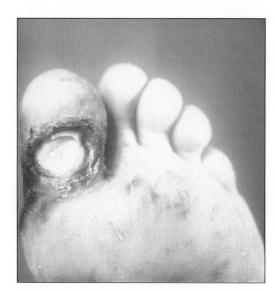

FIGURE 10-12 Trophic ulcer of the foot due to tabes dorsalis. Tabes dorsalis refers to demyelination of the posterior columns of the spinal cord, dorsal roots, and dorsal root ganglia usually seen 20 to 25 years after the initial syphilitic infection. In advanced stages, loss of vibratory, positional, and temperature sensation may develop. Traumatic ulceration of the lower extremities may subsequently develop. (*Courtesy of* the Centers for Disease Control and Prevention.)

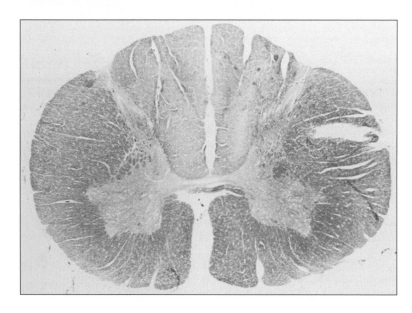

FIGURE 10-13 Spinal cord section demonstrating degeneration of the posterior columns of spinal cord in tabes dorsalis. Tabes dorsalis is characterized by degeneration of the posterior columns of the spinal cord, dorsal root ganglia, and dorsal roots. (Myelin stain.) (*From* Farrar WE, Wood MJ, Innes JA, Tubbs H: *Infectious Diseases: Text and Color Atlas*, 2nd ed. London: Gower Medical Publishing, an imprint of Times Mirror Int Publ Ltd; 1992; with permission.)

Neurosyphilis and HIV Infection

Early neurosyphilis in HIV infection

May be presenting symptom/sign of HIV infection

May appear when CD4 cell count is only modestly reduced

Likely to occur in patients who have received a recommended course of benzathine penicillin in last 3–12 mos

Progresses from asymptomatic to symptomatic meningitis to cranial nerve abnormalities to cerebrovascular accident in the absence of treatment

FIGURE 10-14 Early neurosyphilis in HIV infection. In the prepenicillin era, if therapy was not given for a significant length of time or as a significant dose, the patient would present with an early form of neurosyphilis called *neurorecurrence.* An analogy may be drawn between the use of relatively poor antimicrobial therapy (*eg,* neoarsphenamine plus bismuth) in presumably normal hosts as happened in the past and the use of excellent antimicrobial therapy (penicillin) in immunologically compromised hosts during the AIDS era. Prevention of central nervous system disease seems to require both excellent therapy and intact host defenses. (Stokes JH, Beerman H, Ingraham NR: *Modern Clinical Syphilology,* 3rd ed. Philadelphia: W.B. Saunders; 1944:617–618.)

Presenting manifestations in 42 reported cases of neurosyphilis in HIV infection	
Manifestation	**Cases, _n_**
Asymptomatic meningitis	5
Abnormal CSF	
CSF VDRL, reactive serum RPR	
Meningitis	9
CN abnormalities	15
Retinitis (CN II), auditory and/or vestibular disease (CN VII), facial palsy (CN VII or V)	
Stroke	11
Polyradiculopathy	1
General paresis	1

CN—cranial nerve; CSF—cerebrospinal fluid; RPR—rapid plasma reagin; VDRL—Veneral Disease Research Laboratory.

FIGURE 10-15 Presenting manifestations of neurosyphilis in HIV infection. *Treponema pallidum* is clearly not eradicated during latency in HIV-infected persons and, in fact, persists after seemingly successful antimicrobial therapy. For example, *T. pallidum* can be isolated from lymph nodes of persons with latent infection or those who appear to be cured by treatment with neoarsphenamine or penicillin; organisms can also be found in rabbits that have received enormous doses of penicillin after experimental infection. Because late neurosyphilis appears in < 10% of persons who were not treated for syphilis, in only 1% to 2% of those who were treated with neoarsphenamine, and virtually never in patients after treatment with penicillin, one might presume that the host plays an ongoing role in keeping the infection suppressed. Cases of early neurosyphilis reported in the medical literature in the 1980s fell into the categories described in this figure. Of the 42 patients in this study, several patients who presented with frank meningitis also had cranial nerve abnormalities, and many of those presenting with cranial nerve abnormalities also had an abnormal cerebrospinal fluid examination indicating meningitis; there is overlap between these categories. (Musher DM, Hamill RJ, Baughn RE: Impact of human immunodeficiency virus (HIV) infection on the course of syphilis and the response to treatment. *Ann Intern Med* 1990, 113:872–881.)

Cerebrospinal fluid abnormalities in early neurosyphilis in HIV-infected persons			
CSF parameter	**% Abnormal**	**Median value**	**Range**
Leukocytes*	85	173/mm^3	8–2000
Protein	85	125 mg/µL	46–1000
Glucose	35	37 mg/µL	11–42
VDRL	80	1:4	WR–1:16

*Majority of leukocytes are usually lymphocytes.
CSF—cerebrospinal fluid; VDRL—Veneral Disease Research Laboratory; WR—weakly reactive.

FIGURE 10-16 Cerebrospinal fluid (CSF) abnormalities in early neurosyphilis in patients with HIV infection. As these data show, CSF abnormalities are not distinctive in neurosyphilis. In fact, the Venereal Disease Research Laboratory (VDRL) test may be nonreactive in a seemingly proven case. (Note that the rapid plasma reagin test is done only on serum; VDRL is the nontreponemal test performed on CSF.) This set of findings is not different from those made in non–HIV-infected persons in the preantibiotic era.

Response to treatment of syphilis in HIV-infected patients		
	Ceftriaxone (_n_=44)	**Penicillin** (_n_=13)
Stage of syphilis		
Proven latent	6	0
Presumed latent	30	13
Neurosyphilis	8	0
Response		
Response	29(66%)	8(62%)
Serofast	5(11%)	1(8%)
Relapse	9(20%)	2(15%)
Failure	1(2%)	2(15%)

FIGURE 10-17 Response to treatment of syphilis in HIV-infected persons. Persons without active lesions of syphilis or neurologic symptoms who have a reactive rapid plasma reagin and microhemagglutination assay for *Treponema pallidum* and who submit to lumbar puncture may be proven to have neurosyphilis by cerebrospinal fluid (CSF) abnormalities, including a positive Venereal Disease Research Laboratory test, or may be judged to have latent syphilis based on an entirely normal CSF. Such distinctions are never absolute, because even in the preantibiotic era, one might have had neurosyphilis with an entirely normal CSF. If a lumbar puncture is not done, the patient is presumed to have late latent syphilis. As shown in this figure, Dowell and colleagues treated HIV-infected patients with intravenous ceftriaxone, 1 or 2 g daily for 10 to 14 days (no differences were detected among the dosing schedules) and found a substantial number of failures. A more recent, prospective study by Gordon and colleagues found similar results in 11 patients treated with 18 to 24 MU of intravenous penicillin daily. These results illustrate that 1) the principal problem with the response of neurosyphilis to therapy in HIV-infected patients is the host, not the antibiotic schedule, and 2) there is no antibiotic regimen to definitively treat this condition. (Dowell ME, Ross PG, Musher DM, *et al.*: Response of latent syphilis or neurosyphilis to ceftriaxone therapy in persons infected with human immunodeficiency virus. *Am J Med* 1992, 93:481–488. Gordon SM, Eaton ME, George R, *et al.*: The response of symptomatic neurosyphilis to high-dose intravenous penicillin G in patients with human immunodeficiency virus infection. *N Engl J Med* 994, 331:1469–1473.)

Therapy for Neurosyphilis

CDC-recommended treatment of neurosyphilis

Not HIV-infected	
Procaine penicillin G	1.2 MU/d im × 10 days
or	
Benzathine penicillin G	2.4 MU/wk im × 3 doses total
HIV-infected	
Procaine penicillin G	1.2 MU/d im × 10 days
or	
Ceftriaxone	1–2 g/d iv × 10–14 days
or	
Aqueous crystalline penicillin G	18–24 MU/d iv × 10–14 days

im—intramuscularly; iv—intravenously.

FIGURE 10-18 Centers for Disease Control and Prevention (CDC)–recommended treatment of neurosyphilis. The clinician should be warned that the response of HIV-infected patients to therapy for latent or tertiary syphilis is uncertain, with a substantial rate of relapse or failure. The treatment of neurosyphilis in any patient is controversial, and data are lacking. The CDC recommends aqueous crystalline penicillin G, 18 to 24 MU intravenously daily, or procaine penicillin G, 2.4 MU intramuscularly daily (plus probenecid, 500 mg orally four times daily) for the treatment of neurosyphilis in HIV-infected persons. One must closely monitor patients with neurosyphilis after treatment, and the appearance of headache or cranial nerve abnormalities may indicate the reappearance of neurosyphilis. Serum nontreponemal tests should be repeated at specified intervals. If cerebrospinal fluid (CSF) pleocytosis was initially present, the CSF should be reexamined every 6 months until the abnormality resolves. If the CSF cell count is not entirely normal by 2 years after treatment, retreatment should be strongly considered. (Centers for Disease Control and Prevention: 1993 Sexually transmitted disease treatment guidelines. *MMWR* 1993, 42(RR-14):36–37.)

CARDIOVASCULAR SYPHILIS

Principal cardiovascular manifestations of late syphilis

Asymptomatic aortitis
Aortic insufficiency
Coronary ostial stenosis
Aortic aneurysm
Gummatous myocarditis

FIGURE 10-19 Principal cardiovascular manifestations of late syphilis. Infection with *Treponema pallidum* affects the heart and great vessels in several ways. Organisms are thought to disseminate to these sites early in infection, but clinically apparent damage does not occur for 20 or more years. Aortic insufficiency occurs in about 20% of patients with syphilitic aortitis, and coronary ostial stenosis is seen in about 25% of such patients. Aortic aneurysm produces symptoms in about 5% to 10% of patients with aortitis. The formation of syphilitic gummas in the heart is extremely rare. (Clark EG, Danbolt N: The Oslo study of the natural history of untreated syphilis. *J Chron Dis* 1955, 2:311–344. Heggtveit HA: Syphilitic aortitis: A clinicopathologic autopsy study of 100 cases, 1950–1960. *Circulation* 1964, 19:346–355.)

Major clinical manifestations of cardiovascular syphilis in 100 patients at autopsy

Postmortem diagnosis	Asymptomatic	Precordial pain	Congestive heart failure	Systolic murmur	Diastolic murmur
Aortitis	30%	19%	44%	36%	0%
Aneurysm	4%	48%	52%	57%	9%
Aortic insufficiency	0%	33%	83%	83%	33%
Ostial stenosis	9%	45%	64%	73%	0%

FIGURE 10-20 Major clinical manifestations of cardiovascular syphilis in 100 patients at autopsy. Results of a retrospective chart review of patients autopsied at King County Hospital (Seattle, Washington) in the 1950s show the subtlety of presentation in patients with severe cardiovascular disease. Even in those patients found to have aortic insufficiency at autopsy, a diastolic murmur had been recognized in life in only 33%. Stenosis of the ostia of the coronary arteries was significantly associated with anginal symptoms. (Heggtveit HA: Syphilitic aortitis: A clinicopathologic autopsy study of 100 cases, 1950–1960. *Circulation* 1964, 19:346–355.)

Aortic Involvement

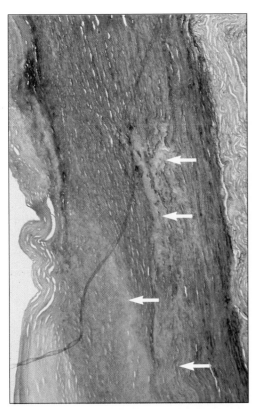

FIGURE 10-21 Histologic features of syphilitic aortitis. *Treponema pallidum* spreads to the vasa vasorum early in the disease and produces an obliterative endarteritis of these nutrient vessels. There is subsequent medial necrosis with destruction of elastic tissue and scarring. In this figure, a decrease in the total amount of elastin fibers (stained brown), some of which are fragmented, and areas of scar formation (*arrows*) can be seen. This kind of weakening of the aorta predisposes to aneurysmal dilatation. (Elastin stain; original magnification, × 100.)

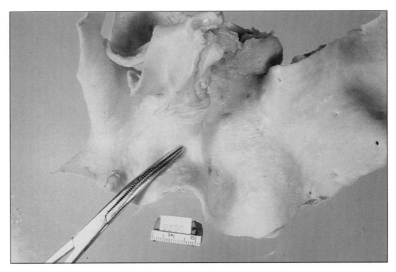

FIGURE 10-22 Gross pathologic specimen showing syphilitic aortitis. Scarring of the media produces wrinkling of the intima, which appears grossly as cross-striations, seen here to the right of the hemostat tip. It has been said that "treatment, with healing sclerosis," may actually exaggerate the process. Atherosclerotic plaques may overlie syphilitic aortitis, and the combination of processes distorts the intima, giving rise to a tree-bark appearance. (Stokes JH, Beerman H, Ingraham NR: *Modern Clinical Syphilology*, 3rd ed. Philadelphia: W.B. Saunders; 1944:901.)

FIGURE 10-23 Sites of involvement of syphilitic aortic aneurysms. The overall distribution of syphilitic aneurysms differs distinctly from that associated with atherosclerotic aneurysms, the great majority of which occur distal to the renal arteries. The distribution of syphilitic aneurysms is thought to occur because of the greater number of vasa vasorum in the ascending aorta. In syphilitic aortic aneurysms, more than one site may be involved in a given patient. For example, both the ascending and transverse arches of the aorta are involved in 8% of autopsy cases, and the entire arch is involved in 6%. (Heggtveit HA: Syphilitic aortitis: A clinicopathologic autopsy study of 100 cases, 1950–1960. *Circulation* 1964, 19:346–355.)

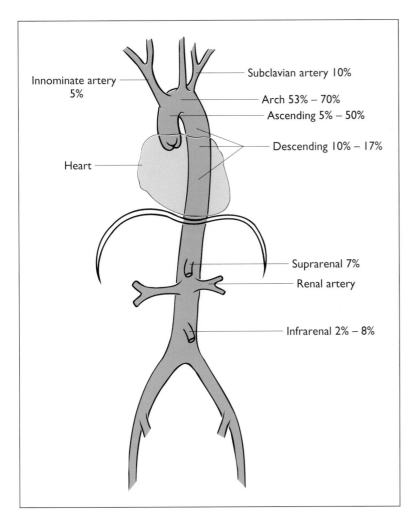

Innominate artery 5%

Subclavian artery 10%

Arch 53% – 70%

Ascending 5% – 50%

Descending 10% – 17%

Heart

Suprarenal 7%

Renal artery

Infrarenal 2% – 8%

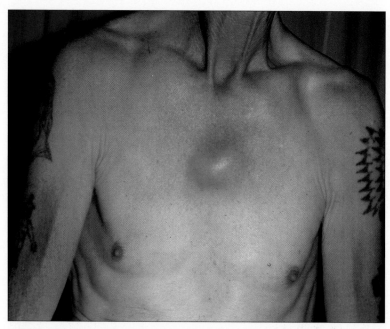

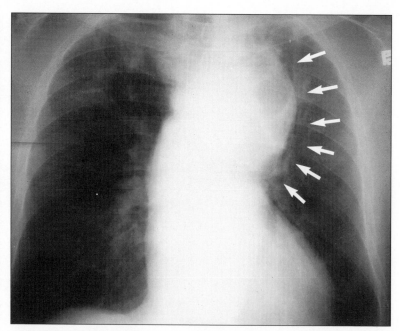

FIGURE 10-24 Syphilitic aneurysm of the ascending aorta eroding through the sternum. In the preantibiotic era, cardiovascular syphilis was two to four times more common in men than in women. Syphilitic aneurysm usually involves the proximal ascending aorta and rarely dissects, probably because the scarring that results from the infectious process may serve to strengthen the aorta near the aneurysm. When symptoms occur, they usually result from direct pressure of the aneurysm on adjacent structures. Most cases of cardiovascular syphilis are asymptomatic. Thus, although autopsy studies from the early 1900s found cardiovascular involvement in 70% to 97% of syphilitics, the diagnosis was made during life in only 16% to 40% of patients from the same period. Syphilitic aortic aneurysms may, however, rupture with dramatic catastrophic results. (Stokes JH, Beerman H, Ingraham NR: *Modern Clinical Syphilology*, 3rd ed. Philadelphia: W.B. Saunders, 1944:896.) (*Courtesy of* the Department of Dermatology, University of Virginia.)

FIGURE 10-25 Admission chest radiograph showing a large aneurysm of the ascending aorta. A 54-year-old man presented with substernal chest pain on exertion that radiated down his left arm. His rapid plasma reagin titer was 1:8, and his fluorescent treponemal antibody absorbed test was reactive. He gave a history of a generalized rash some 30 years previously but denied having genital lesions. He had a grade II/VI diastolic decrescendo murmur at the left sternal border, and the electrocardiogram suggested ischemia. The chest radiograph revealed a large aneurysm of the ascending aorta (*arrows*).

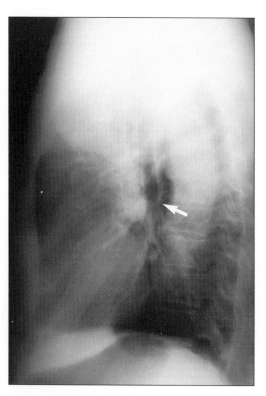

FIGURE 10-26 Lateral chest radiograph showing the ascending aortic aneurysm as an upper lobe density. In the same patient as seen in Fig. 10-25, some fine, "eggshell" calcification is seen within the descending aorta (*arrow*); this finding is observed in 20% of cases of syphilitic aortitis as well as in atherosclerotic disease. Observing linear calcification in the *ascending* aorta should raise the question of syphilitic aortitis, because in the absence of syphilis, such calcifications are rare in that location (although they may be seen in severe atherosclerotic disease). (MacFarlane WV, Swan WGA, Irvine RE: Cardiovascular disease in syphilis: A review of 1330 patients. *BMJ* 1956, 1:827–832. Higgins CB, Reinke RT: Nonsyphilitic etiology of linear calcification of the ascending aorta. *Radiology* 1974, 113:609–613.)

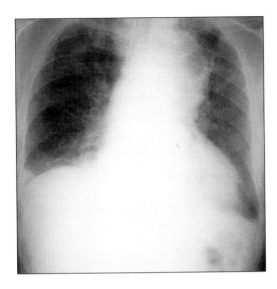

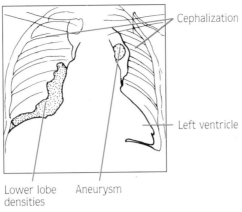

FIGURE 10-27 Follow-up chest radiograph showing stable aneurysm but progression of other cardiovascular disease. The patient (*see* Figs. 10-25 and 10-26) was managed conservatively for his cardiac disease. Cerebrospinal fluid was completely normal, and the Venereal Disease Research Laboratory test was nonreactive. He was treated with benzathine penicillin G, 2.4 MU intramuscularly, administered weekly for a total of three doses. He returned 6 years later complaining of dyspnea on exertion and two-pillow orthopnea. The electrocardiogram now revealed evidence of left ventricular hypertrophy. A chest radiograph at that time revealed an increase in left ventricular size, lower lobe densities consistent with congestive heart failure, and cephalization. The aneurysm had not changed.

Aortic Valvular Disease

Causes of syphilitic aortic insufficiency in cardiovascular syphilis	
Widened aortic valve ring	28%
Distorted aortic valve leaflets	41%
Both	31%

FIGURE 10-28 Causes of aortic insufficiency in cardiovascular syphilis. Aortic insufficiency is common in cardiovascular syphilis, and the finding of a typical murmur was the common mode of detecting this disease in the preantibiotic era. Aortic insufficiency is caused by distortion of the aortic valves, with thickening and curling of the leaflets, which prevents their closure. The process of medial necrosis and weakening may also involve the valve ring, resulting in dilation, further inhibiting apposition of the leaflets. A review of adequate autopsy material on 40 of 100 patients with syphilitic aortitis at King County Hospital (Seattle, Washington) revealed that the two processes were equally important and often occurred together. Interestingly, only 23 of 100 cases had a documented prior history of syphilis. (Heggtveit HA: Syphilitic aortitis: A clinicopathologic autopsy study of 100 cases, 1950–1960. *Circulation* 1964, 19:346–355.)

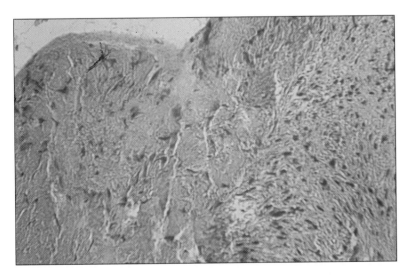

FIGURE 10-29 Histologic specimen showing syphilitic involvement of the aortic valve. The aortic valve leaflets are often involved in the syphilitic process, with thickening and rolling of the cusps. This process leads to aortic insufficiency. In this figure, edema of the leaflet, evidenced by separation of the nuclei, and scarring in the center of the specimen can be seen. Widening of the aortic valve ring also contributes to aortic insufficiency. (Hematoxylin-eosin stain; original magnification, × 400.)

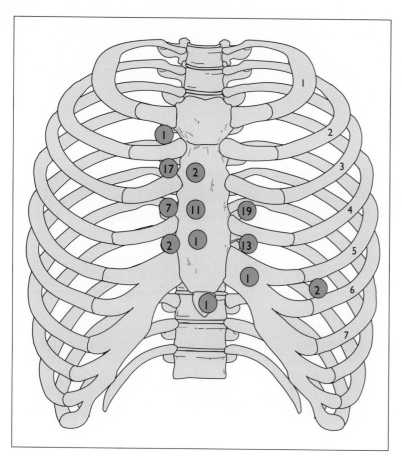

FIGURE 10-30 Auscultation of aortic insufficiency murmur in cardiovascular syphilis. In most forms of aortic valvular disease, the point of maximum intensity of the aortic insufficiency murmur is usually along the left sternal border, particularly in the third and fourth intercostal spaces. Distortion of the aortic root by the syphilitic process may favor a murmur heard loudest along the right sternal border. In a study by Harvey and colleagues, a predominantly right-sided murmur was observed in 58 of 801 cases (7.2%) of aortic insufficiency of any etiology, and syphilitic aortitis was diagnosed in 27 of these 58 cases (47%). In this same study, however, the murmur of syphilitic aortic insufficiency was heard loudest at the left sternal border in 33 of 77 (42.9%) cases. The *circled numbers* indicate those cases of cardiovascular syphilis in which the point of maximal intensity occurred at each location. (Harvey WP, Corrado MA, Perloff JV: Right-sided murmurs of aortic insufficiency (diastolic murmurs better heard to the right of the sternum rather than the left). *Am J Med Sci* 1963, 245:533–542.)

Other Manifestations of Cardiovascular Syphilis

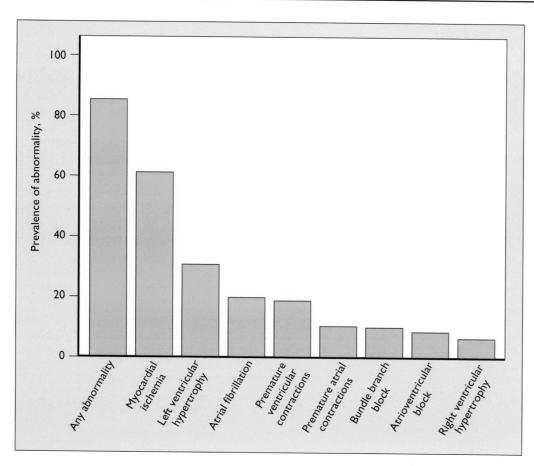

FIGURE 10-31 Prevalence of electrocardiographic abnormalities in cardiovascular syphilis. As shown in this autopsy series, electrocardiographic abnormalities are common in severe cardiovascular syphilis. Ischemia most likely results from inflammatory occlusion of the coronary ostia and decreased coronary perfusion during diastole. Some of the conduction disturbances may result from syphilitic myocarditis. Treponemal invasion of the myocardium is uncommon, but scarring from ischemia was found in 10% to 25% of patients with cardiovascular syphilis. Rarely, gummas may be seen in heart muscle. (Heggtveit HA: Syphilitic aortitis: A clinicopathologic autopsy study of 100 cases, 1950–1960. *Circulation* 1964, 19:346–355. Stokes JH, Beerman H, Ingraham NR: *Modern Clinical Syphilology*, 3rd ed. Philadelphia: W.B. Saunders; 1944:903.)

Prognosis in Cardiovascular Syphilis

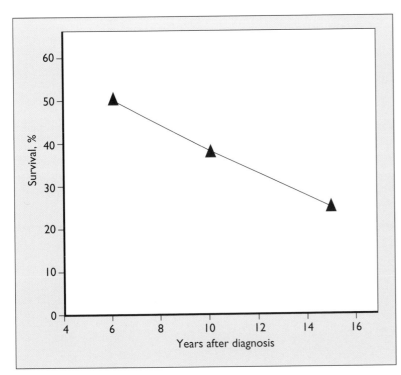

Five-year survival in cardiovascular syphilis	
Always asymptomatic	80%
Asymptomatic at diagnosis	72%
Symptomatic now	45%
Congestive cardiomyopathy	
None ever	78%
None at diagnosis	50%
Present now	15%

FIGURE 10-33 Five-year survival rates in cardiovascular syphilis. Although the medical management of coronary artery disease and congestive heart failure has improved dramatically during the past several decades, cardiovascular syphilis remains a lethal complication of the infection. In an older study by Webster and colleagues, the 5-year survival was predicted on the basis of clinical presentation. The onset of any symptoms after the diagnosis, particularly of congestive cardiomyopathy, was a bad prognostic sign. Antimicrobial therapy is given to arrest disease progression but may not reverse already existing pathology. (Webster B, Rich C Jr, Densen PM, *et al.*: Studies in cardiovascular syphilis: III. The natural history of syphilitic aortic insufficiency. *Am Heart J* 1953, 46:117–145. St John RK: Treatment of cardiovascular syphilis. *J Am Vener Dis Assoc* 1976, 3:148–152.)

FIGURE 10-32 Prognosis in cardiovascular syphilis (during the 1940s). Crude survival rates in cardiovascular syphilis prior to 1950 are shown. Data compiled in the early 1950s indicate the poor prognosis of the disease. Survival is only about 50% by 6 years after diagnosis, and thereafter it appears to decrease linearly with time. It is unclear if penicillin therapy has had much effect on the survival of patients with established cardiovascular syphilis. (Webster B, Rich C Jr, Densen PM, *et al.*: Studies in cardiovascular syphilis: III. The natural history of syphilitic aortic insufficiency. *Am Heart J* 1953, 346:117–145.)

TREATMENT OF LATE BENIGN AND CARDIOVASCULAR SYPHILIS

Treatment of late syphilis (excluding neurosyphilis)	
Recommended regimen	
Benzathine penicillin G	7.2 MU total, given as 3 doses of 2.4 MU intramuscularly, at 1-wk intervals
Penicillin-allergic patients (nonpregnant)	
Doxycycline	100 mg orally 2 times a day × 4 wks
or	
Tetracycline	500 mg orally 4 times a day × 4 wks

FIGURE 10-34 Treatment of late syphilis (excluding neurosyphilis). The term *late* or *tertiary syphilis* refers to patients with gumma and/or cardiovascular syphilis but without neurosyphilis. Patients with symptomatic late syphilis should undergo examination of the cerebrospinal fluid, because the presence of coincident neurosyphilis would dramatically alter the therapeutic approach. Penicillin-allergic pregnant patients represent a special case and should be managed in consultation with an expert. The efficacy of the cephalosporins in this setting is undefined but is probably high. Late benign syphilis usually responds dramatically to therapy. (Centers for Disease Control and Prevention: 1993 Sexually transmitted diseases treatment guidelines. *MMWR* 1993, 42(RR–14):34–35.)

SELECTED BIBLIOGRAPHY

Gjestland T: The Oslo study of untreated syphilis. *Acta Derm Venereol* 1955, 35(suppl 34):1–368.

Jackman JD, Radolf JD: Cardiovascular syphilis. *Am J Med* 1989, 87:425–433.

Musher DM: Syphilis. *In* Gorbach SL, Bartlett JG, Blacklow NR (eds.): *Infectious Diseases*. Philadelphia: W.B. Saunders; 1992:822–828.

Musher DM, Hamill RJ, Baughn RE: Impact of human immunodeficiency virus (HIV) infection on the course of syphilis and the response to treatment. *Ann Intern Med* 1990, 113:872–881.

Rolfs RT: Treatment of syphilis, 1993. *Clin Infect Dis* 1995, 20(suppl 1):523–538.

CHAPTER 11

Congenital Syphilis

Laura T. Gutman

EPIDEMIOLOGY

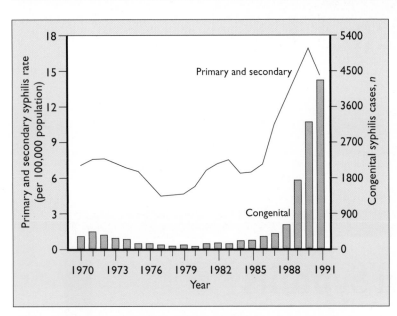

FIGURE **11-1** Incidence of primary, secondary, and congenital syphilis between 1970 and 1991. Approximately one case of congenital syphilis occurs for every 80 cases of primary or secondary syphilis in women of child-bearing age. There has been an increase in cases of congenital syphilis accompanying the current epidemic of early syphilis in adults. (*Courtesy of* the Centers for Disease Control and Prevention.)

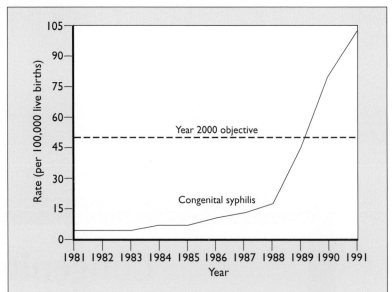

FIGURE **11-2** Incidence of congenital syphilis per 100,000 live births between 1981 and 1991. The rates of congenital syphilis have increased rapidly since 1988. Although some proportion of the increase is due to changes in the case definition of congenital syphilis from the Centers for Disease Control and Prevention, most of the increase is due to increased exposure and disease. (*Courtesy of* the Centers for Disease Control and Prevention.)

Maternal factors associated with increased rates of early syphilis in pregnant women

---

HIV infection
Adolescent or unmarried mother
History of sexually transmitted diseases
Drug use, especially cocaine
Inadequate prenatal care
Prostitution or promiscuity
Specific populations or geographic areas
Treatment of gonorrhea with ciprofloxacin or spectinomycin

FIGURE **11-3** Maternal factors associated with increased rates of early syphilis in pregnant women. The increases in case rates of congenital syphilis can be attributed in large part to the rising incidence of other sexually transmitted diseases, drug use, sex-for-drugs prostitution, early initiation of unprotected and high-risk sex among adolescents, and the failure of public health programs in major cities. (Webber MP, Lambert G, Bateman DA, Hauser WA: Maternal risk factors for congenital syphilis: A case control study. *Am J Epidemiol* 1993, 137:415–432.)

Prenatal care and the occurrence of congenital syphilis in infants		
	Study	
	Mascola 1984 (*n*=50)	**Coles 1995 (*n*=318)**
No prenatal care	56%	46%
First prenatal test negative; testing not repeated in late pregnancy	6%	14%
Medical mismanagement	6%	10%
Failure of conventional prenatal syphilis therapy of mother	8%	5%
Negative maternal syphilis test at delivery	14%	—
Infection late in pregnancy or no prenatal care until late in pregnancy	—	20%
Mother not tested	8%	3%
Laboratory error	2%	—

FIGURE 11-4 Prenatal care as a factor contributing to the occurrence of congenital syphilis in infants of infected women. The identified circumstances surrounding the development of congenital syphilis in two groups of women are listed. The study by Mascola and colleagues was published in 1984 and comprised women in Texas, whereas the study by Coles and colleagues was published in 1995 and comprised women in New York State. In both studies, lack of prenatal care was the primary factor that has inhibited recognition and treatment of infected women. In addition, serologic testing for syphilis must be performed during both early gestation and late gestation and, if the mother is at high risk, at delivery. The results must be made known to the infant's clinicians. Women who acquire syphilis near the time of delivery may not have developed measurable antibody to *Treponema pallidum* at the time of testing. Only careful epidemiologic tracing of case contacts (partners of infected women) allows such circumstances to be recognized. In both studies, infected infants were born to mothers who had developed syphilis late in pregnancy and who had received appropriate therapy more than 1 month prior to delivery. Studies are currently being undertaken to determine which infants born to mothers who were infected and treated late in pregnancy will nonetheless fail therapy. (Mascola L, Pelosi R, Blount JH, *et al.*: Congenital syphilis: Why is it still occurring? *JAMA* 1984, 252:1719–1722. Coles FB, Hipp SS, Silberstein GS, Chen J-H: Congenital syphilis surveillance in upstate New York, 1989–1992: Implications for prevention and clinical management. *J Infect Dis* 1995, 171:732–735.)

SEROLOGIC TESTING AND CASE RECOGNITION

1993 Sexually transmitted diseases treatment guidelines
"No infant should leave the hospital without the serologic status of the infant's mother having been documented at least once during pregnancy. Serologic testing also should be performed at delivery in communities and populations at risk for congenital syphilis."

Comparison of clinical specimens for serologic screening for congenital syphilis at delivery	
3306 Liveborn newborns, Bronx, 1990	
73 (2.2%) had positive sera:	
Maternal sera positive	68/72 (94%)
Neonatal venopuncture sera positive	43/68 (63%)
Cord sera positive	30/60 (50%)

FIGURE 11-5 Testing guidelines for sexually transmitted diseases. A statement of recommendations regarding the prevention of congenital syphilis is highlighted from the 1993 Sexually transmitted diseases treatment guidelines of the Centers for Disease Control and Prevention. Implementation of this policy is an extremely important component of the efforts to recognize and treat exposed infants. This aspect of the prevention of syphilis is the one most likely to be controlled by individual clinicians, especially pediatricians and obstetricians. Each clinician who is responsible for the welfare of delivering mothers and newborns should ensure that his or her institution is implementing or making provisions to begin implementing this policy. Early and very early discharge from the hospital after delivery represents a challenge to the successful maintenance of this policy, and it may require that clinicians advocate for the needs of their patients. (Centers for Disease Control and Prevention:1993 Sexually transmitted diseases treatment guidelines. *MMWR* 1993, 42(RR-14):1–102.)

FIGURE 11-6 Comparison of clinical specimens for serologic screening for congenital syphilis at delivery. The single specimen that most accurately identifies an infant who is at risk of congenital syphilis is maternal serum taken at delivery. Cord blood, which represents baby blood, is accepted in many states and hospitals for screening for congenital syphilis but is a much less accurate reflection of maternal infection than is maternal serum. It may fail to reflect the maternal infection, in part because passive transfer of antibody to the infant is marginal or because the mother's titer is relatively low. In addition, cord blood may also be contaminated with the gelatinous extracellular material found in the umbilical cord (Wharton's jelly), leading to technical errors during the assay. (Chabra RS, Brion LP, Castro M, *et al.*: Comparison of maternal sera, cord blood and neonatal sera for detecting presumptive congenital syphilis: Relationship with maternal treatment. *Pediatrics* 1993, 91:88–91.)

Serologic tests for syphilis

VDRL (Venereal Disease Research Laboratory) and RPR (rapid plasma reagin)
  Titers rise and fall with disease state
  May be falsely-positive in other diseases
  Inexpensive and easy to perform

MHA-TP (microhemagglutination assay–*Treponema pallidum*)
  Can be quantified
  Positive for life after infection
  Sensitive and specific

FTA-ABS (fluorescent treponemal antibody absorption)
  Quantification inaccurate
  Positive for life after infection
  Most sensitive and specific
  Expensive and difficult

FIGURE 11-7 Serologic tests for syphilis. The Venereal Disease Research Laboratory (VDRL) and rapid plasma reagin (RPR) tests are used in screening and to follow the course of therapy, because titers they measure rise and fall with the clinical condition and most patients serorevert following successful therapy. In contrast, the treponemal tests—fluorescent treponemal antibody absorption (FTA-ABS) and microhemagglutination assay for antibodies to *Treponema pallidum* (MHA-TP)—are used to confirm an initial diagnosis but provide scant information about the adequacy of therapy or reinfection. The VDRL test is the only test suitable for detecting central nervous system syphilis. (*See also* Chapter 8.)

A. Rationale for development of antitreponemal IgM antibody assays

Biologic justification for developing assays:
  IgG crosses the placenta. Tests assaying IgG antibody (VDRL, FTA-ABS, most others) cannot distinguish between passively transferred maternal antibody and infant antibody.
  IgM does not cross placenta. IgM found in infant blood was produced by the infant.
  IgM may be produced by infants as early as the 3rd month of gestation.

Situations causing false-negative results in antitreponemal IgM assays:
  Infant infected very late in pregnancy, and IgM antibody not yet produced.
  Maternal IgG antibody may competitively extinguish IgM test.
  Infant may produce IgM antibody against maternal IgG.

FTA-ABS—fluorescent treponemal antibody absorption; VDRL—Venereal Disease Research Laboratory.

B. Investigational assays for IgM antibody in diagnosis of congenital syphilis

Assay	Results in symptomatic infants	Results in asymptomatic infants at high risk of syphilis
IgM capture ELISA	17/19 (90%)	16/18 (80%)
FTA-ABS 19S IgM	14/18 (77%)	13/18 (73%)
IgM Western immunoblot	5/6 (83%)	28/36 (78%)

ELISA—enzyme-linked immunosorbent assay; FTA-ABS—fluorescent treponemal antibody absorption.

FIGURE 11-8 Assays for antitreponemal IgM antibody. **A,** Rationale for development of antitreponemal IgM antibody assays. Considerable efforts have gone into finding alternative means to diagnose congenital syphilis that improve on the rates possible by assaying antitreponemal IgG antibody. All assays for antitreponemal IgM antibody are, at this time, investigational or provisional and not approved for use in the diagnosis of disease. There have been a variety of reasons for difficulties in developing these IgM antibody assays. It should be noted that passively transferred antibody will slowly decline and should usually be absent from the noninfected infant by about 3 to 4 months after birth. **B,** Results of investigational assays for IgM antibody in diagnosis of congenital syphilis. The results of three investigational studies in the application of antitreponemal IgM antibody assays to the evaluation of infants with confirmed and presumed congenital syphilis are summarized. The major failure of these assays is falsely negative results. Because of this shortcoming, it is not yet possible to distinguish exposed infants who are in a serologically prereactive phase of disease from exposed infants who are truly noninfected. Thus, it is recommended that all exposed infants with presumed congenital syphilis should be treated. (Bromberg K, Rawstron S, Tannis G: Diagnosis of congenital syphilis by combining *Treponema pallidum*–specific IgM detection with immunofluorescent antigen detection for *T. pallidum. J Infect Dis* 1993, 168:238–242. Meyer MP, Eddy T, Baughn RE: Analysis of Western blotting (immunoblotting) technique in diagnosis of congenital syphilis. *J Clin Microbiol* 1994, 32:629–633. Schmitz JL, Gortis KS, Mauney C, *et al.*: Laboratory diagnosis of congenital syphilis by immunoglobulin M (IgM) and IgA immunoblotting. *Clin Diag Lab Immunol* 1994, 1:32–37. Stoll BJ, Lee FK, Larsen S, *et al.*: Clinical and serologic evaluation of neonates for congenital syphilis: A continuing diagnostic dilemma. *J Infect Dis* 1993, 167:1093–1099.)

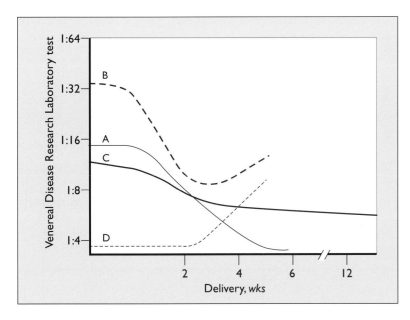

FIGURE 11-9 Patterns of nontreponemal serologic findings in infants born to women who are antitreponemal antibody positive. Interpreting the clinical significance of assays in clinically asymptomatic infants whose mother may have syphilis is fraught with difficulties. Antibody pattern *A* in the illustration represents the assay results over time in infants who have acquired antibody through passive transfer of maternal antibody and who are noninfected. Passively transferred maternal antibody has a half-life of about 2 to 3 weeks and will disappear gradually after delivery. Pattern *B* is that for a child who received maternal antibody and, in addition, is in the incubating phase of disease at delivery. Pattern *C* shows the serologic response of a child who receives passive transfer of antibody from the mother and who may also have incubating infection. Pattern *D* represents the results for infants born to mothers who are infected late in pregnancy; these infants therefore do not receive maternal antibody and manifest disease weeks after delivery. This latter pattern is a very common one. Of note, all children who are evaluated for possible congenital syphilis should have serial serologic assays performed. If they still manifest antibody on a nontreponemal test at age 3 to 4 months and have not already been treated, a course of therapy should be initiated. (*From* Gutman L: Syphilis. *In* Feigin RD, Cherry JD (eds.): *Textbook of Pediatric Infectious Diseases*, 3rd ed. Philadelphia: W.B. Saunders; 1992: 560; with permission.)

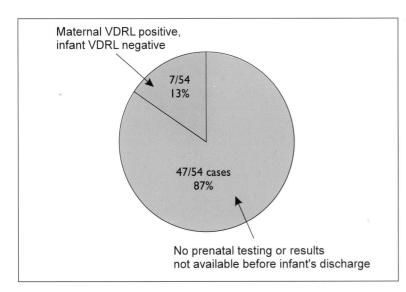

FIGURE 11-10 Factors contributing to the failure to recognize asymptomatic congenital syphilis at delivery. In a study of 54 cases of missed diagnosis in infants with asymptomatic congenital syphilis at delivery, seven cases were missed because the infant's Veneral Disease Research Laboratory (VDRL) test was negative and the mother's positive VDRL was overlooked or not acted upon, a result which emphasizes the importance of testing maternal blood rather than infant blood as a specimen in the diagnosis of congenital syphilis. The more important factor, however, was failure to perform assays or the discharge of infants before results were returned, leading to compromised medical care. (Cohen DA: Congenital syphilis. *N Engl J Med* 1991, 324: 1063–1064.)

Centers for Disease Control and Prevention surveillance case definition for congenital syphilis

Confirmed
  Treponema pallidum identified from lesions, placenta, umbilical cord, autopsy

Presumptive
  Infant's mother untreated or inadequately treated, *or*
    Infant had positive STS and any of:
      Positive physical findings
      Positive CSF VDRL
      CSF cells or protein abnormal
      Osteitis on long-bone radiographs
      Infant's STS titer 4 × mother's
      FTA-ABS 19S-IgM positive

CSF—cerebrospinal fluid; FTA-ABS—fluorescent treponemal antibody absorption; STS—serologic testing for syphilis; VDRL—Veneral Disease Research Laboratory.

FIGURE 11-11 Centers for Disease Control and Prevention surveillance case definition for congenital syphilis for 1988 and 1993. In 1988, the case definition of congenital syphilis was revised so that a child no longer was required to have symptoms of disease or serologic evidence of syphilis. Because passive transfer of maternal antibody occurs, prior to 1988 serologic evidence of infection had required either a rising titer of antibody or the presence of antisyphilitic IgM antibody from the infant. Often, these requirements could only be met if an infant underwent multiple serologic assays, leading to loss to follow-up and emergence of disease during the observation period. In 1988, the case definition was simplified to include either symptoms of disease in the infant or birth to a mother who was untreated or inadequately treated. The definition of inadequate maternal treatment was amplified in 1993 (*see* Fig. 11-13). (Centers for Disease Control and Prevention: 1993 Sexually transmitted diseases treatment guidelines. *MMWR* 1993, 42(RR-14):1–102.)

EVALUATION AND TREATMENT

Treatment of pregnant women with primary or secondary syphilis to eradicate congenital syphilis

HIV-negative women
Benzathine penicillin G — 2.4 MU intramuscularly in 1 dose
Repeat in 1 wk

HIV-positive women
Aqueous crystalline penicillin G — 12–24 MU/d, given as 2–4 MU every 4 hrs intravenously × 15 days, *or*
Procaine penicillin — 2–4 MU/d intramuscularly × 15 days, plus
Probenecid — 500 mg orally 4 times daily × 10–14 days

FIGURE 11-12 Treatment of pregnant women with primary or secondary syphilis. Adequate treatment of mothers with primary or secondary syphilis should eradicate congenital syphilis in the infant with considerable reliability. However, any regimen may fail, and follow-up serologic assays are indicated at 1-month intervals throughout the pregnancy. Some experts recommend additional therapy (*eg*, second dose of benzathine penicillin, 2.4 MU intramuscularly) 1 week after the initial dose, particularly for those women in the third trimester of pregnancy and for women who have secondary syphilis during pregnancy. Therapy should be modified as indicated for women who are HIV infected. Therapy for women who cannot tolerate penicillin should be individualized with the advice of an expert in the treatment of sexually transmitted diseases. (Centers for Disease Control and Prevention: 1993 Sexually transmitted diseases treatment guidelines. *MMWR* 1993, 42(RR-14)31–102.)

Treatment of syphilis in pregnant women that may fail to prevent congenital syphilis of the infant

Treatment during the month before delivery
Treatment in an HIV-infected woman with a regimen ineffective against neurosyphilis
Serial posttherapy assays of maternal nontreponemal antibody titers not performed
Serial posttherapy assays of maternal antibody titers indicate failure to eradicate infection, reinfection, or relapse (< 4-fold decrease in titers)
Treatment with a nonpenicillin regimen
History of maternal treatment was not well documented

FIGURE 11-13 Factors leading to inadequate treatment of syphilis in pregnant women. In certain women who are treated for syphilis, the treatment is inadequate for the reliable eradication of syphilis in the infant. In these circumstances, the diagnosis fulfills the case definition of presumed congenital syphilis, and the infant should receive a full course of therapy for congenital syphilis following delivery.

Clinical findings in infants born to mothers with syphilis

Infant findings	Maternal treatment		
	None (*n*=72)	Inadequate (*n*=31)	Adequate (*n*=45)
Clinical disease	3	0	0
Positive CSF VDRL	7	4	0
Abnormal bone radiograph	6	0	0
Stillbirth	6	0	0
Total (any abnormality)	22 (31%)	4 (13%)	0

CSF—cerebrospinal fluid; VDRL—Veneral Diseases Research Laboratory.

FIGURE 11-14 Clinical findings in infants born to mothers with syphilis, according to maternal treatment. Clinical evaluations were done on 148 infants born to mothers who had positive tests for syphilis, and the findings were grouped according to whether mothers had been untreated, had received inadequate treatment, or had received adequate treatment. Treatment in these cases had been carried out according to current therapeutic recommendations. This study supports the recommendations that children who are born to mothers whose therapy for syphilis was inadequate (*see* Fig. 11-13) should be treated for presumed congenital syphilis. In this population, 13% of such infants had findings indicative of congenital neurosyphilis. A similar proportion of infants of untreated women had neurosyphilis. It should be noted that a primary goal of the current regimens for treatment of congenital syphilis is the eradication of infection of the infant's central nervous system. (Reyes MP, Hunt N, Ostrea EM, George D: Maternal/congenital syphilis in a large tertiary-care urban hospital. *J Infect Dis* 1993, 17:1041–1046.)

Prevention of congenital syphilis

Quantitative dilutions of prenatal and perinatal serologic assays
  for syphilis
More testing in pregnancies of HIV-infected mothers
Careful monitoring in mothers with documented syphilis

FIGURE 11-15 Prevention of congenital syphilis. Mothers who are
at increased risk for syphilis or for a poor response to therapy for
syphilis (*eg*, those who are HIV infected) should be tested frequently.
Those who have been treated for syphilis should be monitored clinically and serologically with great care. *Any* evidence of reinfection or
relapse should elicit a full evaluation and retreatment.

Efficacy of therapy for gonorrhea in the eradication of incubating syphilis

Regimen	Efficacy in incubating syphilis
Ceftriaxone 250 mg intramuscularly	Efficacy uncertain
Spectinomycin 2 mg intramuscularly	Not efficacious
Ciprofloxacin 500 mg orally	Not efficacious
Penicillin 4.8 MU intramuscularly	Efficacious
Amoxicillin 3 g orally	Efficacious

FIGURE 11-16 Efficacy of therapy for gonorrhea in the eradication of
incubating syphilis. Several therapeutic regimens that are commonly
used for the treatment of gonorrhea may fail to eradicate incubating
syphilis. For ciprofloxacin, spectinomycin, and ceftriaxone, the
patient must return 3 to 6 months after the therapy and undergo
repeat serologic assessment for syphilis. These regimens should be
avoided if the patient is pregnant, and if used, particular care in
subsequent evaluations for syphilis is indicated.

A. Evaluation of the mother

Evaluate maternal history for prior syphilis or risk factors for
  syphilis
If mother received treatment for syphilis, evaluate course of
  therapy for adequacy
Evaluate current maternal status with nontreponemal test
  (*eg*, RPR) and treponemal test (*eg*, MHA-TP)

MHA-TP—microhemagglutination assay for antibodies to
Treponema pallidum; RPR—rapid plasma reagin.

FIGURE 11-17 Initial evaluation of an infant for suspected early
congenital syphilis. **A**, Evaluation of the mother. **B**, Medical evaluation of the infant. An infant may be suspected of having contracted
early syphilis because of presenting illness or because the epidemiologic or serologic status of the mother indicates that the infant was
exposed. Screening medical evaluations for asymptomatic infants
include the physical examination, chest and long-bone radiographs,
cerebrospinal fluid evaluation including Veneral Disease Research
Laboratory, fluorescent treponemal antibody absorption, and
complete blood count. However, congenital syphilis may have a
great variety of presentations (*see* Fig. 11-21). Any indication of
organ system dysfunction should be thoroughly evaluated.

B. Medical evaluation of the infant

Asymptomatic infant
  Physical examination
  Chest radiograph
  Long-bone radiograph
  CSF evaluation
   VDRL
   Protein, glucose
   Cells
  IgM-FTA-ABS (if available)
  Complete blood count with differential
  Pathologic examination of placenta or amniotic cord, including
   staining with specific fluorescent antitreponemal antibody

Symptomatic infant
  As above, plus evaluation of involved organ systems as
   indicated (liver, adrenal, ophthalmic, etc.)

CSF—cerebrospinal fluid; FTA-ABS—fluorescent treponemal antibody
absorption; VDRL—Venereal Diseases Research Laboratory.

Evaluation for congenital neurosyphilis by CSF assays

Reactive CSF VDRL

  or

Elevated CSF white blood cell count (> 5–25 cells/mm³)

  or

Elevated CSF protein (> 40–150 mg/dL)

CSF—cerebrospinal fluid; VDRL—Venereal Disease Research
Laboratory.

FIGURE 11-18 Evaluation for congenital neurosyphilis by cerebrospinal fluid (CSF) assays. The primary findings from CSF assays
supporting the diagnosis of neurosyphilis in a newborn infant are
shown. Note that the ranges of normal for leukocytes and protein
are very wide, presumably reflecting effects of the delivery which
may have been traumatic. Consequently, there is considerable
uncertainty about the interpretation of borderline findings. In addition, there is no evidence that normal findings rule out neurosyphilis
in the newborn. Thus, all infants with confirmed or presumed
syphilis should receive a standard course of therapy that is planned
to be adequate in the treatment of syphilitic central nervous system
infection. Because of extreme paucity of prospective studies of the
late outcomes of children with treated congenital syphilis, efficacy
of the current treatment regimen in preventing later neurologic
manifestations is not known.

Recommended treatment regimens for infants with confirmed or presumed congenital syphilis	
Crystalline penicillin G	100,000–150,000 U/kg/d, given intravenously in divided doses every 8–12 hrs × 10–14 days
or	
Procaine penicillin G	50,000 U/kg/d given intramuscularly every day × 10–14 days

FIGURE 11-19 Recommended treatment regimens for infants with confirmed or presumed congenital syphilis. The recommended treatment schedules have been the subject of considerable controversy. A central problem is that studies on the long-term efficacy of all regimens have been inadequate, and consequently outcomes are uncertain. Currently recommended is a 10- to 14-day course of parenteral therapy for all infants who fulfill criteria for confirmed or presumed congenital syphilis (*see* Fig. 11-10). That recommendation pertains to all children born to mothers whose therapy or response to therapy may have been inadequate (*see* Fig. 11-13). Note that the entire course of therapy to the infant must be delivered uninterrupted; if a day of therapy is missed, the course should be restarted. Penicillin G may be used in the treatment of infants even if the mother is allergic to penicillin because IgE does not cross the placenta.

Recommended follow-up evaluations for children with treated congenital syphilis
Serologic assays
Nontreponemal testing at 3-mos intervals through age 15 mos, then at 6-mos intervals until titer is negative or stable at low titer
Repeat cerebrospinal fluid evaluation at 12 mos if initial evaluation indicates neurosyphilis
Developmental evaluations through early childhood (age 5 yrs)
Yearly evaluation for developmental progress
Vision testing yearly
Auditory evaluation yearly

FIGURE 11-20 Recommended follow-up evaluations for children with treated congenital syphilis. Early serologic evaluations should be used to ensure that the nontreponemal antibody titers are falling and remaining low. Failure to serorevert is an indication for reevaluation and possible repeat therapy. Developmental evaluations may allow early remedial intervention and are also a means of detecting inadequately treated disease.

CLINICAL PRESENTATIONS

Early Congenital Syphilis

Findings in 310 cases of early congenital syphilis	
Findings	**Patients, *n***
Hepatomegaly	100
Skeletal abnormalities	91
Birth weight < 2500 g	51
Skin lesions	45
Hyperbilirubinemia	40
Pneumonia	51
Splenomegaly	56
Severe anemia, hydrops, edema	50
Snuffles, nasal discharge	27
Painful limbs	22
Pancreatitis	14
CSF abnormalities	21
Nephritis	11
Failure to thrive	10
Testicular mass	1
Chorioretinitis	1
Hypoglobulinemia	1

CSF—cerebrospinal fluid.

FIGURE 11-21 Prevalence of findings in early congenital syphilis. These findings, from recent reports, represent acute disease during the first weeks to months after onset of infection. Most infants with early congenital syphilis present either at delivery or within approximately 3 to 7 weeks after delivery. Children almost invariably have hepatosplenomegaly and rash. Other very common manifestations include pneumonia, skeletal abnormalities, and severe anemia. The skin lesions in untreated children are infectious, harboring large numbers of organisms, and clinicians should wear gloves while examining a child with dermal or mucosal lesions. (Dorfman DH, Glaser JH: Congenital syphilis presenting in infants after the newborn period. *N Engl J Med* 1990, 323:1299–1302.) (*From* Gutman LT: Syphilis. *In* Feigin RD, Cherry JD (eds.): *Textbook of Pediatric Infectious Diseases*, 3rd ed. Philadelphia: W.B. Saunders; 1992: 552–563; with permission.)

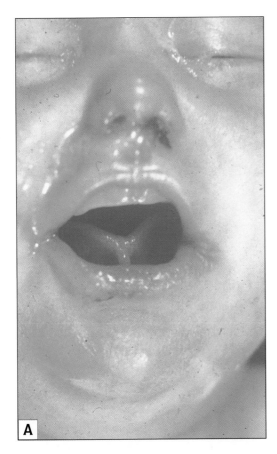

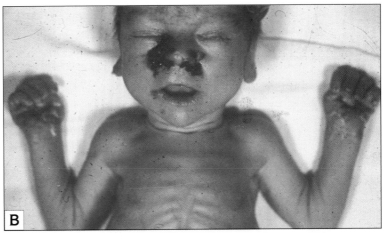

FIGURE 11-22 Snuffles (syphilitic rhinitis). **A**, Early snuffles. A mucopurulent discharge from the nose is seen in an infant with early congenital syphilis. The nasal discharge contains a large number of *Treponema pallidum* organisms and should be considered highly contagious. Darkfield examination of the discharge is frequently diagnostic, revealing motile spirochetes. **B**, Hemorrhagic snuffles. As the process progresses, the discharge becomes increasingly serous or serosanguineous, resulting in "hemorrhagic snuffles," as seen in this prematurely born infant with florid congenital syphilis. These lesions result from vascular necrosis of the mucosa of midline structures of the face. As with other mucosal lesions, the discharge should be considered highly infectious. (*Courtesy of* the Centers for Disease Control and Prevention.)

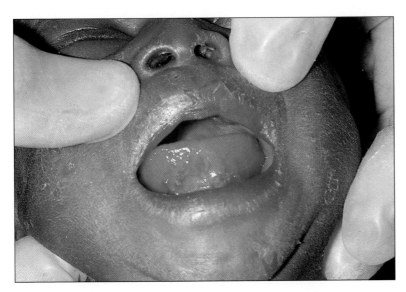

FIGURE 11-23 Syphilitic plaques on lips and buccal mucosa. This term infant developed clinical signs of congenital syphilis at 3 weeks of age. Syphilitic lesions are seen along the margins of the lips, on the tongue, and on the buccal mucosa.

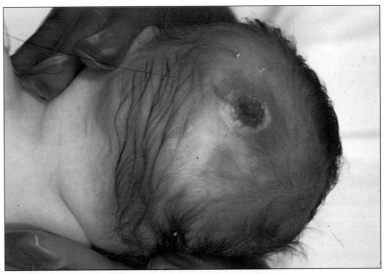

FIGURE 11-24 Primary chancre of syphilis on the occiput. This term infant developed a chancre at age 4 weeks. The lesion was positive for motile treponemas by darkfield microscopy. The mother's rapid plasma reagin had been negative at the time of delivery, presumably because she was experiencing primary syphilis. The mother's chancre was on the vaginal wall and consequently not noted by her. This child presumably had acquired syphilis rather than congenital syphilis. The distinction may be of importance clinically, because in acquired syphilis the inoculum is relatively small and the child may develop defenses during early incubation, whereas congenital disease presents as a bacteremia and is multisystemic from the outset. (*See also* Fig. 11-32.)

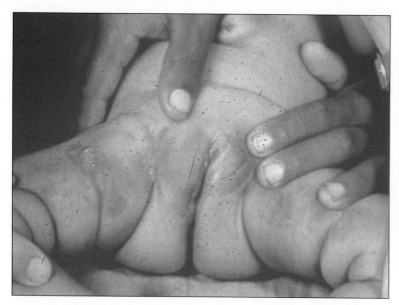

FIGURE 11-25 Syphilitic mucosal lesions. This term infant had dermal lesions at delivery. Lesions were most prominent on moist surfaces, on mucosa, and in folds. Note that the examiner was not wearing gloves and would have been at risk for acquired syphilis if the child had not been treated. (*Courtesy of* the Centers for Disease Control and Prevention.)

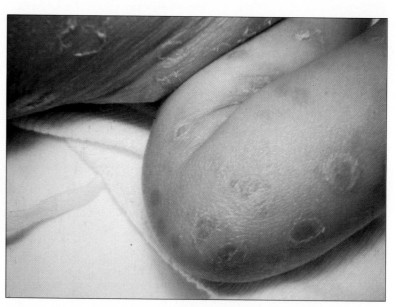

FIGURE 11-26 Plaquelike dermal lesions of congenital syphilis. This child developed signs of congenital syphilis at 5 weeks of age. Plaquelike lesions, which were scaly, rough, pigmented, and round, appeared on all external skin surfaces.

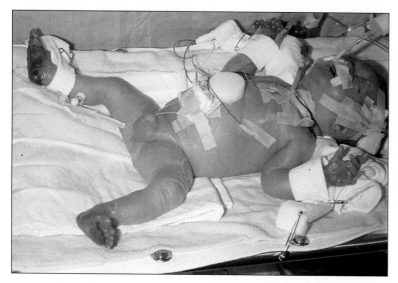

FIGURE 11-27 Hemorrhagic dermal lesions of congenital syphilis. A premature infant with congenital syphilis developed an *Escherichia coli* bacteremia. Coinfection with other pathogens occurs relatively often in children with congenital syphilis. There are also hemorrhagic lesions on the hands and feet. Coinfecting organisms have included *E. coli*, *Yersinia enterocolitica*, *Staphylococcus aureus*, *Klebsiella* spp, *Candida albicans*, Cytomegalovirus, and HIV.

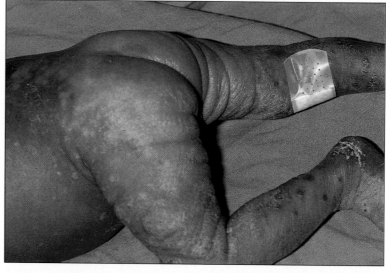

FIGURE 11-28 Hypertrophic dermal lesions of congenital syphilis. This term infant developed symptomatic disease at age 6 weeks. Hypertrophic lesions can be seen on the extremities, and denuded skin is seen in moist areas. Maculopapular lesions develop a coppery color. Healing may be associated with scarring and formation of fissures.

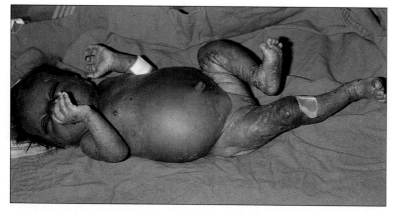

FIGURE 11-29 Dermal lesions and ascites in congenital syphilis. Ascites associated with a chronic hemolytic process is apparent. The hemolytic process seen with congenital syphilis is not fully understood and has been the subject of relatively little research. At least one aspect of the disorder is the production of Forssman antibodies. Forssman hapten is a naturally occurring glycolipid coupled to a ceramide lipid and is widely distributed on mammalian membranes, including circulating erythrocytes and precursors. Following damage by treponemal infection, antibody to Forssman may be produced and directed toward the host tissues. Children with hemolytic processes of congenital syphilis characteristically continue to exhibit chronic hemolysis for an extended period (months) after treatment of syphilis has been completed.

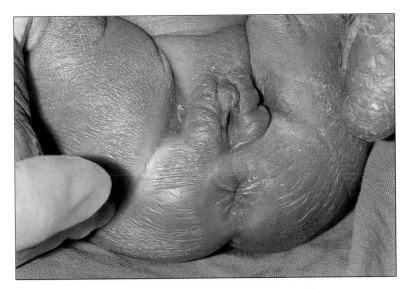

FIGURE 11-30 Perianal lesions of congenital syphilis. Hemorrhagic perianal lesions are evident and result from syphilitic vasculitis. Bullous lesions follow vesicular eruptions of the mucous membranes, palms, and soles. Infancy is the only age in which syphilitic lesions are vesicular or bullous.

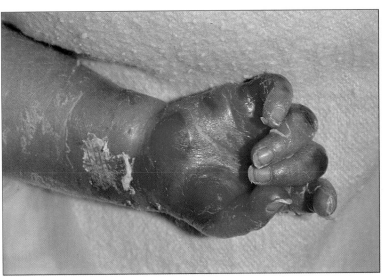

FIGURE 11-31 Hemorrhagic bullous lesions of the hand. Congenital syphilis is one of the few conditions in which there occurs vesicular, bullous, and hemorrhagic lesions of the hands and feet, especially involving the palms and soles.

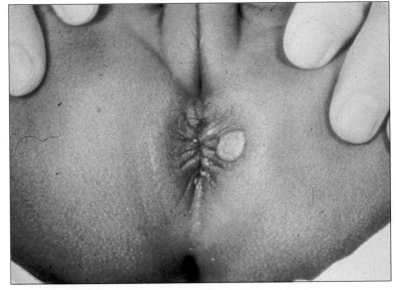

FIGURE 11-32 Primary genital chancre of acquired syphilis in a child aged 2 months. A primary syphilitic chancre of acquired syphilis is seen on the genitalia of a child aged 2 months who had been sexually abused. The lesion presented similarly to those of sexually active adults. Children can acquire syphilis at a very young age, and so the clinician must not assume that all positive serologic assays in infants represent congenital infection. The data must be evaluated and the means of transmission established (congenital, intrapartum, or acquired). (*Courtesy of* D. Ingram, MD.)

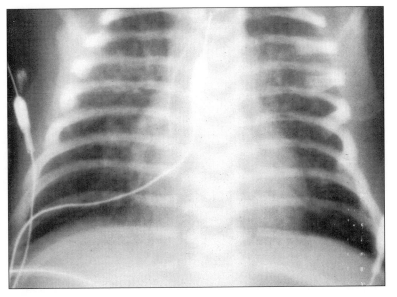

FIGURE 11-33 Pneumonia in congenital syphilis. Pulmonary disease of early congenital syphilis is termed *pneumonia alba.* Histologically, the disease shows interstitial fibrosis and collapse of alveoli.

FIGURE 11-34 Bony lesions in early congenital syphilis. Periosteal new bone formation (*arrow*) is seen at the metaphyseal region. Epiphysitis is seen at the ends of both humerus and ulna. Irregular demineralization of the metaphyses and focal areas of cortical atrophy have occurred. These lesions are painful and cause the child to avoid motion, leading to the appearance of paralysis (pseudoparalysis).

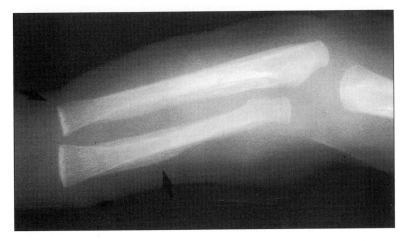

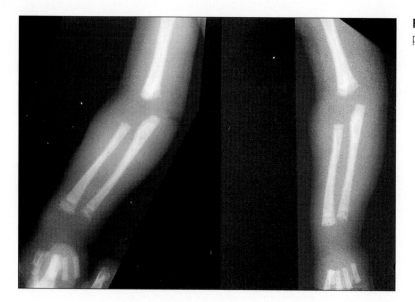

FIGURE 11-35 Bony lesions of early congenital syphilis. Note the patchy necrosis of epiphyses.

Late Congenital Syphilis

Stigmata of late congenital syphilis

	Total patients, %
Frontal boss of Parrott	87
Short maxilla	84
High palatal arch	76
Hutchinson triad	75
Hutchinson teeth	63
Interstitial keratitis	9
Eighth nerve deafness	3
Saddle nose	73
Mulberry molars	65
Higouménakis sign	39
Relative protuberance of mandible	26
Rhagades	7
Saber skin	4
Scophoid scapulae	0.7
Clutton joint	0.3

FIGURE 11-36 Prevalence of findings in late congenital syphilis. These findings represent the late results of syphilitic vasculitis, necrosis, scarring, and fibrosis. Most of these structural findings are first recognized in adolescence and early adulthood, and the earlier pediatric precursor conditions have not received much recognition. Several of the findings (*eg*, Hutchinson's teeth, saddle nose, short maxilla) are accentuated with increasing maturity. (*From* Gutman LT: Syphilis. *In* Feigin RD, Cherry JD (eds.): *Textbook of Pediatric Infectious Diseases*, 3rd ed. Philadelphia: W.B. Saunders; 1992: 552–563; with permission.)

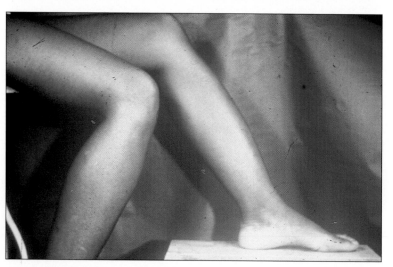

FIGURE 11-37 "Sabre shins" in a survivor of congenital syphilis. Sabre shins, or anterior tibial bowing, results from chronic periosteal inflammation of untreated early congenital syphilis. As new bone is continuously deposited over areas of chronic inflammation, the normal contour of the bone is distorted. The area of maximal involvement is in the midshaft leading to the hypertrophy of bony deposition at that area. (*Courtesy of* the Centers for Disease Control and Prevention.)

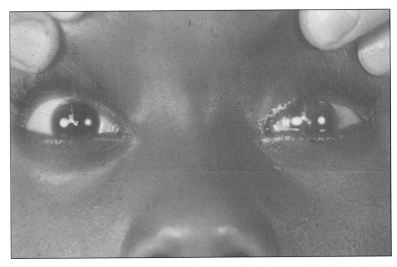

FIGURE 11-38 Syphilitic interstitial keratitis. Interstitial keratitis is the most common of the late manifestations of congenital syphilis. It may present at any age and is one of the three components of "Hutchinson's triad" (interstitial keratitis, Hutchinson's teeth, and eighth nerve deafness).

Hutchinson's triad
Interstitial keratitis
Eighth nerve deafness
Hutchinson's teeth

FIGURE 11-39 Hutchinson's triad. Interstitial keratitis presents as corneal clouding and progresses to glaucoma. It often begins unilaterally but eventually involves both orbits. Eighth nerve deafness appears to be caused by osteochondritis, leading to cochlear degeneration. The child may also experience a conductive deficit. The condition often begins with loss of appreciation of high frequency sounds and slowly progresses to loss of both cochlear and vestibular function. Hutchinson's teeth involve both incisors and molars. The incisors are tapered because of failure to lay down enamel at the center of the dental papilla. Permanent teeth are involved. The molars show poor enamelization and abnormally small cusps.

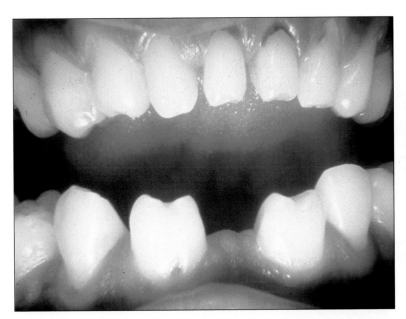

FIGURE 11-40 Hutchinson's teeth. Congenital syphilis causes abnormalities of the teeth, which are manifested by the small size of affected teeth, defective enamelization, and apical notching of incisors. The incisors of this child aged 6 years demonstrate notching.

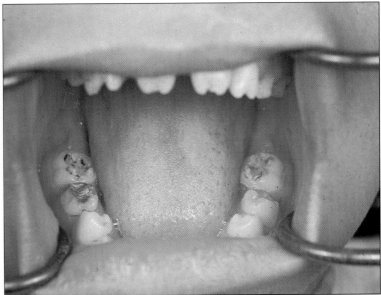

FIGURE 11-41 Hutchinson's molars. Molars are also affected by congenital syphilis and often demonstrate small size, cracking, early decay, and irregular cuspid formation. All are seen in the permanent molars of this child. These are sometimes termed *mulberry molars.*

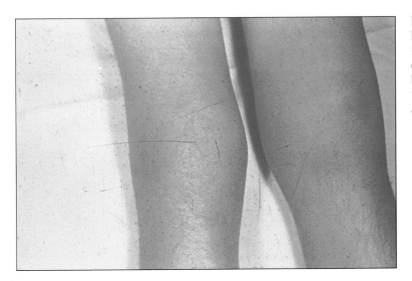

FIGURE 11-42 Clutton's joints. Clutton's joints, symmetrical painless hydrarthroses, were definitely described in 1886. Although usually involving the knees, the condition has also been reported in the elbows, wrists, fingers, or ankles. The process does not involve the bones themselves and probably results from an antigen–antibody reaction. The condition usually appears between 8 and 15 years of age. (*Courtesy of* the Centers for Disease Control and Prevention.)

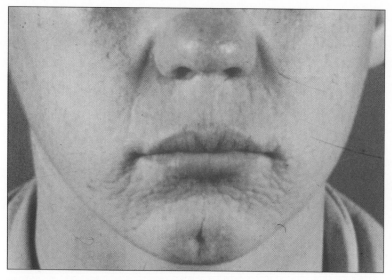

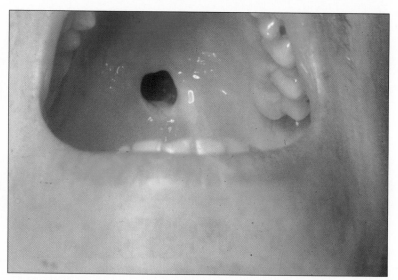

FIGURE 11-43 Rhagades. Rhagades are linear scars radiating from the mouth and nose or, less frequently, the anus and are the result of infiltrative and erosive lesions in infancy. The condition is rare, being seen in about 1% to 2% of early series. (Campmeier RH: *Essentials of Syphiology*. Philadelphia: J.B. Lippincott; 1943; 432.) (*Courtesy of* the Centers for Disease Control and Prevention.)

FIGURE 11-44 Perforation of the palate. Perforation of the palate in an infant should raise the question of congenital syphilis and results from gummatous destruction. Similar lesions are seen in various fungal infections and midline granuloma and possibly in some patients who inhale cocaine. (*Courtesy of* the Centers for Disease Control and Prevention.)

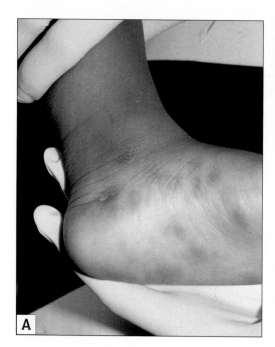

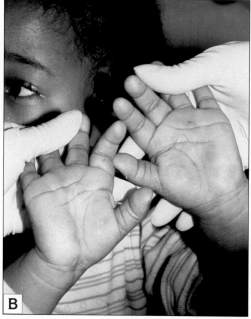

FIGURE 11-45 Dermal lesions in acquired secondary syphilis. **A** and **B**, Dermal lesions are shown in a child aged 2 years with acquired secondary syphilis, which was contracted during abusive sexual contact. This case reflects that the spectrum of modes of transmission of syphilis in young children includes both congenital disease as well as disease acquired postnatally (*Courtesy of* E.D. Everette, MD.)

SUGGESTED BIBLIOGRAPHY

Centers for Disease Control and Prevention: 1993 Sexually transmitted diseases treatment guidelines. *MMWR* 1993, 42(RR-14):1–102.

Gutman LT: Syphilis. *In* Feigin RD, Cherry JD (eds.): *Textbook of Pediatric Infectious Diseases*, 3rd ed. Philadelphia: W.B. Saunders Co., 1992: 552–563.

Ikeda MK, Jenson HB: Evaluation and treatment of congenital syphilis. *J Pediatr* 1990, 117:843–852.

Ingall D, Dobson SRM, Musher D: Syphilis. *In* Remington JJ, Klein JD (eds.): *Infectious Diseases of the Fetus and Newborn Infant*, 3rd ed. Philadelphia: W.B. Saunders Co., 1990: 367–394.

CHAPTER 12

Human Papillomavirus–Associated Diseases

Richard Reid

BASIC BIOLOGY OF HUMAN PAPILLOMAVIRUS

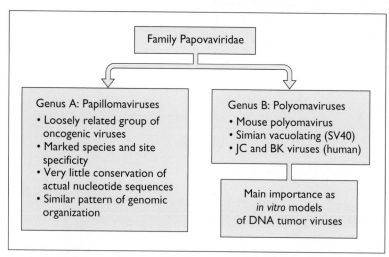

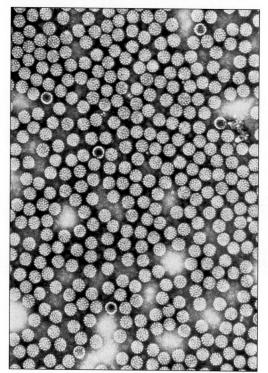

FIGURE 12-1 Taxonomy of the family Papovaviridae. Papillomaviruses are small, double-stranded DNA viruses, classified in the same family as polyomaviruses because of superficial similarities in electron microscopic appearance and biologic properties. However, molecular hybridization studies have shown that the two groups are evolutionarily different. The polyomaviruses served as important laboratory models of a DNA tumor virus but have little role in human disease. Conversely, papillomaviruses cause important diseases in many species, especially humans. All of these viruses alter cell growth and tissue maturation. Although the overall pattern of genomic organization is similar throughout the genus, there is little conservation in actual nucleotide sequence from one virus type to another; hence, papillomavirus infections show profound species and site selectivity.

FIGURE 12-2 Electron micrograph of papillomavirus virions. Each virion is a 55-nm, icosahedral (20-sided) particle composed of a circular, double-stranded, covalently closed DNA molecule, surrounded by a protein capsid. The absence of an outer membrane, such as is found in other viruses, may account for the low antigenicity of papillomavirus infections.

CLINICAL EXPRESSION OF HUMAN PAPILLOMAVIRUS INFECTION

Clinical groupings of HPV-associated diseases

Cutaneotropic—healthy host
  Verrucae (common wart) on nongenital skin
  Plantar warts on nongenital skin
Cutaneotropic—immunodeficient host
  Epidermodysplasia verruciformis
  Skin cancers in transplant recipients
Mucosotropic group
  Anogenital warts, dysplasias, and cancers
  Aerodigestive papillomas and neoplasias

FIGURE 12-3 Clinical groupings of disease associated with the 70 known types of human papillomaviruses (HPVs). The various HPV types can be divided into three main clinical groupings. First, HPVs 1, 2, 3, 4, and 7 are variously associated with plantar or common warts on nongenital skin of healthy individuals. Viruses in this group produce benign warts that are never carcinogenic. Second, about 30 of the known HPV types were isolated from the skin of immunosuppressed individuals. A quarter to one third of these individuals develop skin cancers, usually in sunlight-exposed areas. The two main types associated with oncogenicity are HPVs 5 and 8. Finally, about 35 known HPV types are mucosotropic, affecting either anogenital skin or mucus membranes.

Disease associations of different HPV types

Disease	HPV types	
	Frequent association	Less-frequent association
Plantar warts	1, 2	4, 63
Common warts	2, 1	4, 26, 27, 29, 41, 57, 65
Common warts of meat, poultry, and fish handlers	7, 2	1, 3, 4, 10, 28
Flat warts	3, 10	27, 38, 41, 49
Intermediate warts	10	26, 28
Epidermodysplasia verruciformis	2, 3, 10, 5, 8, 9, 12, 14, 15, 17	19, 20, 21, 22, 23, 24, 25, 36, 37, 38, 47, 50
Condylomata acuminata	6, 11	30, 42, 43, 44, 45, 51, 54, 55, 70
Intraepithelial neoplasia		
Unspecified		30, 34, 39, 40, 53, 57, 59, 61, 62, 64, 66, 67, 68, 69
Low-grade	6, 11	16, 18, 31, 33, 35, 42, 43, 44, 45, 51, 52
High-grade	16, 18	6, 11, 31, 33, 35, 39, 42, 44, 45, 51, 52, 56, 58, 66
Bowen's disease	16	31, 34
Bowenoid papulosis	16	34, 39, 42, 45
Cervical carcinoma	16, 18	31, 33, 35, 39, 45, 51, 52, 56, 58, 66
Recurrent respiratory papillomatosis	6, 11	
Focal epithelial neoplasia of Heck	13, 32	
Conjunctival papillomas and carcinomas	6, 11, 16	
Others		6, 11, 16, 30, 33, 36, 37, 38, 41, 48, 60

FIGURE 12-4 Disease associations of different HPV types. More than 70 different HPV types have been characterized, and many others are recognized. Because the viruses cannot be cultured, typing is based on DNA homology. Each type is site-specific and largely associated with a distinct histopathologic process. (*From* Bonnez W, Reichman RC: Papillomaviruses. *In* Mandell GL, Bennett JE, Dolin R (eds.): *Principles and Practice of Infectious Diseases*, 4th ed. New York: Churchill Livingstone; 1995:1388; with permission.)

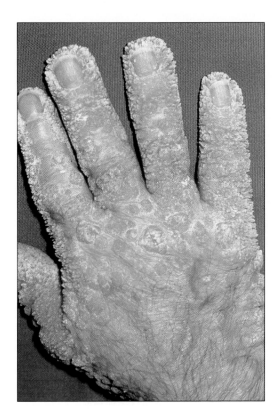

FIGURE 12-5 Extensive verrucae vulgaris of the right hand. Common warts represent up to 71% of all cutaneous warts and are most prevalent among school-aged children. They are believed to be transmitted by close personal contact. (*Courtesy of* R. Ostrow, MD.)

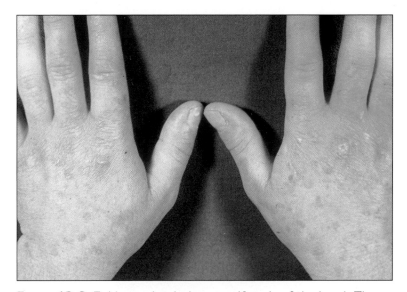

FIGURE 12-6 Epidermodysplasia verruciformis of the hand. The dorsum of the hand shows multiple flat warts that will persist for life in this congenitally immunosuppressed individual. A large invasive squamous cancer (not shown) also has developed in the sunlight-exposed area of the right forehead. Epidermodysplasia verruciformis is rare, probably autosomal dominant condition that is characterized by disseminated cutaneous warts and malignant transformation. It usually appears early in life in persons with depressed cellular immunity. (*From* Pfister H: Relationship of papillomaviruses to anogenital cancer. *Obstet Gynecol Clin North Am* 1987, 4:349–61; with permission.)

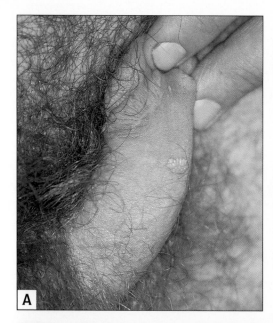

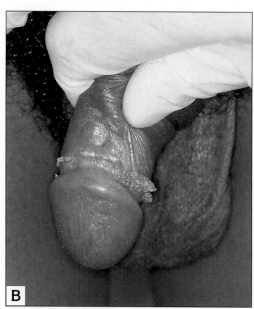

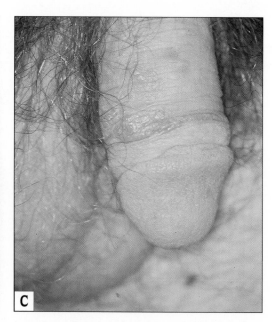

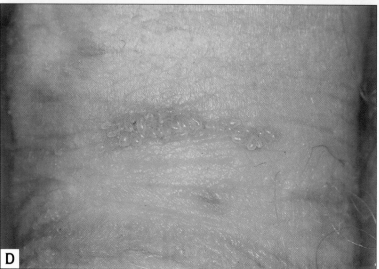

have the typical verrucous appearance seen here, a clinical diagnosis is made easily. The lesions may spread linearly or circumferentially. A smaller lesion is seen distally, just beneath the patient's fingers. **B**, Papilliferous warts of the penis involving the coronal sulcus. The coronal sulcus is a common site for condyloma acuminata in men, perhaps because of the susceptibility of this site to subclinical trauma during intercourse. Here, the warts have spread circumferentially, with the initial lesions to the patient's left. These older lesions have become hyperpigmented. **C**, Flatter, more chronic warts on the penis. These lesions were an incidental finding on a man who presented as an asymptomatic contact to a woman with chlamydial cervicitis. Chronic warts are likely to become keratinized. **D**, Recurrent warts on the penile shaft. This patient had been treated 3 months previously, with complete resolution of visible lesions, but returned with recurrent, tiny lesions. A blush may be seen at the base of some of the individual lesions, which are highly vascular. The appearance of a tiny blood vessel running along the side of a lesion may assist in identifying it as a wart (as opposed to molluscum contagiosum). (Oriel D: Genital human papillomavirus infection. *In* Holmes KK, Mårdh P-A, Sparling PF, *et al.* (eds.): *Sexually Transmitted Diseases*, 2nd ed. New York: McGraw Hill; 1990: 435.) (*Courtesy of* M.F. Rein, MD.)

FIGURE 12-7 Penile warts. **A**, Typical papilliferous wart of the penis in a healthy man. These exophytic lesions are initially soft and fleshy. They occur most frequently on the shaft and coronal sulcus and are commonly found under the prepuce. When lesions

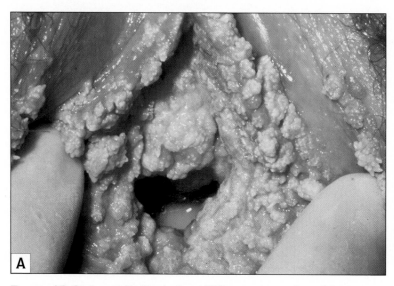

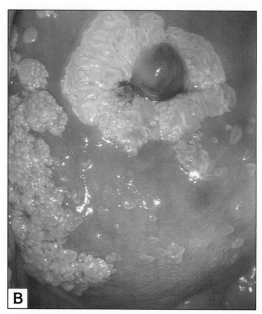

FIGURE 12-8 A and **B**, Typical papilliferous warts (condyloma acuminata) affecting the vulva and vagina (*panel 8A*) and cervix (*panel 8B*) of an immunologically healthy young woman. (*Courtesy of* E. Pixley, MD.)

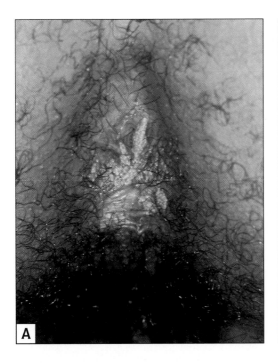 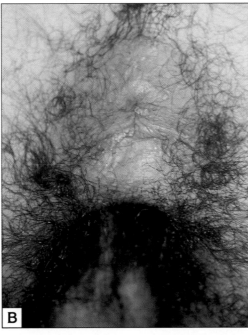

A **B**

FIGURE 12-9 Perianal warts. **A**, This patient was seen in 1977, before the identification of HIV, and was presumably immunologically intact. The presence of such perianal lesions in a man is possible evidence that the patient has engaged in receptive anal intercourse. Such patients should undergo anoscopy to look for internal lesions and should be evaluated for other anorectal sexually transmitted diseases, such as gonorrhea or chlamydial infection. They also should be strongly encouraged to undergo testing for HIV antibody. **B**, Perianal warts, in another homosexual man who practiced receptive anal intercourse, are seen to track into the anus. (*Courtesy of* M.F. Rein, MD.)

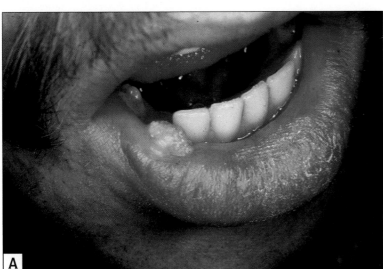 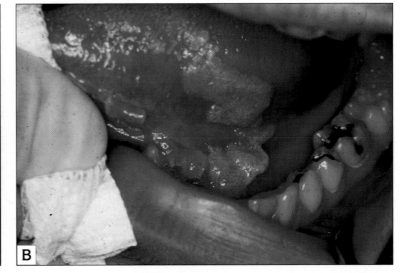

A **B**

FIGURE 12-10 **A** and **B**, Condylomatous lesions affecting the lips (*panel 10A*) and oral mucosa (*panel 10B*) of an immunologically healthy homosexual man.

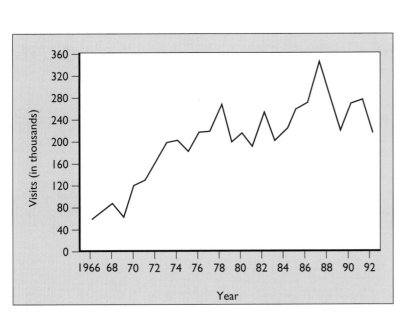

FIGURE 12-11 Annual incidence of HPV-associated genital warts in the United States between 1966 and 1992. The incidence of genital warts has risen dramatically in the past 15 to 20 years. Using data collected by the National Disease and Therapeutic Index, the Centers for Disease Control and Prevention estimate that the number of physicians' office visits related to anogenital warts increased from 169,000 in 1966 to 1.1 million in 1984 in the United States. An estimated half million people each year acquire symptomatic genital warts. (*From* Division of STD/HIV Prevention: *Sexually Transmitted Disease Surveillance, 1992.* Atlanta: Centers for Disease Control and Prevention; 1993:28.)

NATURAL HISTORY AND PATHOGENESIS

Natural History of Genital Human Papillomavirus Infections

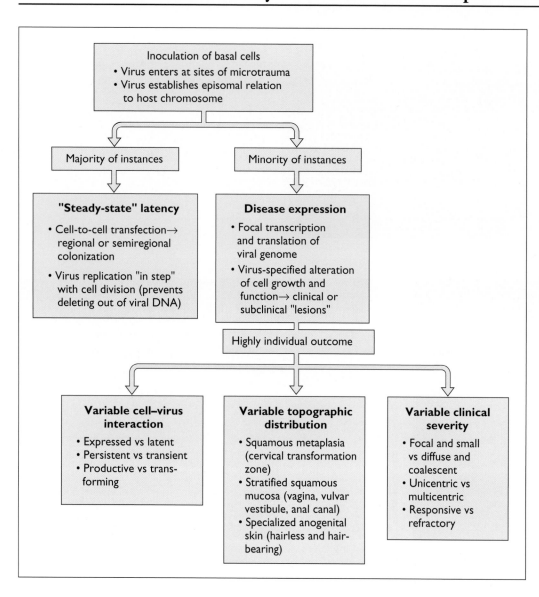

FIGURE 12-12 Individual variation in the natural history of HPV infections. The viral life cycle begins with inoculation of the basal cells at sites of microtrauma. During the incubation phase, the virus establishes an episomal relationship to the host chromosome. In most instances, cell-to-cell transection produces a regional or semi-regional colonization, in which there is no disease expression, and virus exposure can only be detected by molecular hybridization of exfoliated cells. The latency is maintained by the mechanism of virus replication in step with cell division. Conversely, in a minority of instances, focal transcription and translation lead to disease expression. The outcome is highly individual, depending on variations in cell–virus interaction, topographic distribution, and clinical severity.

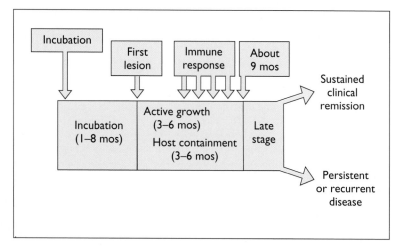

FIGURE 12-13 Stages of HPV infection. After inoculation, there is an incubation period during which the virus establishes itself as a self-replicating, extrachromosomal plasmid throughout the lower genital tract. This is followed by a period of active lesion growth, which typically lasts 3 to 6 months. After a lag time of several months, there is a host-containment phase, during which lesion growth is slowed. In up to 20% of instances, spontaneous regression may occur, even of extensive disease. About 9 months from the time of the first lesion, the lesion growth and host containment come into essential equilibrium. At this point, patients diverge into two groups: those who remain in sustained clinical remission, and those who relapse into continued active disease expression. (*From* Reid R, Dorsey JH: Physical and surgical principles of carbon dioxide laser surgery in the lower genital tract. *In* Coppleson M (ed.): *Gynecologic Oncology*, 2nd ed. Edinburgh: Churchill Livingstone; 1992:1087–1131; with permission.)

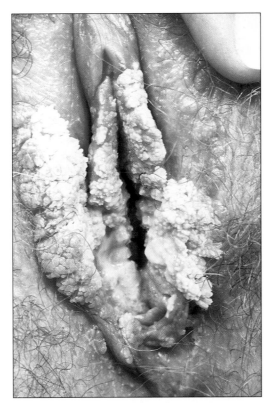

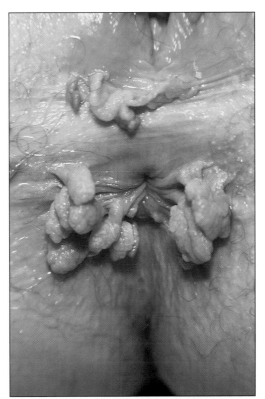

FIGURE 12-14 Active lesion growth. Altered epithelial growth patterns and the proliferation of underlying capillaries produce a diffuse crop of symmetric soft papillomas. The associated vaginal discharge has produced maceration of some of the lesions of the nonglabrous skin. Accumulated clinical experience suggests that perhaps only one in 10 exposed individuals ever develop clinical disease. (*From* Reid R, Campion M: HPV-associated lesions of the cervix: Biology and colposcopic features. *Clin Obstet Gynecol* 1989, 32:157–179; with permission.)

FIGURE 12-15 Papular, pedunculated perianal warts of 4 years' duration. (*From* Reid R: Human papillomavirus-associated diseases of the lower genital tract. *In* Keye WR (ed.): *Laser Surgery in Gynecology and Obstetrics*, 2nd ed. Chicago: Year Book Medical Publishers; 1990:46–99; with permission.)

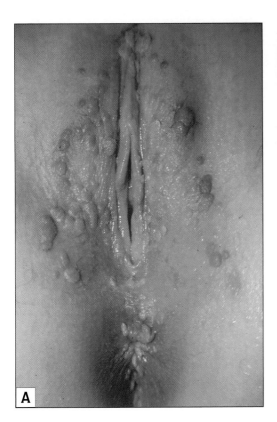

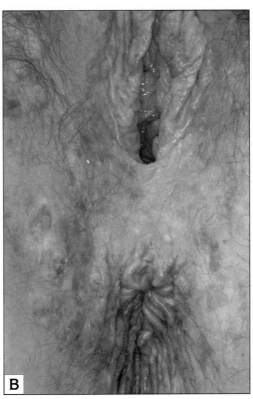

FIGURE 12-16 Persistent or recurrent HPV infection. **A**, Bowenoid papulosis. These pigmented peripheral papules recurred about 2 years after previously "cured" condylomas. Biopsy showed a premalignant epithelium, and virus testing detected HPV 16. Such cases traditionally are called *Bowenoid papulosis* to contrast these peripheral papules with the central macules of classic Bowen's disease. However, both lesions are associated with HPV 16, both have similar histology, and either can progress to invasive cancer. Therefore, the distinction is discouraged and these terms should be abandoned. **B**, Bowen's disease, diffuse macular vulvar intraepithelial neoplasia, grade 3 (VIN 3). In contrast to *panel 16A*, this patient shows the classic macular lesion of Bowen's disease.

Cell–Virus Interactions

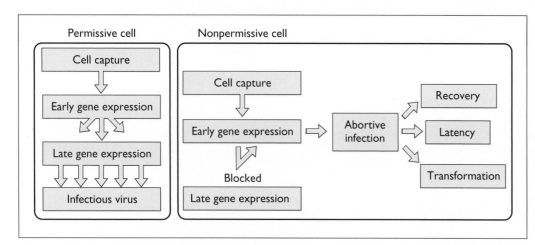

FIGURE 12-17 Outcome of HPV infection in permissive cell vs nonpermissive cell. In the permissive cell, expression of the early viral genes produces cellular proliferation in the basal layers but leads to cell death and virion assembly in the upper layers. In nonpermissive cells, late gene expression fails, leading to an abortive infection from which recovery, persistent latency, or neoplastic transformation may result. (*From* Reid R: Papillomavirus and cervical neoplasia: Modern implications and future prospects. *Colposc Gynecol Laser Surg* 1984, 1:3–34; with permission.)

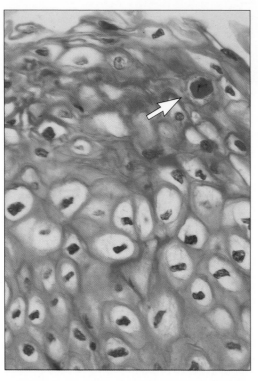

FIGURE 12-18 Tissue micrograph of the upper layers of a productive cell–virus interaction in the cervical epithelium, showing koilocytotic atypia. There is prominent cytopathic effect producing a histologic picture termed *koilocytotic atypia*. The main features are hyperchromatism, nuclear shrinkage and collapse, and perinuclear cytoplasmic vacuolation, which are highly specific findings for HPV infection. One of the cells shows individual cell keratinization (*arrow*).

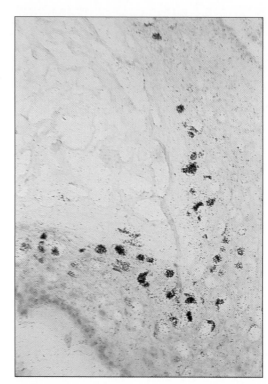

FIGURE 12-19 *In situ* hybridization using ³H-HPV-6 probe to identify replication of viral DNA within cells of a condyloma. Viral replication is indicated by the multiple intranuclear black granules, most prominent at the epithelial surface. (*Courtesy of* A.T. Lorincz, MD.)

Productive Viral Infection

Events in the HPV life cycle	
Viral event	**Histologic reflection**
1. Cell capture (basal layer)	None
2. Early gene expression with "benign transformation" (parabasal layer)	Mitogenic effect (acanthosis, mitoses, hyperchromatism, delayed maturation)
	Viral DNA replication begins
3. Late gene expression begins in maturing cells (intermediate layer)	Initial viral cytopathic effect (mild koilocytosis)
4. Late gene expression in terminally differentiating cells (upper third)	Pronounced nuclear collapse and vacuolization
	Virion assembly begins

FIGURE 12-20 Events in the HPV life cycle with associated histologic reflection. The synthesis of late proteins and production of intact viral particles occur in maturing cells within the intermediate and superficial layers.

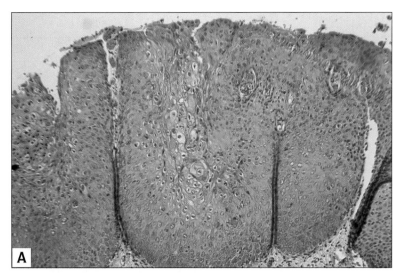

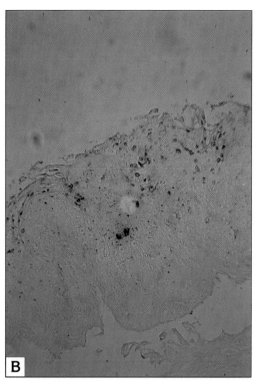

FIGURE 12-21 **A** and **B,** Photomicrographs showing early gene expression in the basal layers (*panel 21A*) and late gene expression at the epithelial surface (*panel 21B*). *Panel 21A* is stained with hematoxylin-eosin and *panel 21B* is an unstained immunoperoxidase preparation of an adjacent section. Cells containing virus-specified capsid protein show intranuclear aggregations of brown staining, seen only in the intermediate and superficial layers.

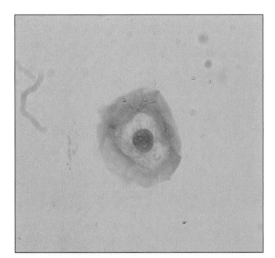

FIGURE 12-22 Classic cytopathic effect seen on Papanicolaou staining of single exfoliated koilocyte. One can see nuclear condensation and the perinuclear clear zone, changes that are highly specific for HPV infection.

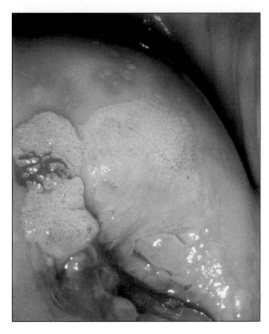

FIGURE 12-23 Colpophotograph showing the prominent upgrowth of HPV-induced capillary proliferation, producing a macroscopically visible condyloma (*left*) and a subclinical aceto-white lesion visible only through the colposcope (*right*).

Human Papillomavirus–Induced Malignant Transformation

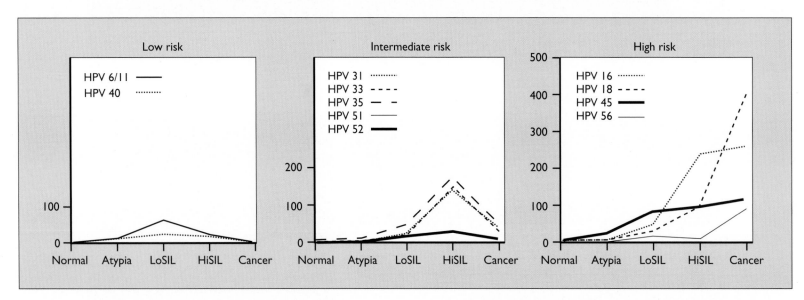

FIGURE 12-24 Odds ratios for low-risk, intermediate-risk, and high-risk HPV types and malignancy. Among the more than 70 types of HPVs that have been identified, certain types, such as 6 and 11, are associated primarily with benign genital warts, but other types, such as 16, 18, and, less frequently, 31, 35, 39, 42 to 45, and 51 to 52, are associated with malignancy of various grades. These graphs display the relative risk of malignancy found in genital infections with various HPV types. Odds ratios were calculated from a series of 2 × 2 contingency tables comparing type-specific virus testing results with histology in a case/control analysis of 2627 women. To test the hypothesis that HPV type was related to histologic grade, contingency tables for atypia of uncertain significance (*n*=270), low-grade

squamous intraepithelial lesion (LoSIL, *n*=377), high-grade SIL (HiSIL, *n*=261), and cancer (*n*=153) were profiled against the table for the control group (*n*=1566). Numerically, HPV 16 is the most important type, being represented in 47% of high-grade SILs and 47% of invasive cancers. HPVs 18, 45, and 56 are overrepresented in invasive cancers and underrepresented in high-grade SILs (27% vs 7%). Conversely, HPVs 31, 33, 35, 39, 51, 52, and 58 are overrepresented in HiSIL but underrepresented in invasive cancer (24% vs 11%). (*From* Lorincz AT, Reid R, Jenson AB: Human papillomavirus infection of the cervix: Relative risk associations of 15 common anogenital types. *Obstet Gynecol* 1992, 79:328–37, with permission.)

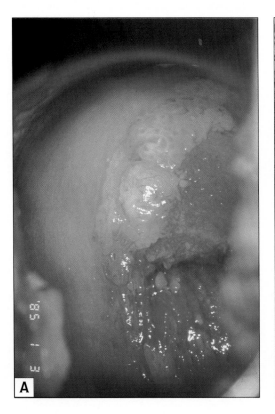

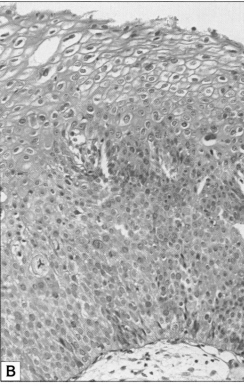

FIGURE 12-25 Low-grade cervical squamous intraepithelial lesion (LoSIL) of doubtful neoplastic potential. **A**, Colpophotograph shows a definite LoSIL at the edge of an extensive immature transformation zone. **B**, Cervical biopsy specimen shows proliferation of atypical basal cells, giving way to partial viral cytopathic effect at the surface. A prominent tripolar atypical mitotic figure is seen in the lower left. (Hematoxylin-eosin stain). Ploidy analysis showed this lesion to be polyploid, reflecting potentially reversible cellular proliferation without definite genetic alteration within the infected epithelium. (Panel 25B *from* Reid R, Fu YS: Is there a morphologic spectrum linking condyloma to cervical cancer? *In Banbury Report No. 21: Viral Etiology of Cervical Cancer.* Cold Spring Harbor, NY: Cold Spring Harbor Laboratory, 1986; with permission.)

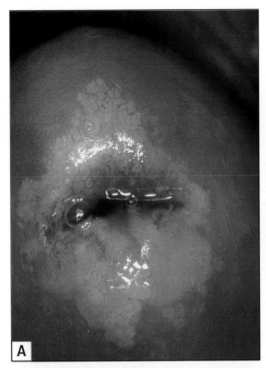

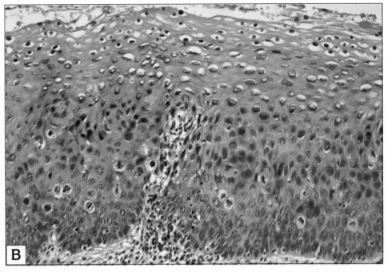

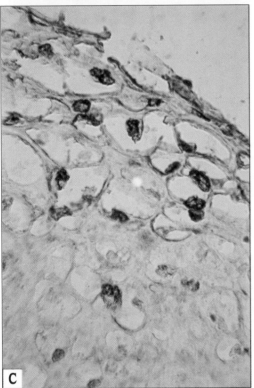

FIGURE 12-26 Low-grade squamous intraepithelial lesion (LoSIL) with undoubted potential for malignant progression. **A**, Colpophotograph shows a flat acetowhite lesion with an irregular peripheral margin, shiny gray color, and a diffuse, fine mosaic pattern. The cervix has been soaked with 5% acetic acid for several minutes, causing HPV-infected areas to become white. On the anterior lip of the cervix, there is an internal demarcation just above the new squamocolumnar junction. Below this demarcation, colposcopic characteristics change; epithelial color changes from a shiny gray to dull white, and vascular pattern changes from fine to coarse. This transition indicates that the lesion is undergoing progression from LoSIL to high-grade SIL (HiSIL). **B**, Directed biopsy shows that the lesion still has the tissue architectural pattern of a low-grade lesion, but within it are prominent cytologic features of developing HiSIL. Cells show hyperchromatism and pleomorphism. Multiple, highly abnormal mitotic figures can be seen throughout the lower half of the epithelium. Surface maturation of these abnormal basal cells results in prominent viral cytopathic effect, showing greater nuclear atypia than seen in most minor-grade lesions. The coarse punctuation seen in the colpophotograph (*panel 26A*) is reflected by the prominent intraepithelial capillary shown in this tissue section. (Hematoxylin-eosin stain.) **C**, Immunoperoxidase preparation shows late gene expression, as manifested by the brown intranuclear staining of virus-specifed capsid protein within the nuclei of some surface koilocytes. Ploidy analysis indicates that this epithelium has undergone permanent premalignant transformation.

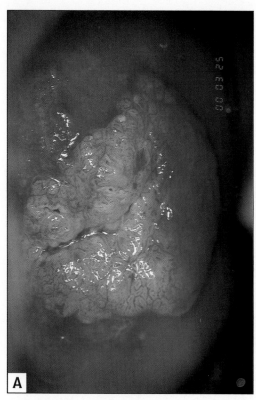
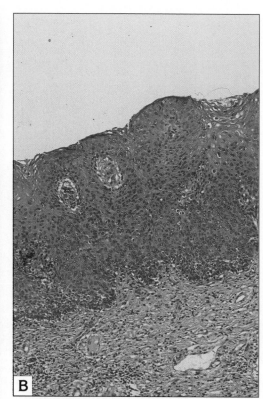
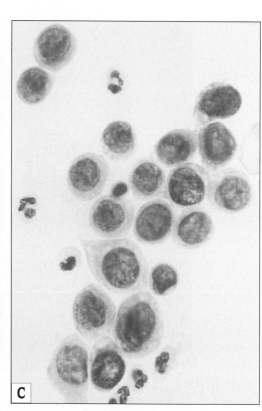

FIGURE 12-27 Diagnostic features of high-grade squamous intraepithelial lesion (HiSIL). **A,** Colpophotograph, following acetic acid soaking of a large abnormal transformation zone, shows a dull premalignant epithelium traversed by a mixture of coarse mosaic and coarse punctuation. **B,** Directed biopsy confirms the presence of a HiSIL, as manifested by full-thickness proliferation of primitive basaloid cells. Minimal focal koilocytotic atypia is seen at the *top left* and *top right*. Also, the mosaic pattern seen at colposcopy is reflected by the horizontal intraepithelial capillaries seen on the tissue section. (Hematoxylin-eosin stain.) **C,** Papanicolaou smear shows a clump of highly abnormal basal cells with increased nuclear-cytoplasmic ratio.

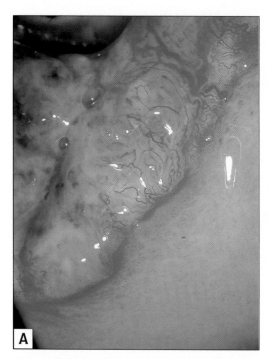
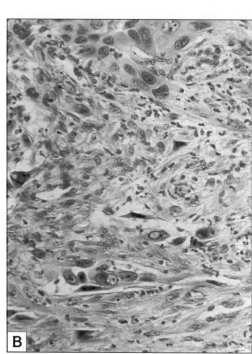
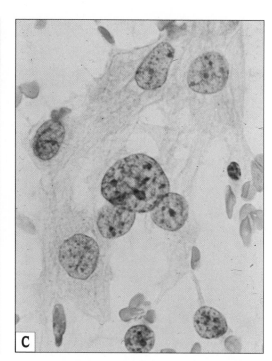

FIGURE 12-28 Diagnostic features of invasive squamous carcinoma of cervix. **A,** Colpophotograph of the right posterior cervical lip shows a rolled epithelial edge, covered by partly necrotic epithelium. Angiogenic factor produced by these metabolically active cells results in prominent neovascularization, as evidenced by the multiple, horizontal atypical vessels growing from the lesion edge toward the necrotic ulcer crater. **B,** Photomicrograph shows bizarre epithelial cells invading the lamina propria of the cervix. Toward the bottom, tumor cells have infiltrated a "capillary-like space." **C,** In a Papanicolaou smear from the same patient, similar bizarre, pleomorphic cells with prominent nucleoli are seen against a "dirty background" (fibrin deposition and erythrocytes). (Panel 28A *courtesy of* E. Pixley, MD.)

Mechanisms of Human Papillomavirus–Induced Malignant Transformation

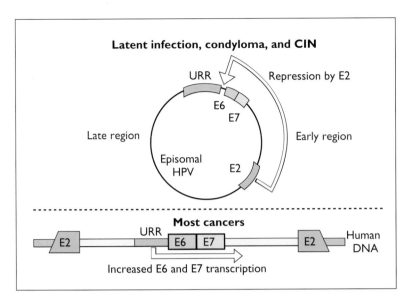

Latent infection, condyloma, and CIN

URR

Repression by E2

E6
E7

Late region

Early region

Episomal
HPV

E2

Most cancers

URR

E2

E6 E7

E2

Human
DNA

Increased E6 and E7 transcription

FIGURE 12-29 Integration of HPV DNA into host genome. The diagram contrasts the episomal relationship seen in latent infection, condyloma, and cervical intraepithelial neoplasia (CIN) (*top panel*) with the integrated pattern of HPV DNA seen in invasive cancers (*bottom panel.*) In the nonintegrated form, the viral DNA exists as a circular plasmid, in which the two transforming genes (E6 and E7) are located just downstream of the "viral brain." In the nonintegrated form, products of the E2 gene down-modulate expression of the E6 and E7 genes. Conversely, as these lesions become invasive, the circular genome of the plasmid splits at about the middle of the E2 gene, producing a linear fragment of viral chromosome in which the late genes and part of the E2 gene are located upstream from the upstream regulatory region (and thus inoperative). However, linearization does preserve the normal function of the two transforming genes, E6 and E7, leading to overexpression of oncogenic proteins. (URR—upstream regulatory region.)

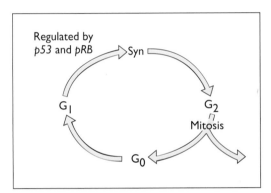

Regulated by
p53 and *pRB* → Syn

G_1

G_2
Mitosis

G_0

FIGURE 12-30 Suspected mechanism by which oncogenic HPVs induce genetic mutation. Within the replicative cycle, cells are normally held in the G_1 phase by two important anti-oncogenes, *p53* and *pRB*, while chromosomal integrity is checked by endonucleases. However, in high-risk HPV infections, the protein specified by the HPV E6 gene blocks *p53* and the protein specified by HPV E7 blocks the retinoblastoma (RB) anti-oncogene. Thus, genetically damaged cells can undergo mitotic division. With time, these genetic errors can amplify to the point of producing the gross chromosomal distortions measured by DNA microspectrophotometry.

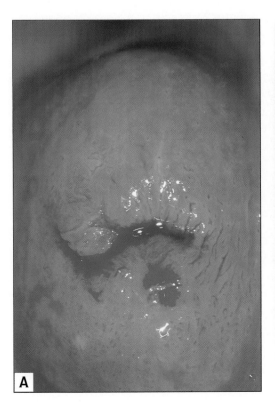

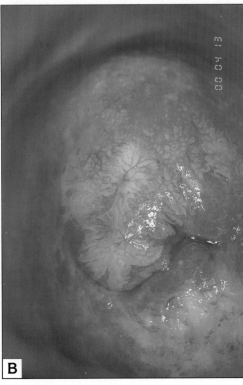

A

B

FIGURE 12-31 Progressive potential depends on HPV type. **A,** Extensive minor-grade colposcopic change is seen in a patient at the enrollment visit of a 4-year natural-history study. Cervical cytology shows atypical squamous cells of uncertain significance. Virus testing isolated HPV 16 at this initial visit. **B,** Colposcopy 7 months later shows diffuse progression to cervical intraepithelial neoplasia, grade 3 (CIN 3), on both anterior and posterior cervical lips.

CLINICAL FEATURES OF HUMAN PAPILLOMAVIRUS–ASSOCIATED VULVAR DISEASE

Distinguishing Expressed Human Papillomavirus Disease From Latent Infection or Nonspecific Mimicry

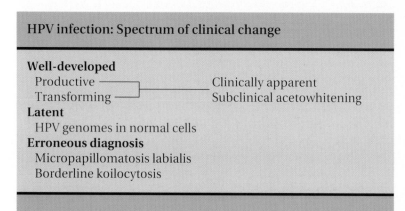

HPV infection: Spectrum of clinical change

Well-developed
  Productive ——————— Clinically apparent
  Transforming ————— Subclinical acetowhitening
Latent
  HPV genomes in normal cells
Erroneous diagnosis
  Micropapillomatosis labialis
  Borderline koilocytosis

FIGURE 12-32 Spectrum of clinical changes seen in HPV infection. Transcription and translation of viral genetic information produces virus-specified proteins that disrupt tissue growth and maturation. In permissive cells, cell–virus interaction results in prolific DNA replication and variable virion assembly, to reinitiate the cycle of infectivity. Conversely, transforming cell–virus interactions lead to premalignant tissue changes, usually associated with cumulative genetic errors within the host chromosome. Both productive and transforming infections can be either clinically apparent (visible to the naked eye) or subclinical (seen through the colposcope as acetowhite change, with or without prominent vascular patterns). In other patients, HPV genomic material can be isolated from morphologically normal keratinocytes; such latent infections presumably represent a cell–virus interaction in which there is insufficient expression of viral genes to disrupt cell growth and maturation. Finally, there is rampant clinical misdiagnosis of nonspecific acetowhitening and micropapillary epithelial change as low-grade HPV infection. Multiple studies have clearly demonstrated that such tissues contain viral genetic material at about the same rate as the normal population.

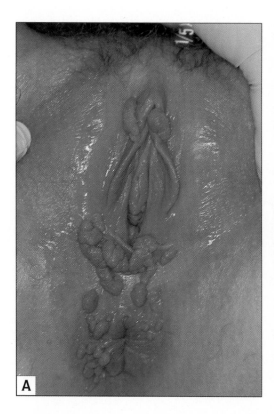
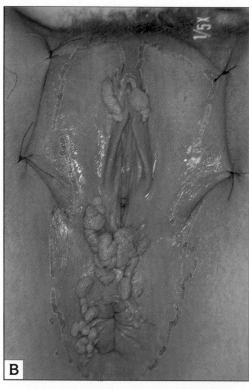

FIGURE 12-33 Acetic acid testing. Application of a 3% to 5% acetic acid solution for up to 3 minutes causes HPV-infected areas to become white, which is useful diagnostic indicator of infection. **A**, Prior to acetic acid application, multiple exophytic (clinically apparent) condylomas are visible. Surrounding skin is slightly erythematous but appears to be unaffected. **B**, After application of acetic acid, the surrounding skin shows a diffuse acetowhite change indicating HPV infection. Histologic changes within the exophytic and subclinical lesions were similar, both showing an equivalent degree of basal proliferation and surface koilocytosis. Southern blot hybridization detected the same type of viral DNA in both the exophytic and subclinical lesions. Both represent productive cell–virus interactions, and both may contain infectious virus particles.

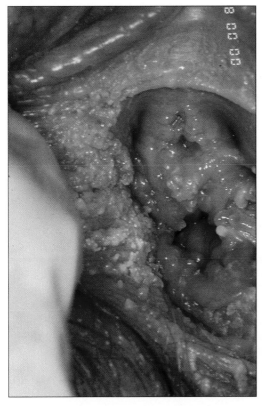

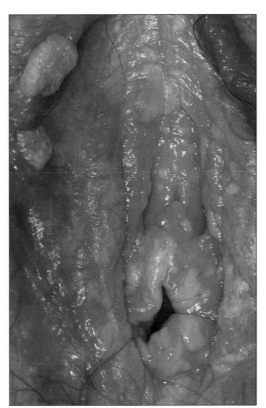

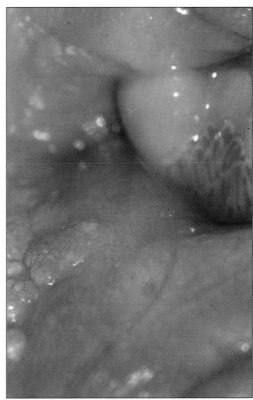

FIGURE 12-34 Micropapillomatosis labialis. Despite the superficial resemblance to condylomas, such micropapillary changes are common in normal women. Whether these appearances represent individual anatomic variation or whether they arise as a result of nonspecific irritation is uncertain. Multiple studies have demonstrated that such patients test negative with HPV DNA hybridization.

FIGURE 12-35 Multiple, slightly elevated, sharply marginated acetowhite lesions with accompanying vascular pattern. Lesions show an asymmetric distribution that crosses anatomic subdivisions of the vulvar epithelium. The patient also has two exophytic condylomas. These appearances contrast sharply with the symmetrical, anatomically confined, micropapillomatous change shown in Fig. 12-34.

FIGURE 12-36 Subtle but genuine condylomas of the vulvar vestibule. One micropapilliferous lesion is growing out of a minor vestibular gland at the hymenal edge. Other lesions are more sessile and show minimal variation in surface contour. In contrast to the pattern of diffuse single papillae seen in micropapillomatosis labialis, the fingerlike extensions on genuine condylomas arise from a central core.

Clinical Presentations of Human Papillomavirus–Associated Vulvar Lesions

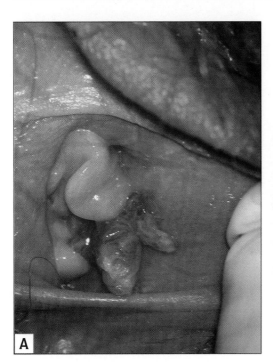

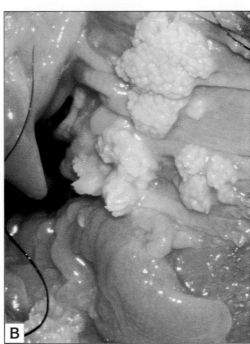

FIGURE 12-37 Mucosal papillomas. **A,** Benign condyloma arising from the Bartholin's duct. The overlying epithelium is thinned and shows minimal acetowhitening. The highly vascularized condylomatous core imparts a diffuse red color to this lesion. By comparison, the edematous flap of hymen just above the condyloma shows the normal deep pink color of the vestibular surface mucosa. **B,** Vestibular condylomas showing very dense acetowhitening, masking both the stromal microcirculation and stem vessels.

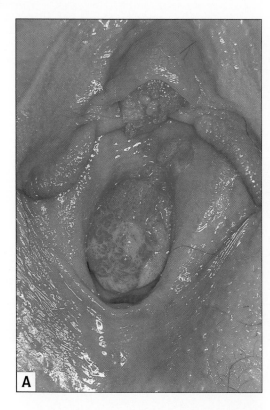

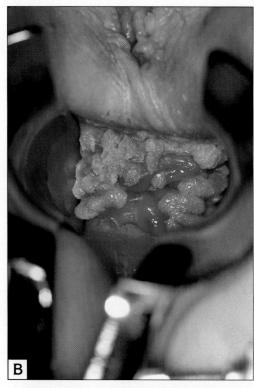

FIGURE 12-38 Condylomas of the urethra and anus. **A**, Very large, vascular condyloma mushrooming out of the external urethral meatus. Some areas have sufficient acetowhitening to hide the vascularity of the underlying microcirculation. Other areas show intensely red vessels highlighted against a suffused deep pink of the well-vascularized stroma. A second condyloma of similar appearance is projecting from beneath the prepuce clitoris. **B**, Densely acetowhite lesions distributed circumferentially within the anal canal of an adult woman. The degree of acetowhitening is sufficient to mask the diffuse red color of the underlying microcirculation but not to hide the stem vessels within the condylomatous core. Isolated anal condylomas can be seen in any infected woman, but this circumferential distribution is suggestive of spread by anal intercourse.

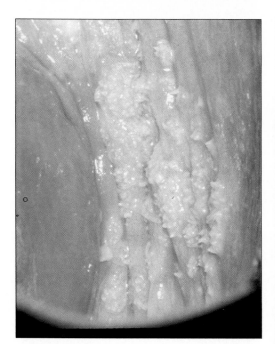

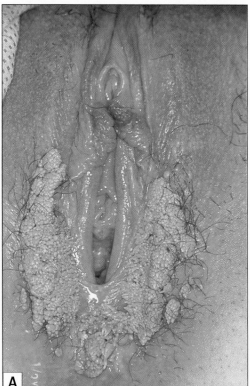

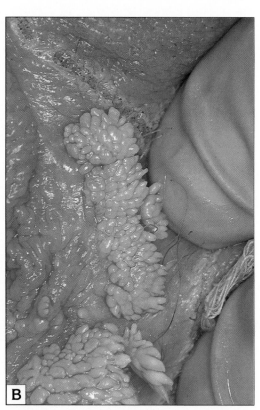

FIGURE 12-39 Condylomas of the vaginal mucosa. A colpophotograph shows a sessile, micropapillary plaque of acetowhite epithelium on the left lateral fornix. The faintly acetowhite edge of a trivial cervical lesion is visible at the far left of this photograph.

FIGURE 12-40 Condylomas of nonglabrous skin. **A**, Classic appearance of recent-onset condylomas within the nonglabrous skin. There is sufficient surface keratosis to make these lesions flesh-colored prior to the application of acetic acid. With vinegar soaking, the lesions are highlighted by prominent acetowhitening, sufficient to mask the underlying vascularity. **B**, The top left portion of the lesion from the same patient, seen at higher magnification.

CLINICAL FEATURES OF HUMAN PAPILLOMAVIRUS–ASSOCIATED CERVICAL DISEASE

Colposcopic grading scheme for HPV-induced cervical disease

Colposcopic sign	0 points	1 point	2 points
Margin	Condylomatous or micropapillary contour Indistinct acetowhitening Flocculated or feathered margins Angular, jagged lesions Satellite lesions and acetowhitening extending beyond transformation zone	Regular lesions with smooth, straight outlines	Rolled, peeling edges Internal demarcations between areas of differing appearance
Color	Shiny, snow white Indistinct acetowhitening	Intermediate shade (shiny gray)	Dull, oyster white
Vessels	Fine-caliber vessels, poorly formed patterns Condylomatous or micropapillary lesions	Absent vessels	Definite punctation or mosaicism
Iodine	Positive iodine staining Minor iodine negativity	Partial iodine uptake	Negative staining of significant lesion

FIGURE 12-41 Colposcopic grading scheme for HPV-associated cervical disease. An index of four statistically independent colposcopic signs, each of which has a morphologic category typical of a low-grade lesion (0 points), a category typical of a high-grade lesion (2 points), and a category intermediate in severity (1 point). Although colposcopic grading is not a formal requirement of the triage process, clinical anticipation of histologic severity adds to physician comfort and patient safety. Many lesions can be adequately managed by conscientious adherence to a triage algorithm, but a sharp eye for colposcopic detail is an important safeguard in subtle cases. (*From* Reid R, Scalzi P: Genital warts and cervical cancer: VII. An improved colposcopic index for differentiating benign papillomaviral infections from high-grade cervical intraepithelial neoplasia. *Am J Obstet Gynecol* 1985, 153:611–618; with permission.)

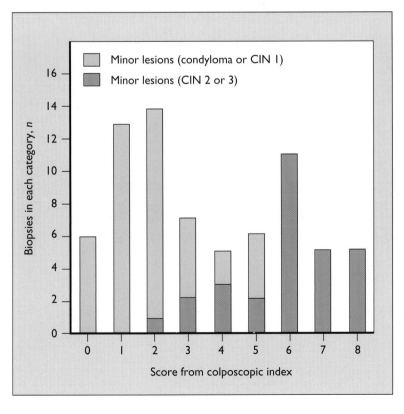

FIGURE 12-42 Bar graph correlating colposcopic score to eventual histology. Scores < 3 almost always correlate with low-grade histology, and scores > 5 almost always correlate with high-grade, aneuploid lesions. Scores between 3 and 5 represent an area of overlap within this continuous morphologic spectrum; in general, such lesions correlate with cervical intraepithelial neoplasia, grade 2 (CIN 2). (*From* Reid R, Stanhope CR, Herschman BR, *et al.* Genital warts and cervical cancer: IV. A colposcopic index for differentiating subclinical papillomaviral infection from cervical intraepithelial neoplasia. *Am J Obstet Gynecol* 1984, 149:815–823; with permission.)

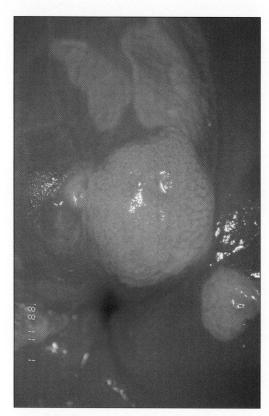

FIGURE 12-43
Colposcopic grading of minor-grade lesions. A colpophotograph of a relatively mature transformation zone shows two sessile exophytic condylomas with shiny snow-white color and fine-caliber punctate vessels. Because the only real difference between exophytic and flat (subclinical) condylomas is whether the vascular scaffolding protrudes above the plane of the surrounding epithelium, subclinical acetowhite lesions would be expected to manifest similar colposcopic changes.

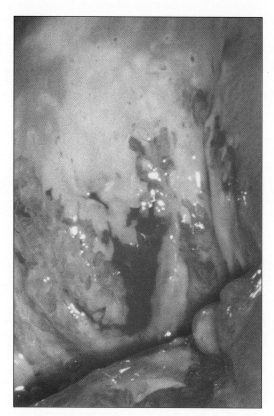

FIGURE 12-44
Colposcopic signs of high-grade lesions. An extensive dull, oyster-white epithelium shows a "peeling" margin (epithelial detachment) on both anterior and posterior lips.

TREATMENT OF HUMAN PAPILLOMAVIRUS–ASSOCIATED GENITAL DISEASE

A. Treatment of vulvovaginal HPV infections: Physical methods

Method	Advantage	Disadvantage	Clinical role
Scissor excision of isolated lesions	Yields tissue for histology or viral typing Removal of large papillomas may allow chemical destruction of remaining smaller lesions	Cumbersome (local anesthesia, suture, instruments) Epithelial denudation and bleeding, if done to excess	Baseline biopsy Removal of large lesions
Localized physical destruction Hot cautery Liquid nitrogen Laser spot welding	Immediate eradication of papillomas	Cumbersome (local anesthesia, special equipment) Time-consuming for physician Local infection or scarring more common than with chemical methods	Destruction of isolated refractory papillomas

FIGURE 12-45 Treatment of vulvovaginal HPV infection. **A.** Physical methods. *(continued)*

B. Treatment of vulvovaginal HPV infection: Chemical methods

Method	Advantage	Disadvantage	Clinical role
Desiccant acids 85% trichloracetic acid in 70% alcohol Bichloracetic acid	Quickest and easiest method Sterile instruments not required Can be used on mucosal surfaces (vagina, rectum, mouth)	Requires weekly or second-weekly office visits Less effective for cutaneous (rather than mucosal) warts; safe during pregnancy	Highly effective for localized mucosal papillomas Moderately effective for localized cutaneous lesions
Crude podophyllin extracts (*eg*, 25% podophyllin in benzoin)	None	Crude, nonstandardized mixture of toxins and active lignans Rare but severe toxicity No more effective than desiccant acids	Obsolete
Podophyllotoxin	Selective destruction of condylomatous areas, with sparing of normal epithelium Self-application regimens more effective than single-dose office therapies	Cannot be used on highly absorptive surfaces (vagina, rectum) Contraindicated during pregnancy	Highly effective for cutaneous condylomas Effective for vulvar mucosal lesions of limited extent
Cytolytic 5-fluorouracil regimens	Nonsurgical method of lesion eradication Can forestall diffuse postoperative recurrence, if therapy begins before extensive papilloma formation	Brutally painful alternative to skilled CO_2 laser photovaporization Potentially teratogenic	Effective for extensive, exophytic vaginal condylomas Valuable postoperative "rescue" strategy
α- or γ-Interferon (as primary therapy)	Biologic substances with documented antiviral and immunomodulatory actions Nonsurgical method of lesion eradication	Primary success rates have been disappointing and unpredictable Intralesional regimens are slow, expensive, and painful Systemic regimens require high dosages, with corresponding side effects	Value as primary therapy not established Valuable as adjuvant

C. Treatment of vulvovaginal HPV infection: Surgical methods

Method	Advantage	Disadvantage	Clinical role
Segmental excision and primary closure	Tissue available for histology, if genuine doubt exists	Tissue removal is fundamentally undesirable	Essentially outmoded by CO_2 laser surgery
Extensive electrodiathermy ("Bovie" destruction)	Equipment readily available	Morbid recovery and unacceptable scarring	Outmoded in western society
Extended laser ablation	Can eradicate any volume of disease epithelium, with negligible scarring Removes entire field of active HPV expression, irrespective of size, shape, or location Anatomic methods of depth control allow destruction of VIN 3 within pilosebaceous ducts	Requires sophisticated laser instrumentation and highly developed physician skills Not appropriate for simpler cases Cannot prevent subsequent reactivation of latent viral reservoir Not an appropriate alternative to simpler methods	Very extensive condylomas (coalescent papillomas occupying ≥ 30% of vulva and perineum) Refractory condylomas (disease not controlled by ≥ 9 mos of office therapy) High-grade intraepithelial neoplasia (VIN 2–3 and PAIN 2–3)

PAIN—perianal intraepithelial neoplasia; VIN—vulvar intraepithelial neoplasia.

FIGURE **12-45** *(continued)* **B**, Chemical methods. **C**, Surgical methods. *(Continued)*

D. Treatment of vulvovaginal HPV infection: Adjuvant therapies

Method	Advantage	Disadvantage	Clinical role
Noncytolytic 5-fluorouracil	Relatively inexpensive Minimal systemic absorption Effective in immunosup- pressed patients	Limited efficacy (especially in simpler cases) Poorly tolerated in patients of fair complexion Distressing side effects (vaginal scarring, vestibular ulcera- tion, possible vulvodynia)	Essential for controlling HPV disease in immuno- suppressed patients
Low-dose adjuvant interferon	Biologic substance with docu- mented antiviral and immunomodulatory actions Adjuvant effect documented in controlled trial (interferon > 5-fluorouracil or surgery alone)	Potential leukopenic and hepa- totoxic effects May not be effective in immunosuppressed patients Theoretical risk of organ rejec- tion in allograft recipients	Probably indicated in immunocompetent patients with disease severe enough to warrant extended laser ablation

Figure 12-45 *(continued)* **D**, Adjuvant therapies (for controlling the residual viral reservoir following primary therapy).

Treatment of external genital and perianal warts

Cryotherapy with liquid nitrogen or cryoprobe
Podophylotoxin, 0.5% solution for self-treatment, applied twice
    daily for 3 days followed by 4 days without therapy
Podophyllin, 10%–25% in compound tincture of benzoin,
    washed off in 1–4 hrs and repeated weekly
Trichloracetic acid, 80%–90%, applied to warts and neutralized
    with talc or sodium bicarbonate
Electrodessication or electrocautery

Figure 12-46 Centers for Disease Control and Prevention recommendations for treatment of external genital and perianal warts. The goal of treatment is the elimination of exophytic warts and the alleviation of signs and symptoms. No therapy has been shown to eradicate HPV. Cryotherapy is relatively inexpensive but requires special equipment and is moderately painful during the procedure. Podophyllotoxin is available by prescription and may be self-applied for up to four cycles. Podophyllin may require multiple treatments and can cause ulceration if applied too liberally or not washed off. Neither podophyllotoxin nor podophyllin should be used in pregnancy. Trichloracetic acid is about as effective as podophyllin, suggesting that 50% of patients will experience complete disappearance of warts. Electrical destruction of warts requires local anesthesia. Data on the efficacy of all of these regimens are limited. Recurrences are common and probably relate to the virus remaining in normal-appearing skin. Treatment with interferon is costly and accompanied by many side effects, and it is not recommended as primary therapy for simple genital warts. (Centers for Disease Control and Prevention: 1993 Sexually transmitted diseases treatment guidelines. *MMWR* 1993, 42(RR-14):83–88.)

Treatment of vaginal warts

Cryotherapy with liquid nitrogen
Trichloracetic acid, 80%–90%, applied to
    warts and neutralized with talc or
    sodium bicarbonate
Podophyllin, 10%–25%, in compound
    tincture of benzoin

Figure 12-47 Centers for Disease Control and Prevention recommendations for treatment of vaginal warts. The use of a cryoprobe in the vagina is not recommended because of the risk of vaginal perforation and fistula formation. Because of concern about potential systemic absorption, some experts caution against the use of podophyllin in the vagina. Podophyllin is contraindicated in pregnancy. (Centers for Disease Control and Prevention: 1993 Sexually transmitted diseases treatment guidelines. *MMWR* 1993, 42(RR-14):83–88.)

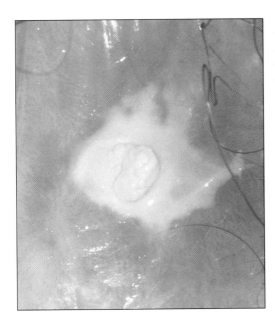

FIGURE 12-48 Vulvar condyloma treated by application of 85% trichloracetic acid.

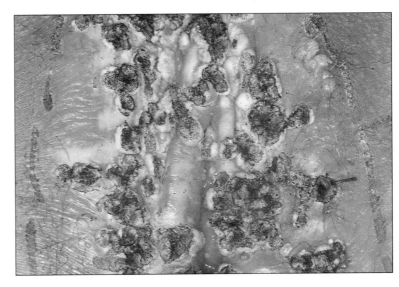

FIGURE 12-49 CO_2 laser "spot welding" of multiple vulvar condylomas. When papilloma density reaches this severity, better results can be achieved from extended laser ablation—meaning en bloc but shallow destruction of both clinically evident and subclinical disease.

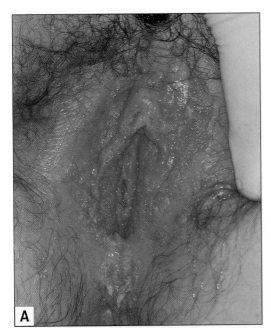

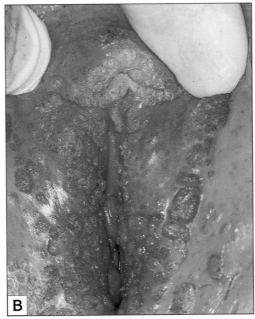

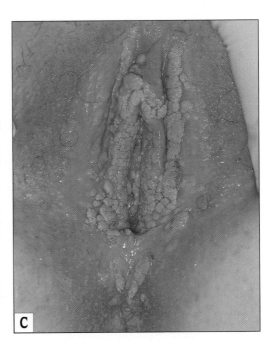

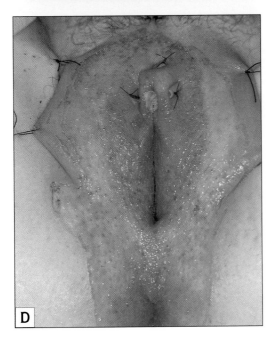

FIGURE 12-50 Treatment of HPV vaginal condylomas by extended laser ablation. **A** and **B**, Pretreatment view of extensive recent-onset condylomas affecting about 80% of the central vulvar epithelium (*panel 50A*), with involvement of the prepuce and glans clitoris (*panel 50B*). **C**, Acetic acid soaking shows extent of subclinical lesions. HPV DNA was detected in both the exophytic and subclinical lesions. **D**, Posttreatment appearance after CO_2 laser to the papillary dermis (second surgical plane). A pledget of Owen's cloth (parachute silk) has been sewn between the glans and prepuce to prevent cross-agglutination during healing.

SELECTED BIBLIOGRAPHY

Bonnez W, Reichman RC: Papillomaviruses. *In* Mandell GL, Bennett JE, Dolin R (eds.): *Principles and Practice of Infectious Diseases*, 4th ed. New York: Churchill Livingstone; 1995:1387–1400.

Campion MJ: Clinical manifestations and natural history of genital human papillomavirus infection. *Obstet Gynecol Clin North Am* 1987, 14:363–388.

Reid R: Biology and colposcopic features of human papillomavirus-associated cervical disease. *Obstet Gynecol Clin North Am* 1993, 20:123–151.

Reid R: Laser therapy of human papillomavirus infections. *In* Keye W (ed.): *Laser Surgery in Gynecology and Obstetrics*, 2nd ed. Chicago: Year Book Publishers; 1989:46–99.

Reid R, Absten G: Lasers in gynecology: Why pragmatic surgeons have not abandoned this valuable technology. *Lasers Surg Med* 1995 (in press).

CHAPTER 13

Ectoparasitic Infestations

Navjeet K. Sidhu-Malik
Michael F. Rein

PEDICULOSIS PUBIS (CRAB OR PUBIC LICE)

Physical findings in pediculosis pubis	
Lice	97%
Nits	80%
Excreta	14%
Maculae ceruleae	1%

FIGURE 13-1 Physical findings in pediculosis pubis. Patients infested with the crab louse, *Phthirus pubis*, are said to have crabs, or pediculosis pubis. Affected individuals usually complain of marked pruritus in the pubic hair region and often see the lice, which are approximately 1 mm long. Patients also may notice the nits attached to the hair shafts or find the crab excreta, which are brownish-red dots, on the skin or underwear. Physical examination reveals the associated findings in a large percentage of patients, although lice and nits many be very few in number and require a diligent search with a hand lens to detect. (Brown S, Becher J, Brady W: Treatment of ectoparasitic infections: Review of the English-language literature, 1982–1992. *Clin Infect Dis* 1995, 20(suppl 1):S104–S109.)

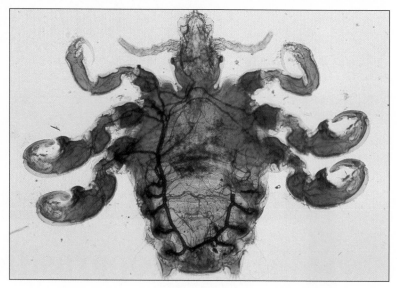

FIGURE 13-2 *Phthirus pubis*, the pubic louse. Lice are wingless, blood-sucking insects with three pair of legs. Pubic lice are 1 to 2 mm long, shorter than head or body lice, with widely spaced legs. Claws on their second and third pairs of legs allow them to grab coarse hairs. A mature female lives for approximately 17 to 28 days, during which time she lays 30 to 50 eggs. Eggs mature in 7 to 8 days, and the louse larva requires a blood meal before undergoing two molts to become a mature adult in 30 days. Unlike the body louse, which is a carrier of several diseases including typhus, the crab louse transmits no known diseases.

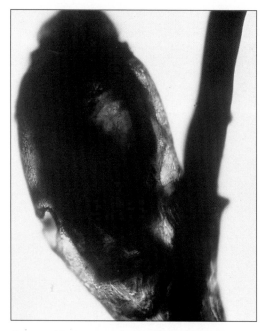

FIGURE 13-3 Pubic louse nit (egg) containing an immature nymph attached to hair shaft. Nits contain the unhatched eggs enclosed in a firm casing, and the empty casings remain attached to the hair after the nymph has hatched. Empty casings appear white. Nits are firmly adherent and cannot readily be pulled off the hairs.

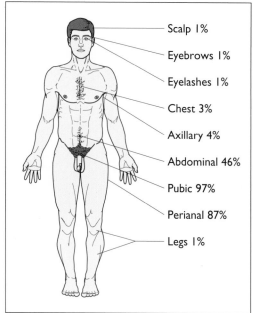

Scalp 1%
Eyebrows 1%
Eyelashes 1%
Chest 3%
Axillary 4%
Abdominal 46%
Pubic 97%
Perianal 87%
Legs 1%

FIGURE 13-4 Sites of infestation with *Phthirus pubis*. *P. pubis* can move up to about 10 cm per day and can also be transported on hands or inanimate objects to other parts of the body. This figure shows the distribution of pubic lice among patients attending a clinic for sexually transmitted diseases. Although pubic lice are usually acquired during sexual contact, they may also be spread by shared clothing or beds, or even by the toilet seat. Patients with pubic lice should be screened for other sexually transmitted diseases. (Billstein S: Human lice. *In* Holmes KK, Mårdh P-A, Sparling PF, Wiesner PJ (eds.): *Sexually Transmitted Disease*, 2nd ed. New York: McGraw-Hill; 1990:467–471. Chapel TA, Katta T, Kusamar T, *et al.*: Pediculosis pubis in a clinic for the treatment of sexually transmitted diseases. *Sex Transm Dis* 1979, 6:257.)

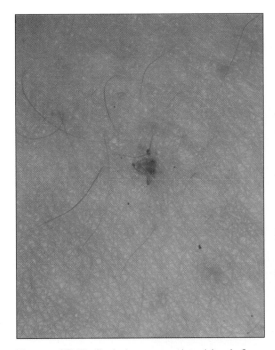

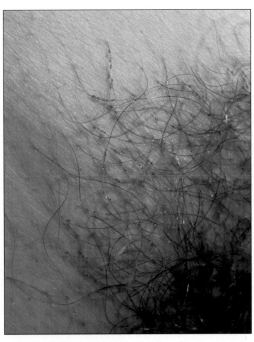

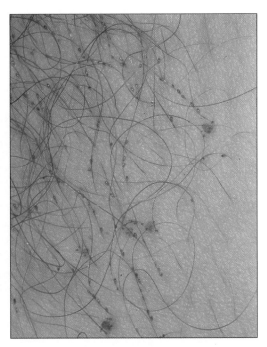

FIGURE 13-5 Crab louse on the skin. Infestation occurs from close body-to-body contact. It is most common in the pubic area, but crabs may also be found in other areas of the body with short hairs, including the axillae, eyelashes, beard, or scalp.

FIGURE 13-6 Pediculosis pubis of groin with a large number of nits attached to the pubic hairs. Human infestation by lice has been reported for thousands of years, with early references noted in the Old Testament of the Bible (Exodus 8:12–15). Lice are insects belonging to the order Anoplura and include the two genera that infest humans, *Phthirus pubis* and *Pediculus humanus*. Of these *P. pubis* is most commonly transmitted by sexual contact.

FIGURE 13-7 Infestation of the pubic hair by crab lice. The crab lice can be seen attached between the hairs, and a large number of nits are attached to the hair shafts. The diagnosis is made by clinical examination of affected areas to detect the adult lice and nits. The crab lice are often found at the base of hairs, with the terminal claws of their legs grabbing the hairs and their heads embedded in the skin. The nits appear as small dots of firm material along the hair shaft.

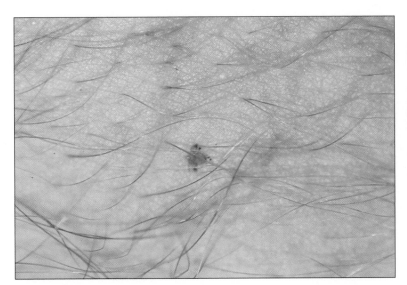

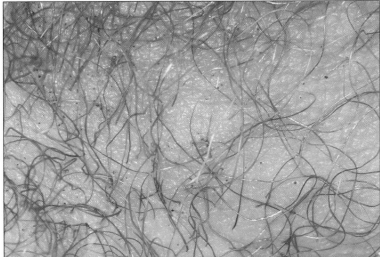

FIGURE 13-8 Crab louse at the base of a hair shaft. Lice can be difficult to see without use of a hand lens. They may appear as small specks or freckles, and only rarely are they found moving.

FIGURE 13-9 Louse feces on skin. The feces are deposited after a blood meal and appear as reddish-brown dots on the affected skin. They may also be found in the underwear by the patient or examiner.

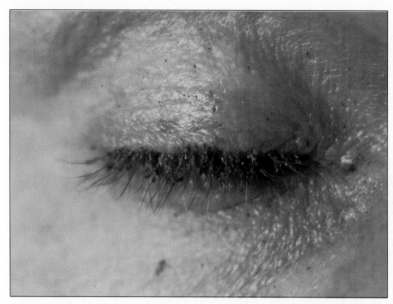

FIGURE 13-10 Louse infestation of the eyelid. A large number of nits are attached to the eyelashes of this patient, and louse feces are observed on the lids.

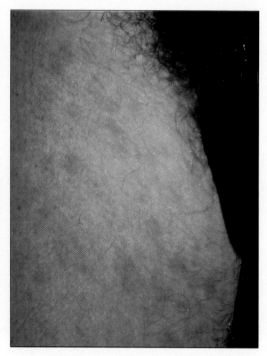

FIGURE 13-11 Maculae ceruleae (blue spots) on the thigh of a patient with pediculosis pubis. Maculae ceruleae are a rare clinical finding that present as slate-gray to blue macules measuring 0.5 to 1 cm in diameter. They are only found in *Phthirus pubis* infestation and are thought to result from the body's reaction to louse saliva, which contains an anticoagulant.

Recommended treatment regimens for pediculosis pubis

Lindane 1% shampoo	Apply for 4 min to all hairy areas of body except for eyebrows and eyelashes, and then thoroughly wash off
or	
Permethrin 1% cream rinse	Apply to affected areas and wash off after 10 min
or	
Pyrethrins with piperonyl butoxide	Apply to affected areas and wash off after 10 min

FIGURE 13-12 Recommended treatment regimens for pediculosis pubis. Three agents used as single applications are recommended by the Centers for Disease Control and Prevention for the treatment of pubic lice. Some experts recommend two applications 4 days apart to kill the hatchlings of any nits surviving the initial treatment. None of these regimens appears toxic when application is limited to the recommended intervals. Clinical data on the effectiveness of these regimens are severely limited, and practitioners have tended to extrapolate from data on pediculosis capitis. (Centers for Disease Control and Prevention: 1993 Sexually transmitted diseases treatment guidelines. *MMWR* 1993; 42(RR-14):94-95.)

Considerations in the treatment of pediculosis pubis

Pregnant or lactating women should not be treated with lindane

Bedding and clothing should be decontaminated or removed from the body for 72 hrs

Fumigation of living areas is not necessary

Sexual contacts within the past month should be epidemiologically treated

The regimens should not be applied to the eyes

FIGURE 13-13 Considerations in the treatment of pediculosis pubis. Pediculosis of the eyelids should be treated with the application of an occlusive ophthalmic ointment to the margins of the eyelids twice daily for 10 days. Bedding and clothing should be decontaminated by machine washing and drying on hot cycle or by dry cleaning, or it should be removed from body contact for at least 72 hours. Pregnant or lactating women should be treated with permethrin or pyrethrins with piperonyl butoxide. Epidemiologic treatment refers to the practice of treating sexual partners even before the disease is clinically manifest or the diagnosis confirmed; it is based on the observed high incidence of disease among sexual partners.

SCABIES

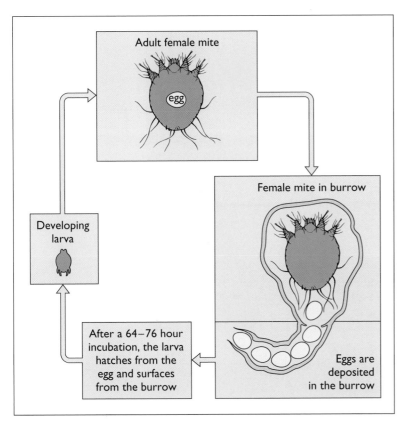

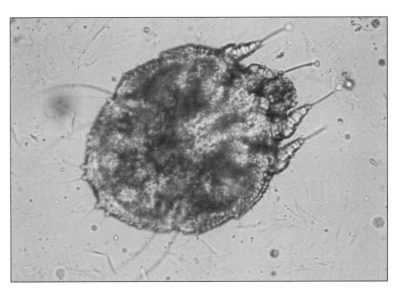

FIGURE 13-15 Adult *Sarcoptes scabiei*, the scabies mite. The adult mite is about 0.35 mm long and has four pairs of legs. The nymphs have three pairs of legs. The mite is an obligate human parasite that can survive away from human hosts for only about 2 days. The mite is extremely contagious via body-to-body contact, and scabies is usually transmitted by sexual contact, although nonvenereal (nosocomial) scabies is well described in nursing homes and child-care centers. The organism can be transmitted via shared clothing.

FIGURE 13-14 Life cycle of *Sarcoptes scabiei* var *hominis*. The adult gravid female scabies mite seeks out moist thin skin where she burrows into the stratum corneum. She is able to lay two to three eggs per day for 30 days. Each egg hatches after 3 to 4 days' incubation, and the larvae feed, molt, and become mature adults in 9 to 12 days. The males die quickly, but female mites can live for 4 to 6 weeks. The infestation is referred to as scabies and has a worldwide distribution. The scabies mite is not a vector for other infectious diseases, although other mites can carry such infections as rickettsialpox and scrub typhus.

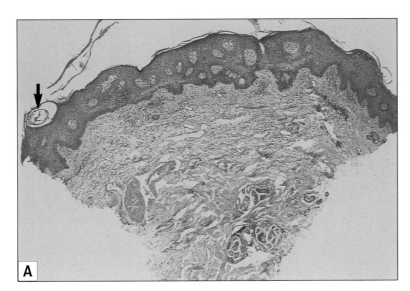

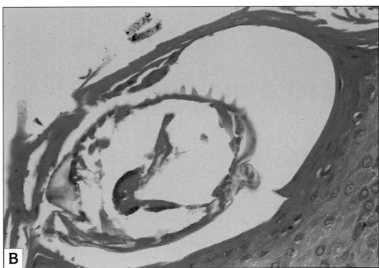

FIGURE 13-16 Burrow containing a scabies mite. **A**, A punch biopsy specimen of skin stained with hematoxylin-eosin reveals a mite burrowed into the superficial stratum corneum. The mite is seen on the left edge of the specimen (*arrow*) on this low-power magnification. **B**, Higher magnification reveals a section of the female mite.

Histologic examination can show the presence of mite, eggs, egg shells, or fecal material. There may be spongiosis surrounding the mite, and a variable dermal infiltrate with eosinophils may be present. (Lever WF, Schamburg-Lever G: *Histopathology of the Skin*, 7th ed. Philadelphia: J.B. Lippincott; 1990:237–238.)

Penile Scabies

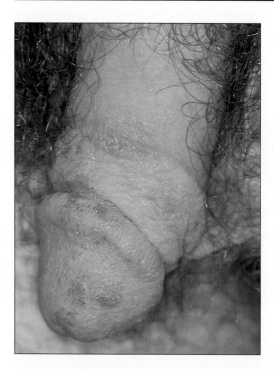

FIGURE 13-17
Penile scabies. Typical lesions in penile scabies are erythematous and scattered over the glans and shaft. The primary symptom of scabies is intense pruritus in the affected areas, and the penis is a prominent site. Itching is typically worse at night or after bathing. In primary infestation, it takes 1 month for sensitization and itching to begin, but in recurrent infestations the itching may begin sooner.

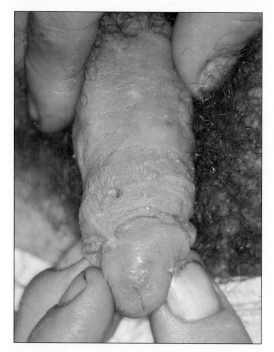

FIGURE 13-18
Penile scabies with weeping lesions. Typically penile lesions are often weepy and crusted. Herpetic lesions also often heal with crusts but are far less pruritic at that stage; in addition, herpetic lesions are often clustered rather than scattered over the penis.

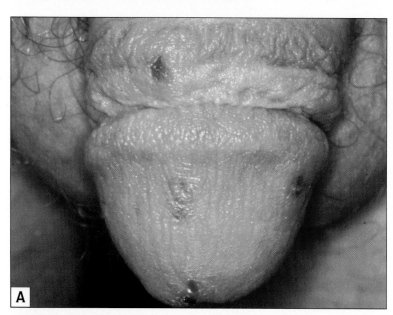

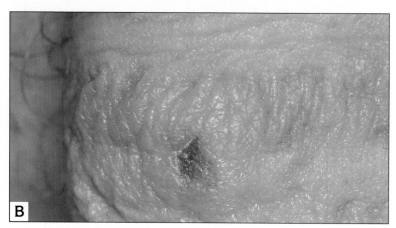

FIGURE 13-19 A and **B.** Penile scabies with crusted, indurated lesions. The lesions of scabies are sometimes slightly indurated. Clinical lesions can include papules, vesicles, nodules, and crusting. Careful examination may reveal a burrow where the mite has buried itself into the skin, but often these are obliterated by scratching.

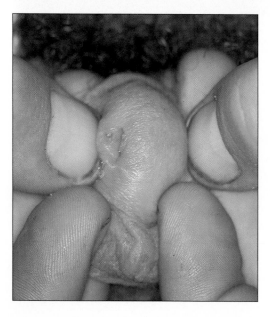

FIGURE 13-20
Perimeatal scabies on the penis. Scabies lesions may be present very near the urethra. This patient suffered from mild dysuria, which resolved when the scabies was treated. Patients with scabies should be screened for coincident sexually transmitted diseases, and dysuria should prompt consideration of an accompanying nongonococcal urethritis.

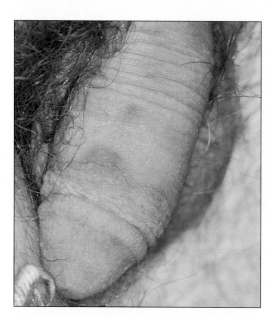

FIGURE 13-21
Penile scabies with nodular lesions. Especially late in infection, the lesions of scabies may be nodular rather than crusted. The nodular variant can be present with active infestation and may persist even after treatment. This variant is thought to represent a persistent inflammatory reaction to the mite.

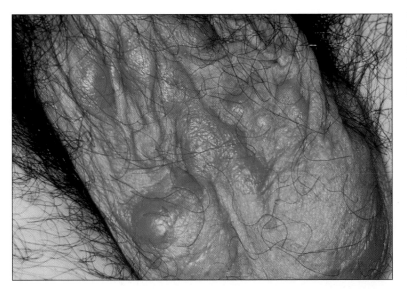

FIGURE 13-22 Scabies of the scrotum. This patient manifests nodular lesions of the scrotum. It may be difficult to demonstrate mites in nodules, particularly if they have been present for several weeks. The nodules may result in part from a hypersensitivity reaction and may persist for months after the infection has been cured.

Extragenital Involvement

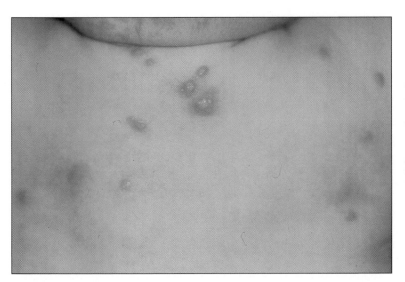

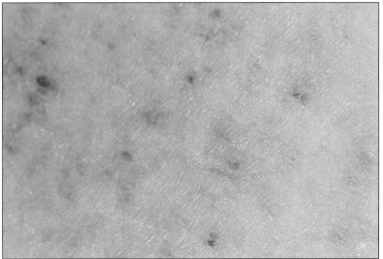

FIGURE 13-23 Nodular scabies on the back of an infected child. Vesicular lesions may be seen in children but are rarely observed in adult cases. In the adult, the upper back is rarely involved, and involvement of the scalp, face, neck, palms, and soles is also quite rare. The presence of lesions in these anatomical sites in adults should suggest a different or additional diagnosis.

FIGURE 13-24 Gluteal skin in scabies. *Sarcoptes scabiei* can travel quickly over human skin (2.5 cm/min), and lesions are frequently found along the belt line and over the pelvic girdle. Typical crusted lesions are seen over the buttocks in this patient. In adults, common sites of involvement include finger webspaces, belt line, genitalia (especially the penis in men), buttocks, and axillae. The head is generally spared. In children, involvement differs in that the head can be affected along with axillae, diaper area, wrists, hands, and feet. (Mellanby K: Biology of the parasite. *In* Orkin M, *et al.* (eds.): *Scabies and Pediculosis.* Philadelphia: J.B. Lippincott; 1977:8–16.)

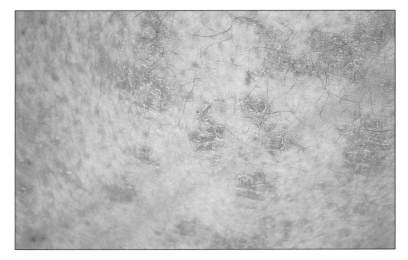

FIGURE 13-25 Scabies involving the thigh. In more chronic cases, the lesions are lichenified and scaly. In occasional patients, urticaria may be the predominant cutaneous manifestation.

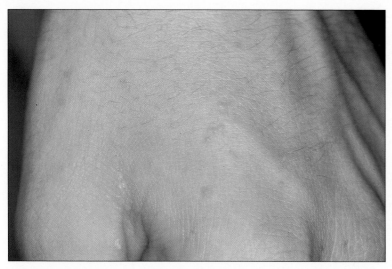

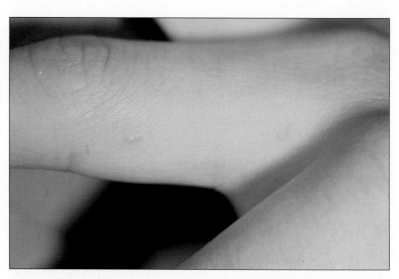

FIGURE 13-26 Scabies of the hand, showing typical moist papules. The hands are commonly involved in venereal scabies and may be the first site of symptoms. The typical moist papules of scabies are seen in this patient. (Orkin M, Maibach HI: Scabies. *In* Holmes KK, Mårdh P-A, Sparling PF, Wiesner PJ (eds.): *Sexually Transmitted Diseases*, 2nd ed. New York: McGraw-Hill; 1990:473–479.)

FIGURE 13-27 Scabies of the hand. Lesions commonly occur along the side of the digits and in the interdigital webs. Here, typical papular lesions are observed near the proximal interphalangeal joint and at the base of the finger.

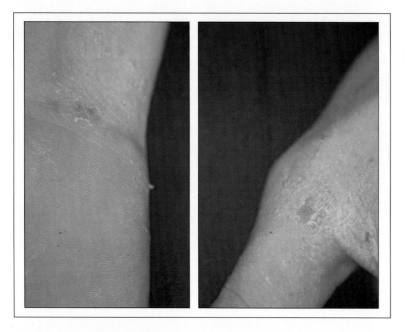

FIGURE 13-28 Scabies of the interdigital web (*right*) and wrist (*left*). The wrist is also commonly involved in scabies. In this patient, scabies involves the hand and wrist with marked excoriation. Severe pruritus of the genital area accompanied by pruritus of the wrists or ankles should suggest the diagnosis of scabies.

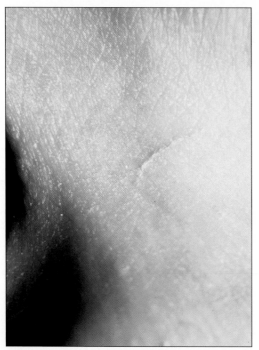

FIGURE 13-29 Scabies burrow on the lateral aspect of the finger. Threadlike burrows, which are pathognomonic for scabies, are most often observed between the fingers or on the wrists and occasionally on the penis. They are frequently obscured by excoriation. Burrows may be better visualized if fountain-pen ink is applied to the skin and wiped off after 5 minutes. The ink may enter the burrow and stain it. Papules at the end of the burrows contain the mites and eggs and are a fruitful area for diagnostic scraping. (Woodley D, Saurat JH: The burrow ink test and the scabies mite. *J Am Acad Dermatol* 1981, 4:715.) (*From* Parlett HW: Scabietic infestations of men. *Cutis* 1975, 16:47–51; with permission.)

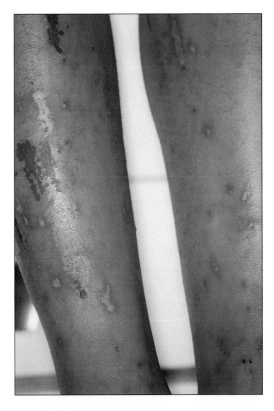

FIGURE 13-30 Scabies involving the legs. Untreated scabies can be chronic, leading to the title "seven-year itch." Here, chronic scratching has led to a reaction resembling prurigo nodularis.

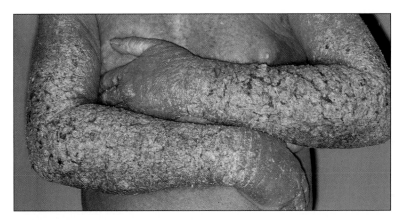

FIGURE 13-31 Norwegian scabies presenting with hyperkeratotic crusting of the arms. Norwegian scabies occurs most commonly in the immunocompromised or neurologically impaired host, with an increasing number of cases reported in HIV-positive patients. Itching may not be present, and burrows are generally not evident on examination. Whereas scabies in the normal host generally represents a minimal mite burden (with estimates in the range of one to 20 mites), in hypertrophic scabies a large number of mites are present. This increased mite load makes treatment difficult, and often multiple treatment applications are necessary for eradication. The scabies in these patients is also very contagious, with high risk of spread to health-care workers and other contacts.

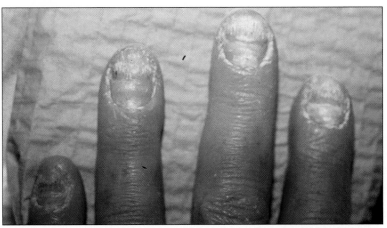

FIGURE 13-32 Norwegian (hypertrophic) scabies with crusting under the fingernails. Crusts in hypertrophic scabies represent a reservoir for mites. In cases resistant to treatment, it is essential to ensure that such "forgotten" areas are treated.

Diagnosis and Treatment

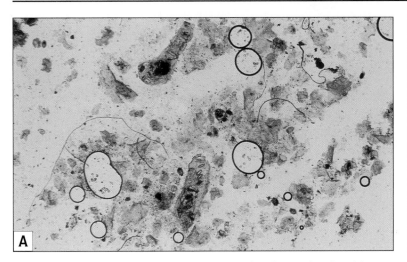

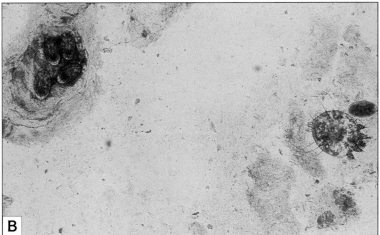

FIGURE 13-33 Microscopic examination in the diagnosis of scabies. Scabies is usually diagnosed clinically from the typical distribution of markedly pruritic lesions. When the diagnosis is in doubt, a fresh lesion may be scraped and the diagnosis of scabies infestation confirmed microscopically by identifying the mite, egg, or feces (scybala). Suspicious burrows or papules are scraped with a #15 blade; a drop of mineral oil or immersion oil on the edge of the blade prevents the scraped material from falling off. The sample is then covered with mineral oil and cover slip and examined under the microscope. The scabies mite is too small to observe without magnification. **A.** This low-power microscopic view reveals a large amount of scale and debris, with several mites in the field. **B.** Higher-power microscopic examination of the same preparation confirms the presence of the mite (*right*) and several unhatched eggs (*left*).

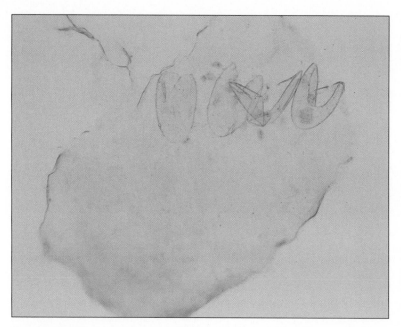

FIGURE 13-34 High-power microscopic view of empty egg casings in scabies.

Recommended regimens for treatment of scabies in adults

Recommended regimens	
Permethrin cream 5%	Apply to all areas of body from the neck down, and wash off after 8–14 hrs
or	
Lindane 1%	Apply 1 oz of lotion or 30 g of cream thinly to all areas of body from the neck down, and wash off thoroughly after 8 hrs
Alternative	
Crotamiton 10%	Apply to entire body from neck down, nightly for 2 consecutive nights, and wash off 24 hrs after the second application

FIGURE 13-35 Recommended regimens for treatment of scabies in adults. Three regimens are recommended by the Centers for Disease Control and Prevention. Permethrin is safe and may be slightly more effective than lindane, but it costs more. Lindane is effective against scabies found in most areas of the United States, but lindane resistance has been reported in some areas of the world, including parts of the United States. Seizures have been reported when lindane was used after bathing or in patients with extensive dermatitis. Aplastic anemia has also been reported following the use of lindane. It is important that patients be cautioned not to wash their hands after applying a treatment. (Taplin D, *et al.*: Comparison of crotamiton 10% cream (Eurax) and permethrin 5% cream (Elimite) for the treatment of scabies in children. *Pediatr Dermatol* 1990, 7:67–73. Centers for Disease Control and Prevention: 1993 Sexually transmitted diseases treatment guidelines. *MMWR* 1993, 42(RR-14):95–96.)

Cure rates in trials comparing lindane and permethrin for treatment of scabies

	Lindane	Permethrin
Schultz, 1990	177/205 (86%)	188/199 (91%)
Haustein, 1989	55/61 (92%)	71/71 (100%)
Taplin, 1989	15/23 (65%)	21/23 (91%)

FIGURE 13-36 Cure rates in trials comparing lindane and pyrethrin treatment of scabies. A trial by Schultz and colleagues included the largest number of participants, randomized the treatments, and ensured treatment of family members. This study found no significant difference in treatment results between agents. Other, smaller, comparative trials have appeared to demonstrate a therapeutic advantage for permethrin. The low cure rate for treatment with lindane suggested by Taplin and coworkers is inconsistent with a higher cure rate demonstrated by the same team in other studies. Although both permethrin and lindane are considered effective therapy for scabies, permethrin may be slightly more effective. (Schultz MW, Gomez M, Hansen RC, *et al.*: Comparative study of 5% permethrin cream and 1% lindane lotion for the treatment of scabies. *Arch Dermatol* 1990, 126:167–170. Haustein UF, Hlawa B: Treatment of scabies with permethrin versus lindane and benzyl benzoate. *Acta Dermatol Venereol* 1989, 69:348–351. Taplin D, Meinking TL, Porcelain SL, *et al.*: Permethrin 5% dermal cream, a new treatment for scabies. *J Am Acad Dermatol* 1986, 15:995–1001.)

Considerations in the treatment of scabies

Infants, young children, and pregnant or lactating women should not be treated with lindane

Bedding and clothing should be decontaminated or removed from the body for 72 hrs

Fumigation of living areas is not necessary

Sexual and close personal or household contacts within the past month should be epidemiologically treated

Pruritus may persist for several weeks following treatment

FIGURE 13-37 Considerations in the treatment of scabies. Clothing can be decontaminated by machine washing or drying using the hot cycle or by dry cleaning. Some experts recommend retreatment for patients who are still symptomatic after 1 week, but others suggest that such retreatment be limited to those patients in whom live mites are persistently demonstrated. Patients not responding to initial treatment should be retreated with a different regimen.

Selected Bibliography

Alexander J: *Arthropods and Human Skin*. Berlin: Springer-Verlag; 1984.

Brown S, Becher J, Brady W: Treatment of ectoparasitic infections: Review of the English-language literature, 1982–1992. *Clin Infect Dis* 1995, 20(suppl 1):S104–S109.

Chapel TA, Katta T, Kusamar T, *et al.*: Pediculosis pubis in a clinic for the treatment of sexually transmitted diseases. *Sex Transm Dis* 1979, 6:257.

Elgart M: Pediculosis. *Dermatol Clin North Am* 1990, 8(2):219–228.

Elgart M: Scabies. *Dermatol Clin North Am* 1990, 8(2):253–263.

CHAPTER 14

Molluscum Contagiosum

Barbara B. Wilson

CLINICAL PRESENTATION

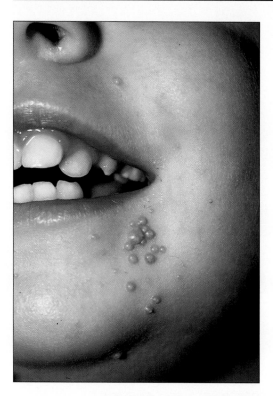

FIGURE 14-1 Cluster of molluscum contagiosum lesions on a child's face. The lesions of molluscum contagiosum typically appear as 1- to 5-mm, solitary or grouped, firm papules and are painless. They are pearly to pink in color, dome shaped, and may be umbilicated. Molluscum contagiosum is caused by a poxvirus. The disease is worldwide in distribution, and its spread may be enhanced by poverty, overcrowding, and poor hygiene. (Epstein WL: Molluscum contagiosum. *Semin Dermatol* 1992, 11:184–189.)

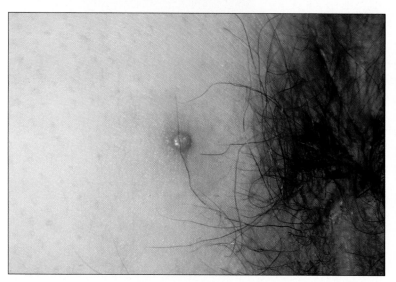

FIGURE 14-2 Solitary lesion of molluscum contagiosum in the perianal region of an adult. Infection in adults is frequently acquired through sexual contact, and lesions are most often found on the lower abdomen, upper thighs, buttocks, and genitalia. (Buntin DM, Rosen T, Lesher JL, *et al.*: Sexually transmitted diseases: Viruses and ectoparasites. *J Am Acad Dermatol* 1991, 25:527–534.)

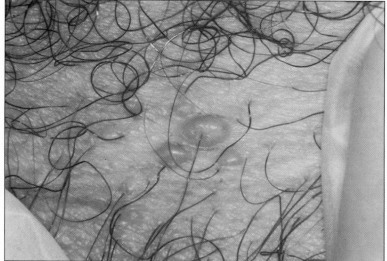

FIGURE 14-3 Molluscum contagiosum lesions in the pubic hair of a 32-year-old woman. Umbilications on the lesions are barely visible. Additional lesions were present on the thighs. (*Courtesy of* M.F. Rein, MD.)

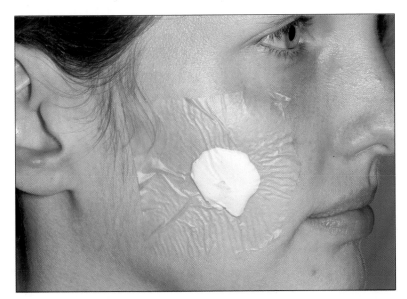

FIGURE 14-17 Topical anesthesia in preparation for curettage or cryotherapy of molluscum contagiosum lesions. Although curettage treatments are well tolerated by adults, children may be incooperative because of pain as well as fear. In such cases, a topical anesthetic cream containing 2.5% lidocaine and 2.5% prilocaine (eutectic mixture of local anesthetics [EMLA]) can be applied under occlusion for 30 minutes before the procedure. (de Waard-van der Spek FB, Oranje AP, Lillieborg S, *et al.*: Treatment of molluscum contagiosum using a lidocaine/prilocaine cream [EMLA] for analgesia. *J Am Acad Dermatol* 1990, 23:685–688.)

SELECTED BIBLIOGRAPHY

Buntin DM, Rosen T, Lesher JL, *et al.*: Sexually transmitted diseases: Viruses and ectoparasites. *J Am Acad Dermatol* 1991, 25:527–534.

Epstein WL: Molluscum contagiosum. *Semin Dermatol* 1992, 11:184–189.

Highet AS: Molluscum contagiosum. *Arch Dis Child* 1992, 67:1248–1249.

Lowy DR: Milker's nodules and molluscum contagiosum. *In* Fitzpatrick TB, Eisen AZ, Wolff K, *et al.* (eds.): *Dermatology in General Medicine*, 4th ed. New York: McGraw-Hill, Inc.; 1993:2606–2610.

Schwartz JJ, Myskowski PL: Molluscum contagiosum in patients with human immunodeficiency virus infection. *J Am Acad Dermatol* 1992, 27:583–588.

CHAPTER 15

Herpes Simplex Virus Infections

Lawrence Corey

PATHOGENESIS OF GENITAL HERPES

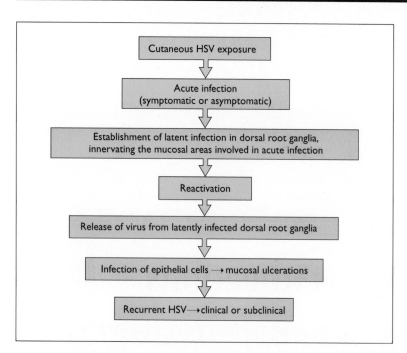

FIGURE 15-1 Pathophysiology of herpes simplex virus (HSV) infection. Acute infection with HSV may be acquired either clinically or subclinically. For orally acquired infections, latency is established in the trigeminal and autonomic nerve root ganglia (superior cervical). For genitally acquired infections, latency is established in sacral nerve root ganglia. Some initial infections are acquired in both anatomic regions simultaneously. Moreover, HSV-2 infections may be acquired in the genital region after previous oral–labial HSV-1 infection. Subclinically acquired infections may be manifest clinically with subsequent reactivation. In addition, persons with clinically symptomatic acute primary infections may also have subclinical reactivation.

Serologic classification of genital infections

| | First episode | | | | Recurrent | |
	Primary HSV-2	Primary HSV-1	Nonprimary HSV-2	Nonprimary HSV-1	HSV-2	HSV-1
Types of virus isolated	HSV-2	HSV-1	HSV-2	HSV-1	HSV-2	HSV-1
HSV Ab, acute serum	0	0	HSV-1	HSV-2	HSV-1 & HSV-2	HSV-1
HSV Ab, convalescent serum	HSV-2	HSV-1	HSV-1 & HSV-2	HSV-1 & HSV-2	HSV-1 & HSV-2	HSV-1

Ab—antibodies.

FIGURE 15-2 Serologic classification of genital HSV infections. Primary HSV infection defines the initial contact with either HSV-1 or HSV-2. As such, the acute sera lack antibodies to either HSV-1 or HSV-2; the convalescent sera show seroconversion to the infecting viral type. Acute primary HSV infection is the most clinically severe form of the infection. Nonprimary first-episode herpes is the acquisition of a new serotype in a person with prior HSV infection; it is usually newly acquired HSV-2 in a person with previous HSV-1. This nonprimary infection is less severe than primary infection because of some cross-protecting host responses. Reactivation of latent HSV-1 and HSV-2 infection occurs in the face of constant levels of antibodies to HSV-1 and/or HSV-2. Persons with recurrent HSV-2 infection possess HSV-2 antibodies in both acute and convalescent sera. Conversely, persons with recurrent HSV-1 infection possess HSV-1 antibodies in both acute and convalescent sera. Many persons are infected with both subtypes and have recurrences with both subtypes, usually HSV-1 in the oral–labial region and HSV-2 in the genital region.

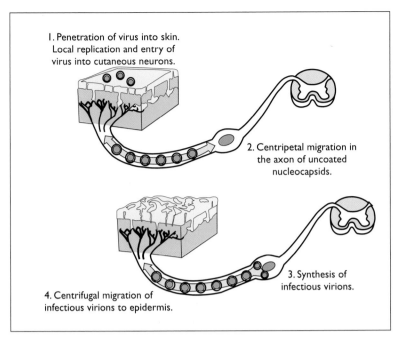

1. Penetration of virus into skin. Local replication and entry of virus into cutaneous neurons.

2. Centripetal migration in the axon of uncoated nucleocapsids.

3. Synthesis of infectious virions.

4. Centrifugal migration of infectious virions to epidermis.

FIGURE 15-3 Pathogenesis of HSV infections. During acute HSV infection, virus penetrates the skin either on a mucosal surface or through a break. Local replication of virus in epithelial cells may occur, but within hours the virus enters axons of peripheral nerves and ascends intraneuronally into the dorsal nerve root ganglia. Acute replication within several ganglia and across the spinal cord occurs in animals. Virus then spreads within neurons back down to the mucosal and epithelial skin area, is released from neural endings and causes the characteristic multiple, bilaterally distributed lesions seen with primary infections. (*From* Corey L, Spear P: Infections with herpes simplex viruses. *N Engl J Med* 1986, 314:686; with permission.)

EPIDEMIOLOGY OF HERPES SIMPLEX VIRUS INFECTIONS

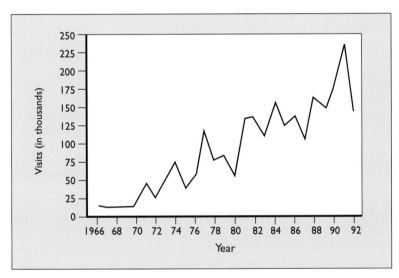

FIGURE 15-4 Incidence of genital HSV infections in the United States between 1966 and 1992. The annual numbers of patients making an initial visit to their physicians' offices with genital HSV infection are recorded. The rates show that an epidemic of HSV-2 infections has occurred in the United States in the past two decades. (Division of STD/HIV Prevention: *Sexually Transmitted Disease Surveillance*, 1992. Atlanta: Centers for Disease Control and Prevention; 1993:28.)

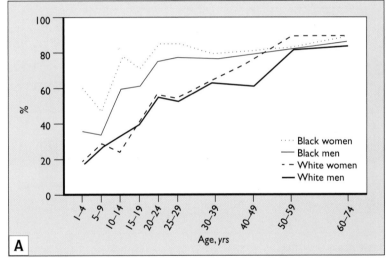

Black women
Black men
White women
White men

A

FIGURE 15-5 Seroprevalence of HSV in the US population during 1978. **A,** Seroprevalence of HSV-1–specific antibody by age, sex, and race. As shown in a 1978 population-based survey of US households, the age-specific seroprevalence of HSV-1 is dropping in the United States. For example, only 50% of white men and women are HSV-1 seropositive at age 20 years, whereas most studies in the early 1950s predicted that 70% to 75% of such persons would be HSV-1 seropositive. Both HSV-1 and HSV-2 seroprevalence rates are higher in lower socioeconomic populations. (*continued*)

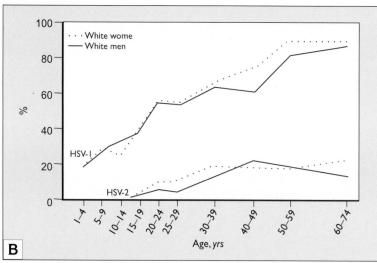

B

FIGURE 15-5 *(continued)* **B.** Age- and sex-specific seroprevalence of HSV-1– and HSV-2–specific antibodies in whites during 1978. An epidemic of HSV-2 infections has occurred in the United States in the past two decades. Women tend to have higher seroprevalence rates than men. In some populations, 75% of persons are HSV-2 infected. (*From* Johnson RE, Nahmias AJ, Magder LS, *et al.*: Seroepidemiologic survey of the prevalence of HSV-2 infection in the United States. *N Engl J Med* 1989, 321:7; with permission.)

Acquisition rates of HSV-1 and HSV-2 in a cohort of Swedish women

Age, *yrs*	HSV-1	HSV-2
15–19	2.9	0.5
20–24	3.5	2.4
25–29	1.5	2.3

FIGURE 15-6 Age and acquisition of HSV in a cohort of Swedish women. In a cohort of European women, very high acquisition rates of HSV-2 were noted in persons aged 20 to 30 years. The overall rate of HSV-2 seropositivity at age 29 years was nearly 30% in these women. Below age 20, 2.4% of women per year acquired HSV-2 infection.

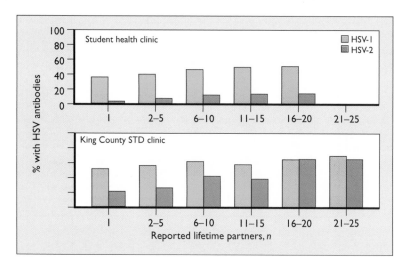

FIGURE 15-7 Seroprevalence of HSV-1 and HSV-2 in women by number of sexual partners. An association between the number of sexual partners and seroprevalence for both HSV-1 and HSV-2 is shown in a comparison of two populations of women—658 college students visiting the student health service and 751 women attending the sexually transmitted diseases (STD) clinic in King County, Washington. However, at equal numbers of lifetime sexual partners, the two populations do differ in their seroprevalence to both viruses. For example, HSV-2 seroprevalence rates approach 50% in women recruited from the STD clinic who had 16 or more lifetime partners. In contrast, only 10% of the university women are HSV-2 seropositive who report similar numbers of partners. (Koutsky LA, Ashley RL, Holmes KK, *et al.*: The frequency of unrecognized type 2 herpes simplex virus infection among women: Implications for the control of genital herpes. *Sex Transm Dis* 1990, 17:90–94.)

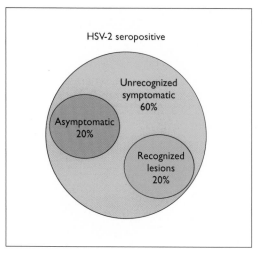

FIGURE 15-8 Rates of clinical versus subclinical episodes of genital herpes. Most HSV-2–seropositive persons do not report genital lesions. However, when patients are screened for HSV-2 antibodies, and HSV-2–seropositive persons identified and subsequently counseled about the clinical manifestations of genital herpes, 60% subsequently report symptomatic infections. Thus, most HSV-2 infections are really symptomatic but are "unrecognized."

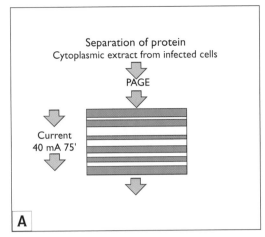

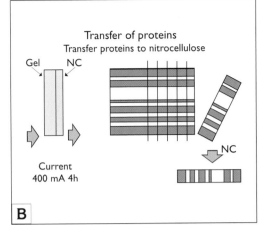

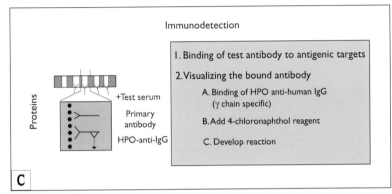

FIGURE 15-9 Western blot assay for detecting HSV-1– and HSV-2–specific antibodies. The Western blot assay is the most accurate and sensitive technique to identify the HSV serotype in human sera. A, Separation of proteins. In this assay, lysates of prototype HSV-1– and HSV-2–specific strains are electrophoresed into polyacrylamide gels (PAGE). B, Transfer of proteins. The denatured viral proteins to HSV-1 and HSV-2 are then transferred onto nitrocellulose (NC) paper, which is cut into thin paper strips to be used with individual sera. C, Immunodetection. Test serum is applied to the paper strip, which is then incubated on a rocker panel to allow binding. Bound antibody is reacted with a horseradish peroxidase (HPO) anti-human IgG. A 4-chloronaphthol reagent is then added that stains bound antibodies dark brown-black.

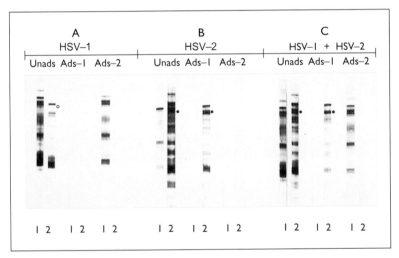

FIGURE 15-10 HSV antibody patterns detected on Western blot. A, Pattern with HSV-1 antibodies only. Many bands are seen within the unadsorbed (*Unads*) HSV-1 strips. When the sera are adsorbed with sepharose beads containing HSV-1 antigen (*Ads-1*) and then re-run, all the antibody is removed. B, Pattern with HSV-2 antibodies only. The dot indicates antibody to gG2, which is an HSV glycoprotein that differs in the HSV-1 and HSV-2 serotypes (gG1 and gG2, respectively). The antibodies to HSV-2 are removed with adsorption to sepharose beads containing HSV-2 antigen (*Ads-2*) but not HSV-1 antigen (*Ads-1*). C, Pattern with antibodies to both HSV-1 and HSV-2. (Ashley RL, Militoni J, Lee F, *et al.*: Comparison of Western blot (immunoblot) and glycoprotein G-specific immunoblot enzyme assay for detecting antibodies to herpes simplex virus types 1 and 2 in human serum. *J Clin Microbiol* 1988, 26:662–667.)

CLINICAL MANIFESTATIONS OF HERPES SIMPLEX VIRUS INFECTIONS

Clinical differences between HSV-1 and HSV-2

Characteristics	HSV-1	HSV-2
Urogenital infection	-(< 30%)	+(90%)
Nongenital infections		
Labialis	+(80%–90%)	-(≤ 5%)
Keratitis	+	-
Whitlow (hand)	+	+
Encephalitis (adult)	+	-
Neonatal infection	-(≈ 30%)	+(≈ 70%)
Transmission (primary route)	Nongenital	Genital

FIGURE 15-11 Clinical differences between HSV-1 and HSV-2. (*Adapted from* Hirsch MS: Herpes simplex virus. *In* Mandell GL, Bennett JE, Dolin R (eds.): *Principles and Practice of Infectious Diseases*, 4th ed. New York: Churchill Livingstone; 1995:1336; with permission.)

Oral–Labial Herpes Simplex Virus Infections

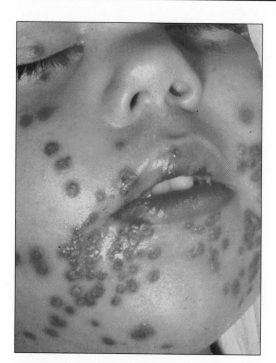

FIGURE 15-12 Primary HSV-1 gingivostomatitis in a child. In a classic case of primary HSV-1 gingivostomatitis, multiple clusters of bilaterally distributed lesions involve both intraoral and external surfaces. Lesions on the eyelids are often seen and indicate likely spread of infection to the ophthalmic region of the trigeminal nerve. Although the child does not have ocular infection with this episode, he will be at risk for subsequent HSV keratitis due to reactivation of infection. Other symptoms included fever and severe pharyngitis. Many physicians would treat this child with oral acyclovir suspension to hasten healing of lesions.

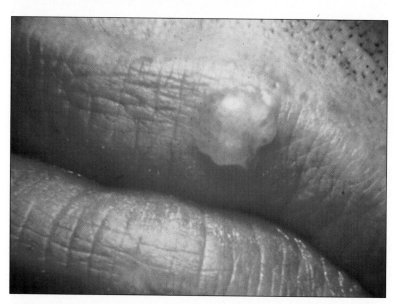

FIGURE 15-13 Recurrent oral–labial HSV-1 infection, showing characteristic fever blister. A characteristic "fever blister" of recurrent oral–labial HSV infection is shown. Almost all reactivation of HSV in the oral cavity is due to HSV-1, with HSV-2 rarely being isolated from recurrent fever blisters. Reactivation of herpes in the oral cavity may be clinically asymptomatic (with shedding of HSV in saliva), may cause lesions on mucosal surfaces, or may result in a pathognomonic fever blister. Fever blisters characteristically involve the vermilion border of the lip. The preexisting host responses localize the infection to mucosal surfaces. Systemic signs and symptoms are uncommon with these reactivations.

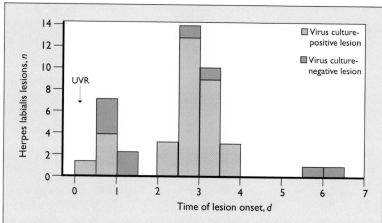

FIGURE 15-14 Time to appearance of herpes lesions on lips after exposure to ultraviolet radiation. There is both an early and late distribution of reactivation of HSV infection after experimental exposure to ultraviolet light (UVR). Similar observations have been made with sunlight exposure. Lesions that appear immediately (within 6–24 hours) after UVR exposure are not prevented by the administration of oral acyclovir. In contrast, later lesions are effectively reduced by the compound. (*From* Spruance SL, Freeman DJ, Stewart JCB, *et al.*: The natural history of UV radiation-induced herpes labialis and response to therapy with peroral and topical formulations of acyclovir. *J Infect Dis* 1991, 163:728; with permission.)

Primary Genital Herpes

Differential diagnosis of genital ulcer–adenopathy syndromes			
Diagnosis	**Etiology**	**Ulcer**	**Nodes**
Herpes	HSV-2 > HSV-1	Painful, soft	Firm, tender
Syphilis	*Treponema pallidum*	Painless, hard	Firm, nontender
Chancroid	*Haemophilus ducreyi*	Painful, soft	Fluctuant, tender
Donovanosis	*Calymmatobacterium granulomatis*	Painless, chronic, spreading	Normal
Lymphogranuloma venereum	*Chlamydia trachomatis*	Usually absent	Fluctuant, tender

FIGURE 15-15 Differential diagnosis of genital ulcers–adenopathy syndromes. Primary genital HSV infection is most common in adolescents and young adults and is usually caused by HSV-2 (in 70%–95% of cases) rather than HSV-1. Primary genital herpes in both sexes may be associated with tender, bilateral inguinal adenopathy and with vesicular lesions that ulcerate rapidly and become tender. Other sexually transmitted diseases may cause similar lesions and adenopathy and must be differentiated.

Most common etiologies of genital ulcers in the United States	
	Reported cases, 1992
Herpes simplex virus type 2	200,000–500,000
Syphilis (*Treponema pallidum*)	33,973
Chancroid (*Haemophilus ducreyi*)	1886

FIGURE 15-16 Most common etiologies of genital ulcers in the United States. In 1992, 33,973 cases of primary syphilis, 200,000 to 500,000 first patient visits for genital herpes, and 1886 cases of chancroid were reported. (Division of STD/HIV Prevention: *Sexually Transmitted Disease Surveillance*, 1992. Atlanta: Centers for Disease Control and Prevention; 1993.)

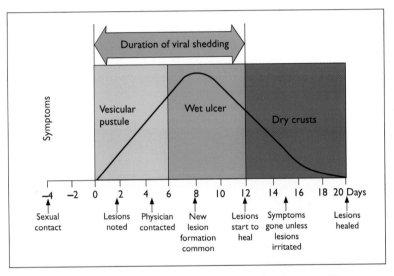

FIGURE 15-17 Clinical course of primary genital herpes. The clinical course of untreated primary HSV infection is depicted. In general, the infection increases in severity over the first 7 to 10 days, peaking between 8 and 10 days after onset. New lesions develop frequently during the early time periods due to centrifugal spread of the virus to the mucosal surfaces and occasionally from autoinoculation of new areas. HSV can be isolated readily from the lesions in high titer (10^5–10^7 virions/mL of vesicle fluid) for the initial 10 to 14 days. As the immune response ensues, HSV excretion is reduced and healing occurs. Systemic symptoms usually occur early. Oral acyclovir therapy reduces the duration of lesions and viral shedding by over 50%.

FIGURE 15-18 Duration of genital herpes lesions and symptoms according to serologic status. The clinical manifestations of mucosal HSV infections differ according to the patient's serologic status. Primary HSV infections last longer than nonprimary first-episode infections, which last longer than reactivation infections. However, there is great variability within each category of disease (as shown by the error bars), making clinical classification very difficult; only "classic" cases can be readily characterized clinically. Patients with genital and oral–labial herpes should have laboratory confirmation of their diagnosis by Western blot assay, cytologic examination, or virus isolation, especially when therapy is being contemplated.

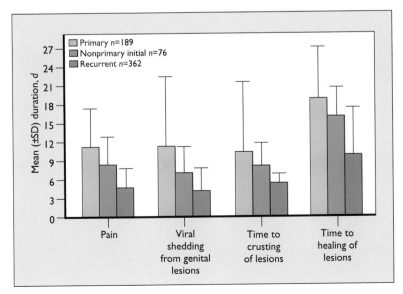

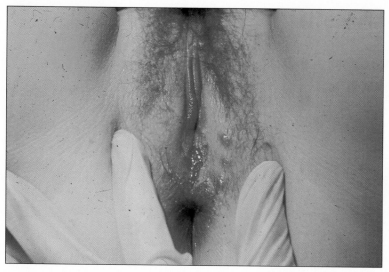

FIGURE 15-19 Primary genital herpes of the vulva. A woman with classic primary genital herpes shows the bilaterally distributed lesions. She complained of headache, malaise, and myalgias and had a low-grade fever. Primary HSV infection also involved the urethra and cervix in this woman, and HSV-2 was isolated from urethral swabs and urine. Clinically, one cannot distinguish primary genital herpes due to HSV-1 from that due to HSV-2; only laboratory assays can distinguish between the two viral subtypes.

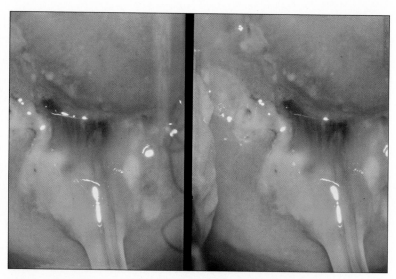

FIGURE 15-20 Colposcopic view of purulent HSV cervicitis. A colposcopic view of the cervix from the patient in Fig. 15-19 shows a characteristic purulent HSV cervicitis. Note the purulent exudates and characteristic erosive lesions on the exocervix. She responded well to treatment with oral acyclovir, 400 mg three times daily (or 200 mg five times daily) for 10 days.

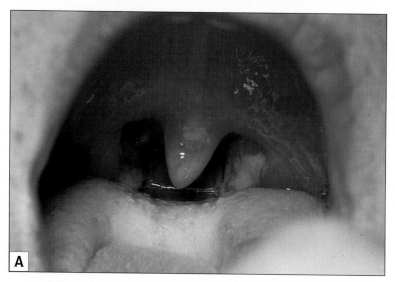

A

FIGURE 15-21 HSV-2 pharyngitis associated with acquisition of primary genital herpes in a woman. **A,** The patient came to the emergency department complaining of pharyngitis and was given ampicillin. She reported oral–genital contact with a partner with a

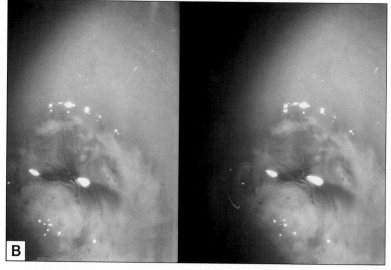

B

genital sore. She returned in 24 hours complaining of genital pain and dysuria. **B,** Pelvic examination showed bilateral genital lesions and a purulent, erosive cervicitis (as shown). Identical isolates of HSV-2 were recovered from oral, genital, and cervical regions.

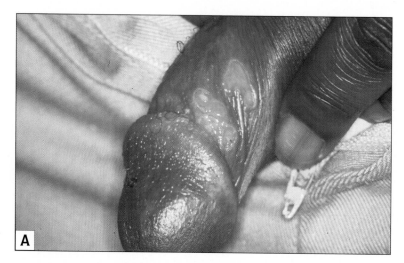

A

FIGURE 15-22 Primary genital HSV infection in a man. **A,** Two clusters of large ulcers are seen on the left side of the penile shaft. Although these appear to be single lesions, each actually is formed from the coalescence of multiple ulcers. (*continued*)

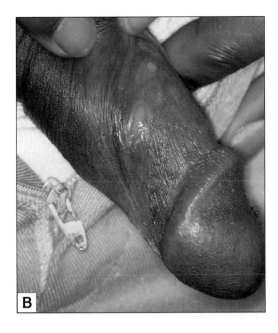

FIGURE 15-22 (*continued*) **B.** A similar coalescence of lesions, as well as a single lesion, is seen on the right side of the penile shaft. Such lesions are tender and nonindurated. Herpetic lesions tend all to be similar in size, whereas lesions of chancroid may vary in size. This patient also had bilateral tender lymphadenopathy of the inguinal nodes and was slightly febrile. He improved on oral acyclovir therapy. (*Courtesy of* M.F. Rein, MD.)

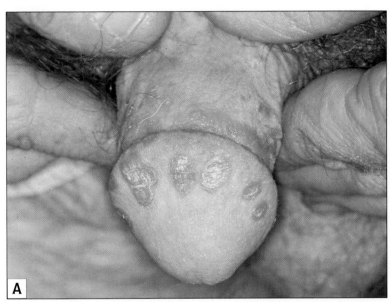

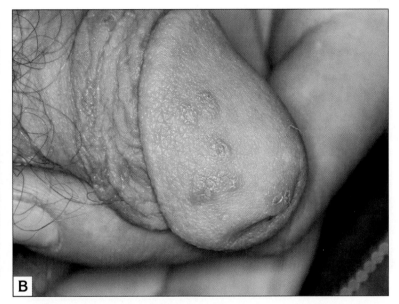

FIGURE 15-23 Healing HSV lesions on the penis. **A,** Herpetic lesions tend to heal by crusting over, as seen on the glans and coronal sulcus in this patient. Culture of material from crusted lesions has a sensitivity of only 27% for the virus. **B,** The pattern of crusts seen on the glans in this patient suggests the clustering of initial lesions, which is characteristic in genital HSV infections. The differential diagnosis of crusted lesions includes scabies, which tend to be scattered rather than clustered, are markedly pruritic, and usually do not involve inguinal adenopathy. (Moseley RC, Corey L, Benjamin D, *et al.*: Comparison of viral isolation, direct immunofluorescence, and indirect immunoperoxidase techniques for detection of genital herpes simplex virus infection. *J Clin Microbiol* 1981, 13:913–918.) (*Courtesy of* M.F. Rein, MD.)

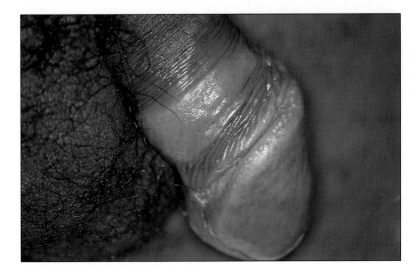

FIGURE 15-24 Atypical primary HSV infection on the penis. In this patient, the larger, denuded areas are formed by the coalescence of many tiny ulcerations, which are visible on close examination. The patient also had bilateral, tender, inguinal lymphadenopathy. Culture of the denuded area was positive for HSV (not serotyped), and the patient responded to oral acyclovir therapy. (*Courtesy of* M.F. Rein, MD.)

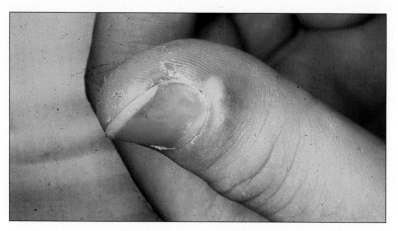

Figure 15-25 Autoinoculation of the thumb (herpetic whitlow) after primary genital herpes. Autoinoculation of distal sites is frequently seen during primary HSV infection, usually during the second week of therapy. Prompt diagnosis and treatment of primary infections reduces the occurrence of this complication. Once latency is established in the hand area, periodic reactivations of herpetic whitlow occur. Both HSV-1 and HSV-2 can be isolated from such lesions.

Recurrent Genital Herpes

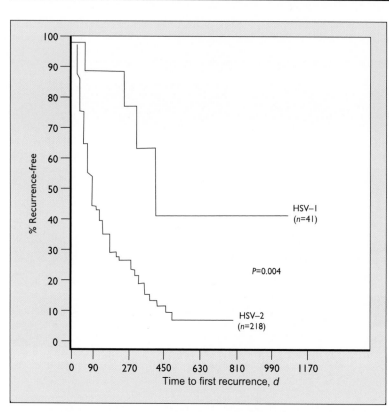

Figure 15-26 Comparison of reactivation rates for HSV-1 and HSV-2 following primary genital herpes. When HSV infection is acquired genitally, reactivation is common: 98% of all patients with genital HSV-2 infection and 50% of those with genital HSV-1 infection have recurrences. Most patients with primary genital HSV-2 infection have at least one recurrence by 12 months after acquisition. Systemic symptoms and local involvement are generally less severe in reactivation than in primary infection.

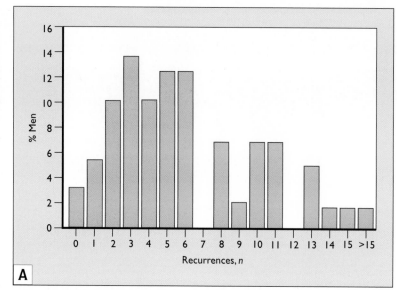

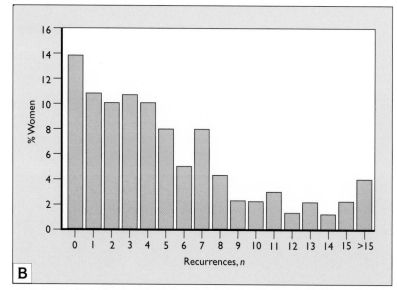

Figure 15-27 Frequency of genital HSV-2 recurrences in men and women in first year after acquisition of infection. **A**, Distribution of recurrences in men. **B**, Distribution of recurrences in women. The graphs show that persons who acquire genital HSV-2 infection have a high number of reactivations, and 20% to 30% will have very frequent recurrences (> 10/yr). The median number of recurrences per year in men and women is five for the first 3 to 4 years after infection. (Benedetti J, Corey L, Ashley R: Recurrence rates of genital herpes after acquisition of symptomatic first-episode infection. *Ann Intern Med* 1994, 121:847–854.)

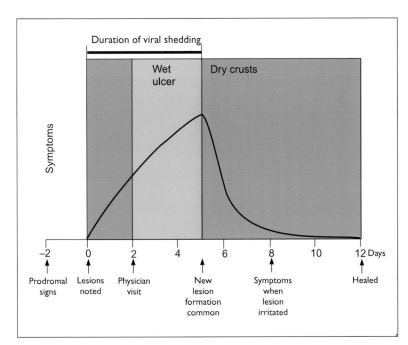

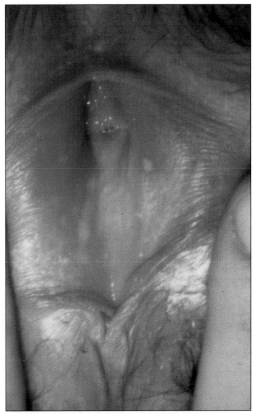

FIGURE 15-29 "Kissing" (autoinoculation) ulcers of the vulva due to HSV-2. Autoinoculation of new areas is rare with reactivation infection, but the figure illustrates two "kissing" ulcers due to HSV-2.

FIGURE 15-28 Clinical course of recurrent genital herpes. The clinical course of reactivated HSV-2 infection differs markedly from the course of primary genital herpes (*see* Fig. 15-17), in that host responses to HSV are present and both memory T-cell and B-cell responses help combat infections. In immunocompetent persons, all HSV reactivations eventually heal without therapy. Virus is isolated for only a short time and generally at 1 to 2 logs lower titer than with primary infections. Healing is more rapid as lesions involute quicker.

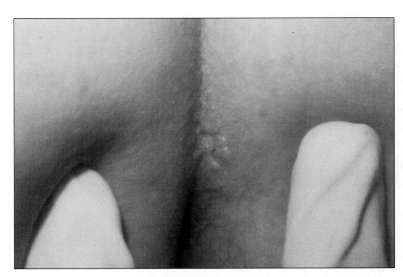

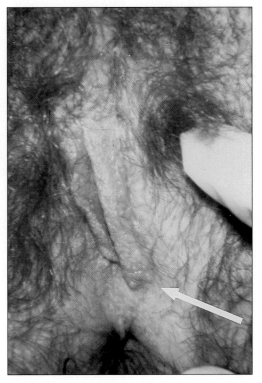

FIGURE 15-31 Recurrent genital HSV-2 infection on the lower labia (*arrow*). The classic occurrence of recurrent genital lesions in women is as grouped, unilateral vesicles. Mild pain and irritation may be present.

FIGURE 15-30 Recurrent vesicular HSV-2 lesions on the buttock. The classic appearance of vesicular lesions clustered in the buttock area is shown. Twenty percent of persons who acquire HSV-2 infection subsequently develop buttock lesions, as buttocks are innervated by sacral nerve roots 3 to 5. Persons with buttock herpes should be counseled about the manifestations of genital herpes and the risk of transmission during subclinical reactivation of infection. (Benedetti JK, Zeh J, Selke S, Corey L: Frequency and reactivation of nongenital lesions among patients with genital herpes simplex virus infections. *Am J Med* 1995, 98:237–242.)

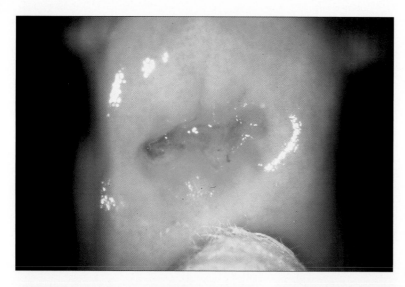

FIGURE 15-32 Subclinical shedding of HSV-2 from a small cervical ulceration during reactivation. HSV infection may reactivate silently in the cervical region or with small unnoticed lesions. Two tiny cervical ulcers can be seen at the lower edge of the cervical os. Recent studies show that one third to one half of all HSV reactivations in the genital area are subclinical and involve such unnoticed lesions. These unnoticed lesions are the predominant means by which HSV is transmitted to others.

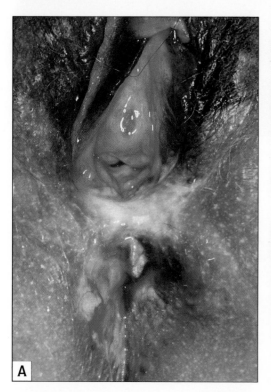

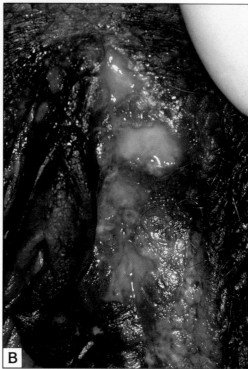

FIGURE 15-33 Recurrent genital herpes lesions in women. **A,** A 31-year-old woman with HIV infection and a 4-year history of recurrent genital herpes presented with a chronic (7-month-old) perianal ulcer that was resistant to treatment with acyclovir. Culture showed acyclovir-resistant herpesvirus. **B,** Multiple recurrent ulcers developed in another HIV-infected woman. Herpetic lesions can become quite large or secondarily infected and assume an unusual appearance in HIV-infected persons. (Panel 33A *courtesy of* K. LaGuardia, MD; panel 33B *courtesy of* T.C. Wright, Jr, MD.)

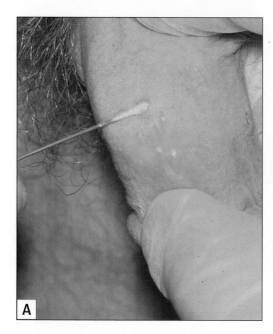

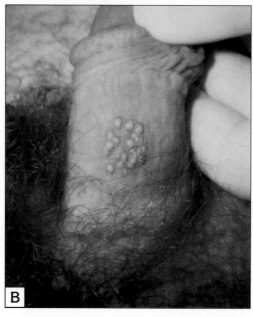

FIGURE 15-34 Recurrent genital HSV lesions on the penis shaft. **A** and **B,** In men, genital herpes recurs as clusters of vesicular lesions on an erythematous base, usually on the penis shaft or glans. This patient reported episodes of exacerbations every other month. He was both HSV-1– and HSV-2–seropositive by Western blot analysis, with HSV-2 being isolated from the genital lesions. He elected to initiate suppressive acyclovir therapy, 400 mg orally twice daily, and did not have any recurrences during the initial year of therapy.

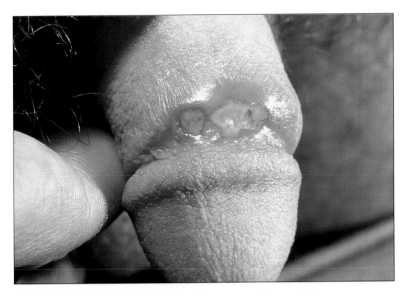

FIGURE 15-35 Atypical genital ulceration due to HSV-2 reactivation on the penis corona. HSV reactivations may be atypical in appearance, as with the chancroidal presentation of this lesion. The lesion was painful, and the patient had only mild lymphadenopathy. Because HSV is the most common cause of genital ulcerations in the United States, all such lesions should be cultured. (*Courtesy of* H.H. Handsfield, MD.)

Other Mucocutaneous Herpes Simplex Virus Infections

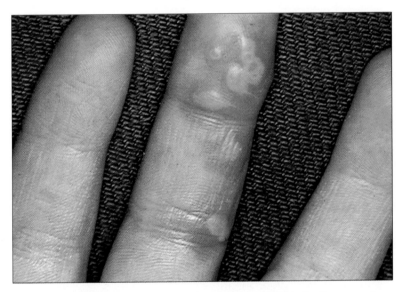

FIGURE 15-36 Recurrent herpetic whitlow. HSV infection may be acquired on the finger, as is sometimes seen in medical personnel. Lesions are painful, often accompanied by lymphadenitis, and often misdiagnosed as bacterial. These lesions respond to oral acyclovir therapy. (*See also* Fig. 15-25.)

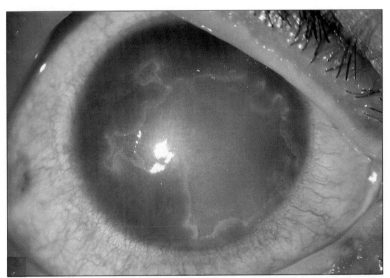

FIGURE 15-37 HSV keratitis. A nonhealing corneal ulcer of the right eye, in a 15-year-old girl with AIDS, was shown by culture to be due to HSV-1. (*Courtesy of* J.L. Davis, MD.)

DIAGNOSIS OF HERPES SIMPLEX VIRUS INFECTIONS

Tests for detecting HSV in genital lesions
Cytology
Isolation
Antigen detection
Genomic detection

FIGURE 15-38 Tests for detecting HSV in genital lesions. Both clinical and laboratory criteria are useful for establishing the diagnosis of HSV infection. Cytologic techniques, including Wright, Giemsa (Tzanck), or Papanicolaou stains, are useful for quick office procedures to confirm diagnosis but are only 60% as sensitive as viral isolation in tissue culture. Antigen detection techniques, such as immunofluorescence or enzyme-linked immunosorbent assays, and DNA hybridization procedures approach the sensitivity of viral isolation but are less reliable in asymptomatic cases. Polymerase chain reaction assays to detect HSV DNA recently have been shown to be more sensitive than viral isolation and are now acknowledged to be the most sensitive assay for detecting HSV in secretions, lesions, tissue, or bodily fluids. Several methods are available for viral subtyping, including the use of monoclonal antibodies to the two HSV subtypes or the use of restriction enzyme digests that differentiate HSV-1 from HSV-2.

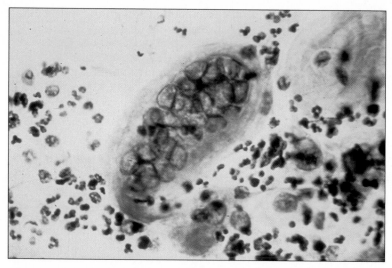

FIGURE 15-39 Multinucleated giant cell in a Papanicolaou smear from a women with HSV cervicitis. For rapid diagnosis of skin or mucous lesions, scrapings or swabs may be stained with Wright, Giemsa (Tzanck preparation), or Papanicolaou stains to demonstrate the characteristic, multinucleated giant cells of HSV infection (although varicella-zoster virus infections also produce such giant cells). Intranuclear inclusions may also be seen on Papanicolaou stain.

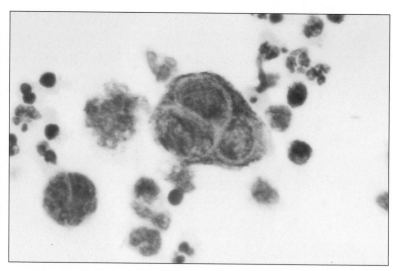

FIGURE 15-40 Tzanck smear of genital HSV lesion with Giemsa staining. (*Courtesy of* the Centers for Disease Control and Prevention.)

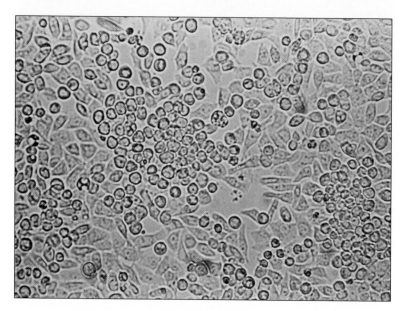

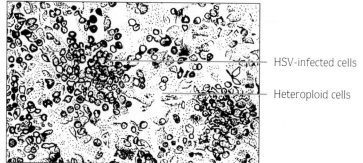

HSV-infected cells

Heteroploid cells

FIGURE 15-41 Cytopathic effect of HSV in HEP-2 cells culture, showing heteroploid cells. On culture, HSV-infected cells become rounded and clump, with rapid progression of the process through the cell monolayer. HSV grows quickly in tissue culture, and most isolates can be identified within 72 hours. Isolation of the virus may be confirmed by reacting the infected cells with monoclonal antibodies to HSV-1 or HSV-2, which confirms identification and serotypes the isolate.

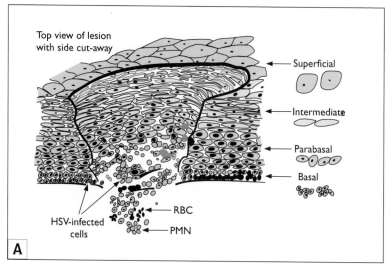

Top view of lesion with side cut-away

Superficial

Intermediate

Parabasal

Basal

RBC

HSV-infected cells

PMN

A

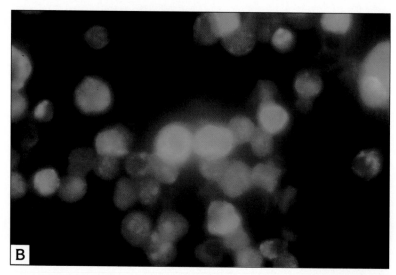

B

FIGURE 15-42 HSV antigen detection assay. **A**, Diagrammatic representation of cell types in HSV ulcer. **B**, Immunofluorescent staining of HSV antigens in a herpetic lesion. Collection of speci-mens for HSV antigen detection should be done by scraping the base of the lesion, where viral-infected cells predominate. (PMN—polymorphonuclear cell; RBC—red blood cell.)

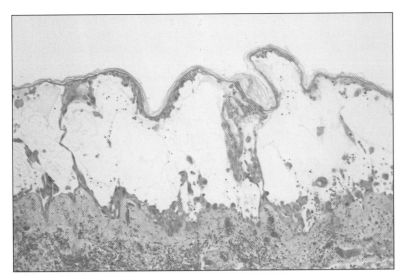

FIGURE 15-43 Histopathologic cross-section from the margin of an HSV ulcer. The empty space is vesicular fluid, and multinucleated giant cells can be seen in the submucosal area. Note the inflammatory response involves both lymphocytes and polymorphonuclear cells. Initially, the lymphocytic infiltrate is predominantly of the CD4 subtype, and later CD8 T-cells are present. (Hematoxylin-eosin stain.)

COMPLICATIONS OF HERPES SIMPLEX VIRUS INFECTIONS

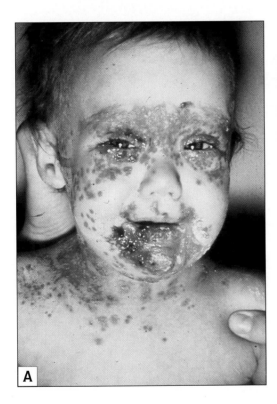

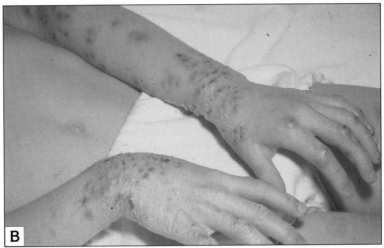

FIGURE 15-44 Eczema herpeticum (Kaposi's varicelliform eruption). **A**, Eczema herpeticum in a child with eczema. **B**, Kaposi's varicelliform eruption in an adult. HSV may spread extensively and rapidly among persons with eczema, because of both the disrupted epithelium and altered host responses. Both of these patients experienced a prompt response to acyclovir therapy. The child was treated with intravenous acyclovir because of his extensive disease and high fever, and the adult received oral acyclovir.

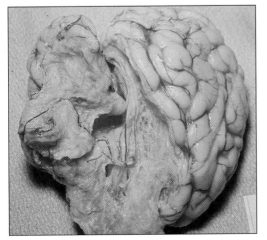

FIGURE 15-45 Severe necrotic HSV encephalitis. HSV encephalitis is the most common form of viral central nervous system infection. HSV encephalitis occurs in both adults and children, with over 95% of cases due to HSV-1. Fever and focal neurologic signs are the most common clinical manifestations of infection. The disease is rapidly progressive and severe unless diagnosed and treated promptly. Brain biopsy previously was the procedure of choice, but now, demonstration of HSV DNA in cerebrospinal fluid by polymerase chain reaction is the most accurate, sensitive, and least invasive approach to diagnosis. Systemic antiviral therapy with acyclovir, 5 mg/kg intravenously every 8 hours, should be initiated promptly in suspected cases. Although encephalitis is rarer with HSV-2, aseptic meningitis is more common, occurring in 55% of women and 11% of men with primary genital herpes in one study. The condition is usually mild and self-limited. HSV-2 may also cause so-called benign recurrent lymphocytic meningitis. (Corey L, Adams HG, Brown ZA, Holmes KK: Genital herpes simplex virus infections: Clinical manifestations, course, and complications. *Ann Intern Med* 1983, 98:958–972. Tedder DG, Ashley R, Tyler K, Levin MJ: Herpes simplex virus infection as a cause of benign recurrent lymphocytic meningitis. *Ann Intern Med* 1994, 121:334–338.)

Incidence of HSV-1 infection in immunosuppressed patients	
Renal transplant	50%–80%
Cardiac transplant	≈ 40%
Bone marrow transplant	50%–80%
Leukemia	20%–40%
Lymphoma	10%–20%

FIGURE 15-46 Incidence of HSV-1 reactivation in immunocompromised patients. Patients compromised by immunodeficiency or immunosuppression, malnutrition, or disorders of skin integrity (*eg*, burns or eczema) are at greater risk of developing severe HSV infections. Both antibody-mediated and cell-mediated immune reactions are clinically important. Immunocompromised patients with defects in cell-mediated immunity experience more severe and extensive HSV infections than those with deficits in humoral immunity (*eg*, agammaglobulinemia).

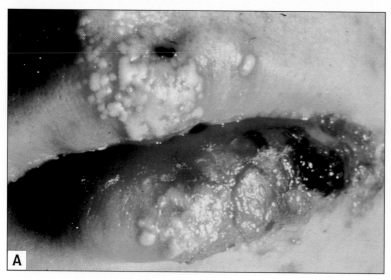

A

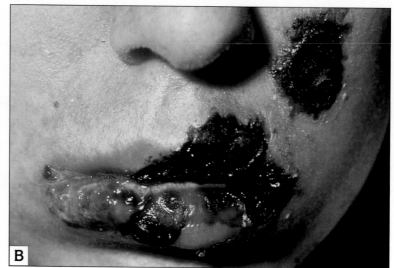

B

FIGURE 15-47 Oral lesions in severe HSV-1 reactivation after bone marrow transplantation. **A** and **B**, HSV reactivations are much more extensive and severe in immunocompromised patients, especially those with reduced T-cell responses. Patients undergoing bone marrow transplantation and chemotherapy may develop extensive herpetic lesions. These ulcerations become rapidly necrotic and may disseminate to the lung and liver. Most HSV reactivations occur within the first 30 days of onset of immunosuppression. Because of the frequent recurrences and extensive morbidity, HSV-seropositive persons who undergo transplantation or chemotherapy receive chronic systemic antiviral therapy to prevent such reactivations.

Neonatal Herpes Simplex Virus Infections

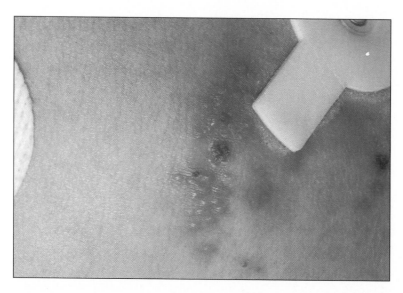

FIGURE 15-48 Classic herpetic lesions in an infant with disseminated HSV-2 infection. Neonatal herpes is the most severe complication of mucosal HSV infection. Clinically, it is manifest by three forms of infection: 1) disease localized to the mucosal area, called skin, eye, and mouth (SEM) disease; 2) primarily central nervous system infection; and 3) disseminated infection. Overlap exists among these forms, and untreated SEM infection in babies may progress to encephalitis or disseminated disease. Untreated, neonatal herpes has a mortality of over 65%. Acyclovir therapy has reduced this mortality, but extensive intravenous therapy is needed for all cases.

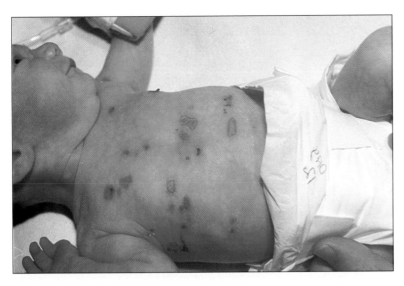

FIGURE 15-49 Classic large vesiculopustular lesions in an infant with neonatal herpes. This child was originally thought to have a staphylococcal infection, but when multiple lesions appeared, HSV was considered. HSV-2 antigen was noted on a skin scraping by direct immunofluorescent staining. His cerebrospinal fluid showed an elevated protein level, mild pleocytosis (12 cells/mL), and HSV DNA on polymerase chain reaction. He was classified as having skin and central nervous system infection. He was treated with acyclovir, 45 mg/kg/day intravenously for 21 days.

Consequences of HSV infections in pregnant women

| Outcome | Type of infection of pregnant women | | |
	First episode, primary	First episode, nonprimary	Reactivation
Spontaneous abortion	++	—	—
Premature rupture of membranes	++	±	—
Intrauterine growth retardation	+	—	—
Intrauterine infection	+	?	—
Neonatal herpes with infection at term	50%	25%	< 1%

FIGURE 15-50 Consequences of HSV infections in pregnant women. Primary HSV infection during pregnancy may result in abortion, premature labor, congenital infection, or growth retardation. Rarely, in third-trimester infections, disseminated disease can occur, with fatal outcome to both mother and fetus. The highest risk for transmitting neonatal herpes from mother to infant occurs when the mother acquires genital herpes near term. The transmission rate to infants from any mother acquiring primary HSV is 50%; among those acquiring nonprimary HSV-2, it is about 25%.

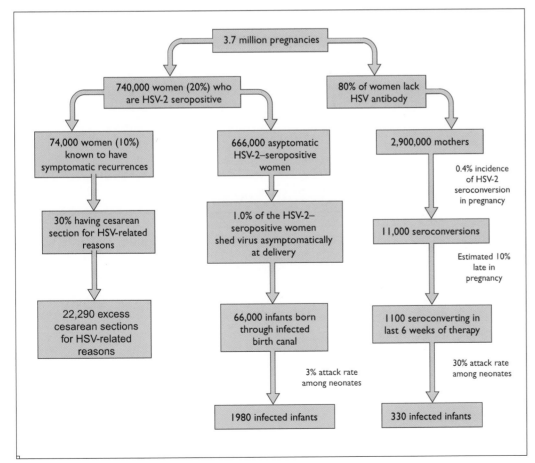

FIGURE 15-51 Morbidity of HSV infections in pregnancy. Most cases of neonatal herpes result from the mother's acquisition of primary genital herpes during pregnancy, with transmission to the infant during delivery through an infected birth canal. Congenital infection also may occur, again usually with mothers who acquire primary HSV infection during pregnancy. The risk of neonatal infection is 10-fold less with reactivated HSV infections, but cesarean delivery is recommended in these cases to avoid exposure of the neonate. Neonatal infection may rarely result from postnatal contact with infected family members or from nosocomial transmission. Infected neonates have a high frequency of central nervous system involvement, resulting in neurologic sequelae in most and mortality in 25% despite therapy.

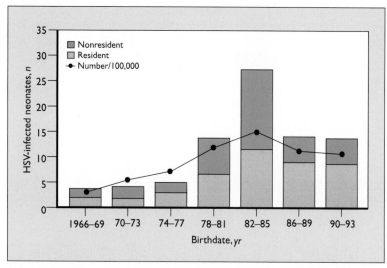

FIGURE 15-52 Incidence of neonatal herpes per 100,000 live births in King County, Washington. The incidence of neonatal herpes is estimated to range from 10 to 50 per 100,000 live births and is higher in premature than in full-term infants. The incidence in King County, Washington, has increased since 1966, peaking at 15 per 100,000 in 1982 to 1985 and reflecting the current epidemic of HSV-2 infection nationwide.

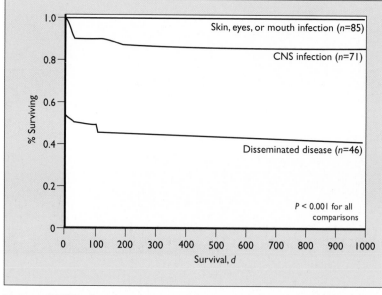

FIGURE 15-53 Survival of infants with neonatal herpes according to form of disease. (CNS—central nervous system.) (*From* Whitley RJ, Arvin A, Prober C, *et al.*: Predictors of morbidity and mortality in neonates with HSV infections. *N Engl J Med* 1991, 324:450–454; with permission.)

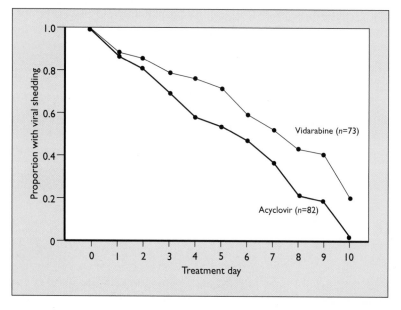

FIGURE 15-54 Cessation of viral shedding during treatment of neonatal herpes. The clearing of HSV from lesions of neonates is better with acyclovir than vidarabine. The slow clearance of virus in the infant illustrates the difficulty in treating this infection. Because occult central nervous system infection is common and response to therapy is prolonged, larger doses of intravenous acyclovir are used to treat infants. Standard therapy for central nervous system and disseminated disease is 45 to 60 mg/kg/day of intravenous acyclovir for 21 days. The drug is given at 8-hour intervals, usually in saline, over a 1-hour period. (*From* Whitley RJ, Arvin A, Prober C, *et al.*: A controlled trial comparing vidarabine with acyclovir in neonatal HSV infection. *N Engl J Med* 1991, 324:444; with permission.)

Herpes Simplex Virus Infection in HIV-Infected Patients

Common clinical manifestations of HSV infection in HIV-infected persons
Recurrent anogenital ulceration
Recurrent oral–labial ulceration
Proctitis
Esophagitis
Acyclovir-resistant disease

FIGURE 15-55 Common clinical manifestations of HSV infection in HIV-infected persons. Severe HSV infections are a prominent feature of AIDS. Progressive perianal ulcers, oral–labial ulcers, colitis, esophagitis, pneumonitis, and neurologic disorders due to HSV have been observed. In addition, genital HSV-2 infection is a risk factor for acquisition of HIV-1 infection among heterosexuals.

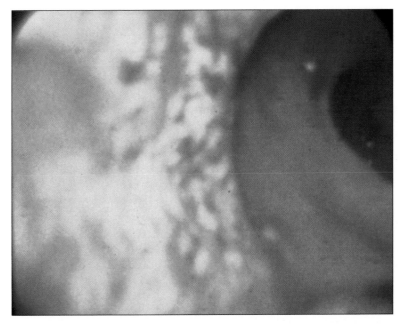

FIGURE 15-56 HSV proctitis. Rectal mucosal infection is a common manifestation of HSV infection among homosexual men. The disease presents with passage of rectal mucus and blood, tenesmus, and often, painful perirectal lesions. Colonoscopy reveals purulent lesions, which on biopsy may show characteristic intranuclear inclusions. Therapy with antivirals shortens the course of infection.

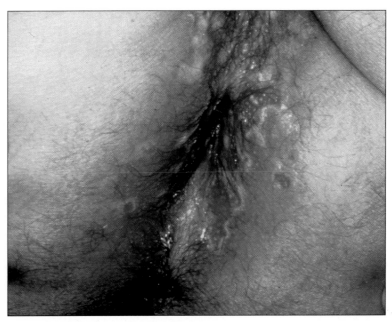

FIGURE 15-57 Severe anogenital HSV infection in a patient with AIDS. Persistent mucocutaneous HSV infection was one of the originally described opportunistic infections in patients with AIDS. HSV infections remain common in persons with HIV infection. As HIV infection progresses, many develop severe, persistent, painful, mucocutaneous lesions. Initially, therapy with antivirals such as acyclovir or famciclovir will result in healing of lesions. Chronic daily therapy may prevent or control lesions effectively. Increasingly, however, persistent lesions may occur that harbor acyclovir- or famciclovir-resistant viruses.

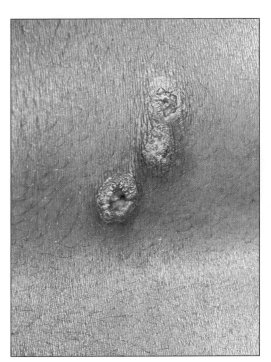

FIGURE 15-58 Chronic hyperkeratotic HSV lesions in a patient with AIDS. Chronic nonhealing herpetic lesions that become hyperkeratotic may be seen in persons with HIV infection. The lesions in this patient were present for 12 weeks and persisted despite chronic daily acyclovir therapy. Acyclovir-resistant virus that lacked thymidine kinase activity was isolated.

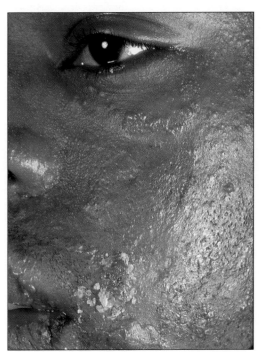

FIGURE 15-59 Recurrent facial HSV infection in an AIDS patient. Recurrent facial infections, due to either HSV-1 or 2, most often involve the lips, oral mucosa, eye, and nose, although any site on the glabrous skin may also be affected. Occasionally, more than one mucocutaneous location may be involved simultaneously. Recurrent herpetic infections in HIV-infected patients tend to occur more frequently, are more severe, and persist longer than in healthy individuals. (*Courtesy of* A.E. Friedman-Kien, MD.)

THERAPY FOR HERPES SIMPLEX VIRUS INFECTIONS

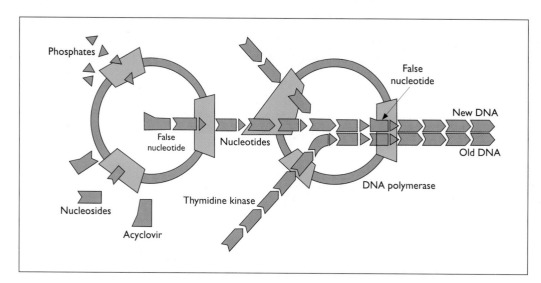

FIGURE 15-60 Chemical structure of acyclovir and famciclovir. Acyclovir is similar in structure to the natural nucleoside guanosine. Because of its acyclic structure, acyclovir induces early chain termination when it is incorporated into viral DNA. HSV-1, HSV-2, and varicella-zoster virus have viral thymidine kinase, which phosphorylates acyclovir to its active triphosphate form. The mechanism of action of famciclovir is similar to that of acyclovir. Famciclovir has been shown to be effective in varicella-zoster infection and in the treatment of first and recurrent episodes of genital herpes (although the Food and Drug Administration has not yet approved a dosage).

FIGURE 15-61 Mechanism of action of acyclovir. Acyclovir is a highly potent and selective inhibitor of HSV replication. Infection of cells with HSV results in the production of viral thymidine kinase, which phosphorylates acyclovir to its monophosphate form. Host cell kinases subsequently convert acyclovir monophosphate to the active triphosphate form, which inhibits HSV DNA polymerase and causes little cellular toxicity. Its incorporation into viral DNA results in early chain termination. Cells not infected with HSV have little thymidine kinase, leading to the selective concentration of acyclovir in HSV infected cells.

Mechanisms of acyclovir resistance

	Virus			
	Lacks TK	TK altered	TK altered	DNA polymerase altered
Phosphorylates thymidine	-	-	+	+
Makes full-length TK polypeptide	-	+	+	+
Phosphorylates acyclovir	-	-	-	+
Neurovirulent	-	?	+	+
LD$_{50}$ reduced	100-fold	100-fold	Some	No

LD$_{50}$—lethal dose for 50% of the test subjects; TK—thymidine kinase.

FIGURE 15-62 Mechanism of acyclovir resistance in HSV mutants. Acyclovir-resistant strains of HSV are being identified increasingly, especially in HIV-infected or immunocompromised patients receiving multiple, intermittent courses. Frequent reactivations and high viral titers in these patients, in combination with medication use, select out resistant strains. Most acyclovir-resistant strains lack thymidine kinase (TK), resulting in low intracellular levels of acyclovir triphosphate. These strains tend to be less neurovirulent in animals. However, occasional strains occur with TK present but with an altered substrate specificity for acyclovir, and these strains are fully neurovirulent. Acyclovir-resistant HSV responds best to foscarnet therapy, which does not require TK for activation and which inhibits the HSV DNA polymerase at a different site from acyclovir or its derivatives.

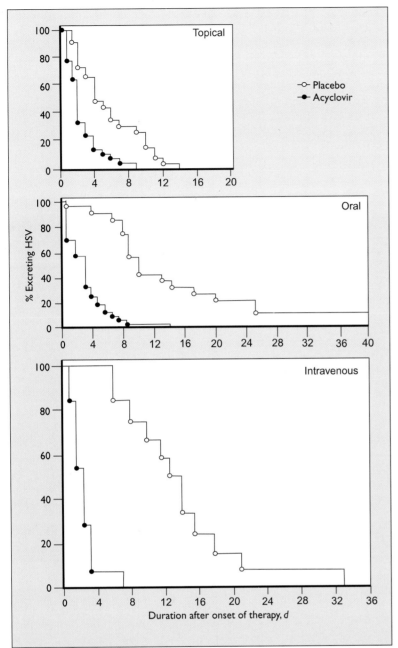

FIGURE 15-63 Comparison of topical, oral, and intravenous acyclovir regimens in primary genital herpes. Acyclovir is effective in shortening the duration of symptoms and lesions of first-episode genital herpes in immunocompetent patients. Oral acyclovir is the treatment of choice. Topical ointment or cream may be beneficial in patients without cervical, urethral, or pharyngeal involvement. Intravenous acyclovir brings about the quickest resolution of lesions but is indicated only for severe, disseminated, or neurologic involvement. (Corey L, Benedetti J, Critchlow C, *et al.*: Treatment of primary first episode genital HSV infections with acyclovir: Results of topical, intravenous and oral therapy. *J Antimicrob Chemother* 1983, 12(B):79–88.)

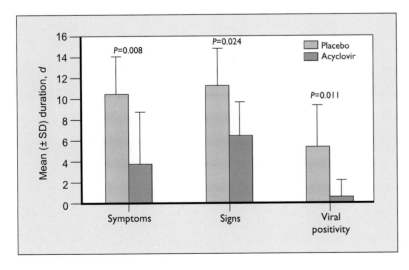

FIGURE 15-64 Acyclovir treatment of herpetic whitlow. Oral acyclovir, 200 mg given five times a day for 7 to 10 days or 400 mg given three times a day for 7 to 10 days, is effective in reducing the duration and extent of herpetic whitlow. Medical workers with active infection should double-glove and refrain from caring for high-risk patients until the lesions are crusted and dry. (Gill MJ, Bryant HE: Oral acyclovir therapy of recurrent HSV-2 infection of the hand. *Antimicrob Agents Chemother* 1991, 35:382–383.)

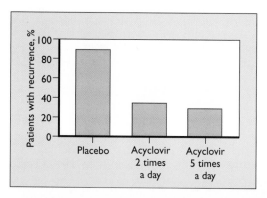

FIGURE 15-65 Suppression of HSV recurrences with daily oral acyclovir. Chronic oral acyclovir, 400 mg twice a day or 200 mg five times a day, will reduce the number of recurrences of symptomatic genital herpes in persons with frequent recurrences. In a double-blind trial comparing acyclovir and placebo, patients receiving chronic daily acyclovir were less likely to have recurrences over a 120-day period of treatment. Chronic suppressive acyclovir therapy does not eliminate latent virus or viral shedding, and lesions will recur after discontinuation of suppressive therapy. (*Adapted from* Douglas JM, Critchlow C, Benedetti J, *et al.*: Prevention of recurrent genital herpes simplex infection with daily oral acyclovir: A double-blind trial. *N Engl J Med* 1984, 310:1551–1556; with permission.)

A. Antiviral chemotherapy for mucocutaneous HSV infections: Genital herpes

First episode	Acyclovir, 200 mg orally 5 times daily × 10–14 days
	Acyclovir, 5 mg/kg intravenously every 8 hrs × 5 days (for severe disease or neurologic involvement)
	Topical acyclovir 5% ointment or cream, 4–6 times daily* × 7–10 days (for localized external lesions only)
	Famciclovir, 500 mg 3 times daily × 7–10 days
Symptomatic recurrences	Acyclovir, 200 mg orally 5 times daily × 5 days, *or*
	Acyclovir, 400 mg orally 3 times daily × 5 days
	Famciclovir, 250 mg (or 125 mg) 3 times daily × 5 days
Suppression of recurrences	Acyclovir, 200 mg capsule 2–3 times daily†
	Acyclovir, 400 mg orally 2 times daily
	Acyclovir, 800 mg orally once daily

*Although approved by the Food and Drug Administration, oral or intravenous acyclovir therapy is recommended.
†Preferred regimen. Famciclovir is not approved for suppression of recurrences.

B. Antiviral chemotherapy for mucocutaneous HSV infections: Oral–labial herpes

First episode	Acyclovir, 200 mg orally 4–5 times daily × 7 days
	Acyclovir suspension is available for children
Recurrences	Oral acyclovir is of minimal benefit
	Topical acyclovir has no benefit
Suppression of recurrences	Acyclovir, 400 mg orally 2 times daily, started before exposure and continued for duration, usually 5–10 days (for severe sunlight exposure)

C. Antiviral chemotherapy for mucocutaneous HSV infections: Other mucocutaneous herpes

Herpetic whitlow	Acyclovir, 200 mg orally 5 times daily × 7–10 days, *or*
	Acyclovir, 400 mg orally 3 times daily × 7–10 days
HSV proctitis	Acyclovir, 400 mg orally 5 times daily
	Acyclovir, 5 mg/kg intravenously every 8 hrs (in immunosuppression or severe infection)
HSV keratitis	Topical trifluorothymidine, vidarabine, idoxuridine, acyclovir, or interferon
Neonatal herpes	Acyclovir, 30 mg/kg/d intravenously × 10 days (for skin, eye, and mouth disease)
	Acyclovir, 45–60 mg/kg/d intravenously × 14–21 days (for CNS or disseminated disease)
	Vidarabine, 30 mg/kg/d intravenously × 14 days (for CNS)

CNS—central nervous system.

FIGURE 15-66 Antiviral chemotherapy for HSV infection. For mucocutaneous HSV infection, acyclovir has been the mainstay of therapy. **A.** Genital herpes. **B.** Oral–labial herpes. **C.** Other mucocutaneous herpes. (*continued*)

D. Antiviral chemotherapy for mucocutaneous HSV infections: Immunocompromised patients

Acute symptomatic first episode or recurrence	Acyclovir, 5 mg/kg intravenously every 8 hrs × 5 days Acyclovir, 400 mg orally 4 times daily × 7–10 days Topical acyclovir 5%, 4–6 times daily (for localized external lesions only)
Suppression of reactivation	Acyclovir, 5 mg/kg intravenously every 8 hrs Acyclovir, 400 mg orally 3–5 times daily (both regimens for use in high-risk periods)
Acyclovir resistance	Foscarnet, 60 mg/kg every 8 hrs until healing (reduced dosage in renal impairment)

Figure 15-66 (*continued*) **D.** Immunocompromised hosts. Recently, famciclovir has been approved for varicella-zoster infection and some aspects of genital HSV infection. (*Adapted from* Corey L: Herpes simplex virus infection. *In* Isselbacher KJ, *et al.* (eds.): *Harrison's Principles of Internal Medicine*, 13th ed. New York: McGraw-Hill; 1994:786; with permission.)

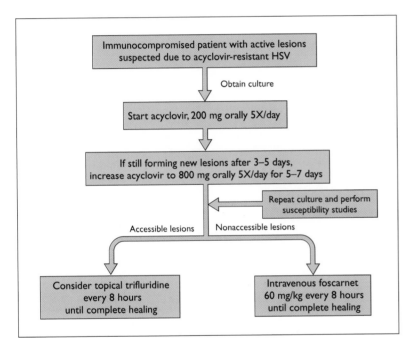

Figure 15-67 Treatment of acyclovir-resistant herpes. Acyclovir resistance is becoming increasingly associated with progressive disease in immunocompromised patients. Because of its lack of toxicity and lower cost, most clinicians initially utilize higher dosages of acyclovir, which may result in clearing of lesions in some patients. For severe acyclovir resistance, intravenous foscarnet is required. Foscarnet is usually reserved for patients with extensive mucocutaneous infections because of its toxicity and cost. (Safrin S, Crumpacker C, Chatis P, *et al.*: A controlled trial comparing foscarnet with vidarabine for acyclovir-resistant mucocutaneous herpes simplex in AIDS. *N Engl J Med* 1991, 325:551–555.)

SELECTED BIBLIOGRAPHY

Corey L: Genital herpes. *In* Holmes KK, Mårdh P-A, Sparling PF, *et al.* (eds.): *Sexually Transmitted Diseases*, 2nd ed. New York: McGraw Hill; 1990:391–408.

Corey L: Herpes simplex virus infection. *In* Isselbacher KJ, *et al.* (eds.): *Harrison's Principles of Internal Medicine*, 13th ed. New York: McGraw-Hill; 1994:782–788.

Corey L, Spear P: Infections with herpes simplex viruses [pts 1 and 2]. *N Engl J Med* 1986, 314:686–691, 749–757.

Dorsky DI, Crumpacker C: Drugs five years later: Acyclovir. *Ann Intern Med* 1987, 107:859–874.

Whitley RJ: Neonatal herpes. *In* Remington JS, Klein JO (eds.): *Infectious Diseases of the Fetus and Newborn Infant*, 3rd ed. Philadelphia: W.B. Saunders; 1990:282–305.

CHAPTER 16

Chancroid

Allan Ronald

EPIDEMIOLOGY

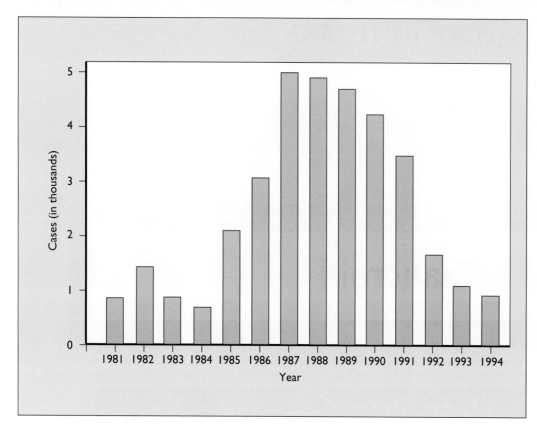

FIGURE 16-1 Reported incidence of chancroid in the United States between 1981 and 1994. After many years of low incidence, chancroid increased greatly in incidence during the 1980s, peaking at just under 5000 cases in 1987. Since then, the annual number of cases has fallen, presumably due to increased efforts to control the disease by treating contacts (particularly prostitutes), case finding, and more adequate treatment regimens. However, a recent study indicates that under-reporting of chancroid is common, and perhaps two to three times more cases are occurring unreported each year in the United States.

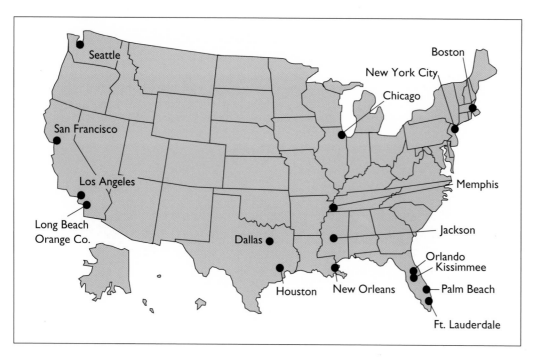

FIGURE 16-2 US cities with confirmed outbreaks of chancroid between 1983 and 1995. Cities having culture-proven or clinically diagnosed cases of chancroid are indicated. In most years, the largest number of cases occurs on the east coast and in the southern states. There also has been one large, extended outbreak in Southern California. Most outbreaks occur in urban slums and appear to be associated recently with crack cocaine use and with women who exchange sex for drugs. (*Courtesy of* G. Schmid, MD.)

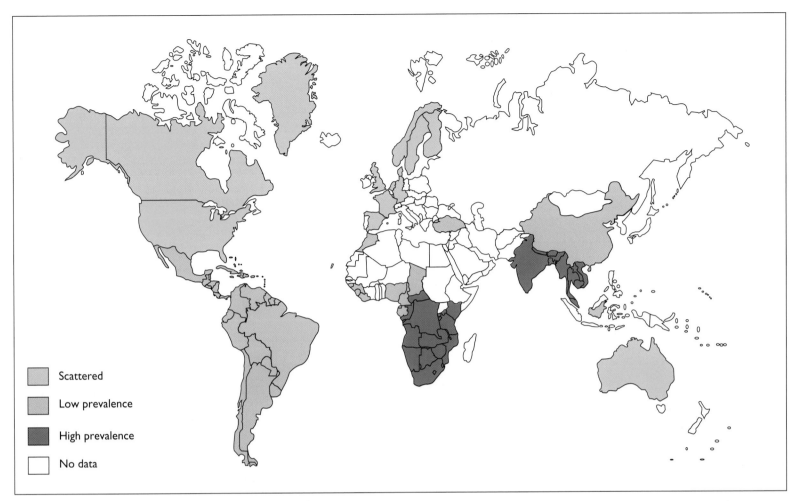

FIGURE 16-3 Estimated worldwide prevalence of chancroid. Central, eastern, and southern Africa, India, and Southeast Asia are areas of particularly high prevalence. (*Courtesy of* G. Schmid, MD.)

Scattered

Low prevalence

High prevalence

No data

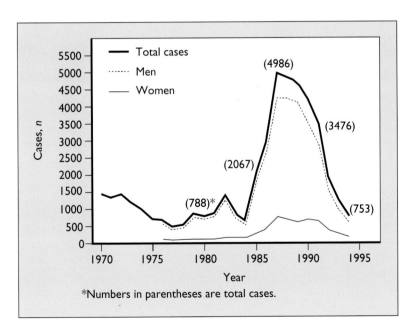

*Numbers in parentheses are total cases.

FIGURE 16-4 Frequency of chancroid in the United States by gender from 1990 to 1994. This graph of the reported incidence of chancroid in men and women documents the overwhelming prevalence of men. The diagnosis of chancroid is often not made in women, even when they present with genital lesions. Also, because most source contacts for men with chancroid are women with many male contacts, each infected woman probably infects five to 10 men. (*Courtesy of* G. Schmid, MD.)

CLINICAL MANIFESTATIONS

Pathogenic stages of chancroid

Papule	1–3 days
Vesicle/pustule	1–3 days
Ulcer	3–60 days
Lymphadenitis	Occurs in 30%–50%, usually within 7 days of onset of illness
Bubo	Occurs in 5%–10%, usually during the second or later weeks of illness

FIGURE 16-5 Pathogenic stages of chancroid. The incubation period for chancroid varies from 1 day to several weeks, with a median of 5 to 7 days. The lesion begins initially as a small papule with surrounding erythema, which soon progresses to a pustule and then erodes to form a painful ulcer. The ulcer has soft, ragged, undermined edges and an erythematous halo; the base is composed of gray or yellow granulation tissue that bleeds easily. Painful, unilateral, regional (inguinal) lymphadenopathy is seen in about half of the patients. Buboes can form and rupture, with formation of inguinal ulcers.

Chancroid in Men

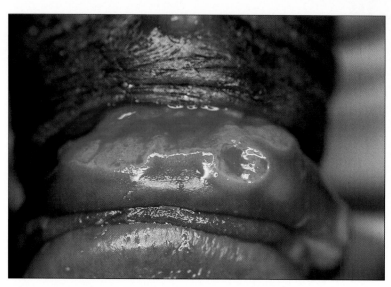

FIGURE 16-6 Classic, purulent chancroid lesion on the distal penis. A purulent, bleeding lesion 2 cm in diameter is seen on the prepuce. This patient had two other smaller lesions on the shaft of the penis. The most common sites of involvement in men are the distal prepuce, the mucosal surface of the prepuce on the frenulum, and the coronal sulcus.

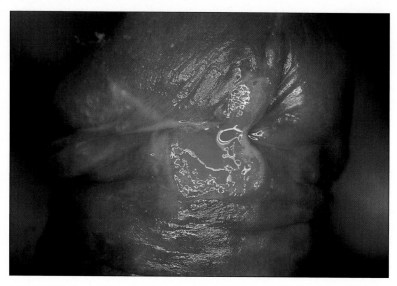

FIGURE 16-7 Irregular chancroid lesion on the frenulum. This lesion has been present for 2 weeks, and its site makes it very painful and obvious to the patient.

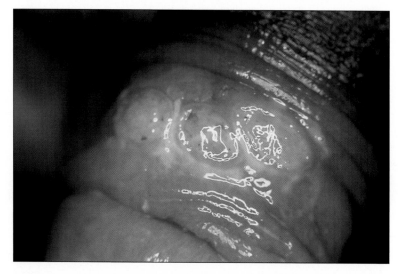

FIGURE 16-8 Multiple chancroid lesions on the coronal sulcus. The coronal sulcus is a very common site for chancroid, particularly in uncircumcised patients, and often the lesions merge to form an entire ring around the circumference of the penis.

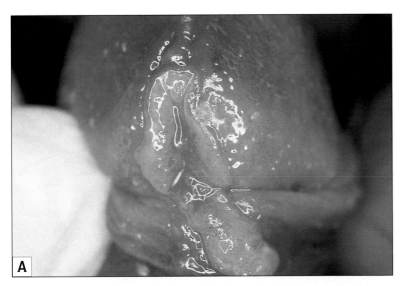
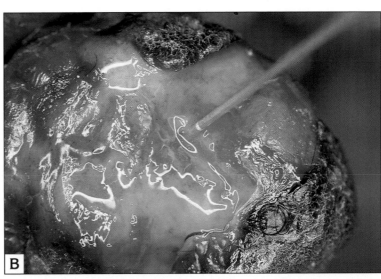

Figure 16-9 Penetrating chancroid ulcers leading to urethral fistulas. **A** and **B**, In both patients a destructive untreated lesion eroded through penile tissue, and ultimately the patient presented because of urination through the fistula. Treatment resulted in healing of the ulcer, and over the course of about 2 weeks, both patients had resolution of the fistula.

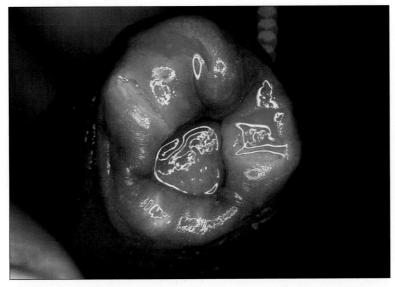

Figure 16-10 Ring of ulcers on the distal prepuce. This ulceration is associated with considerable edema of the prepuce and other ulcers on the inner aspect. In uncircumcised men, almost one half of ulcers occur on the prepuce.

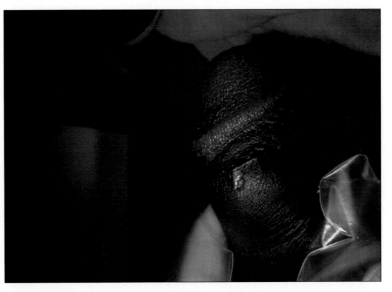

Figure 16-11 "Septic sore" presentation of chancroid. This presentation of chancroid is not well described in textbooks, but in Kenya, about 5% of men present this way. Pus is trapped in the skin of the shaft or prepuce. There may be no obvious ulcer. Usually, the septic sore can be drained readily with probing, and several milliliters of pus will be expressed. The pus almost invariably shows pure *Haemophilus ducreyi* on culture. Frequently, the overlying skin breaks down, and classic ulceration results unless treatment is given.

Figure 16-12 Ruptured right inguinal bubo. The patient had had a small subpreputial bubo that had not been recognized. *Haemophilus ducreyi* were grown from the ulcerated bubo. With treatment, this "growing abscess" responded readily to cure and 1 week later had almost resolved.

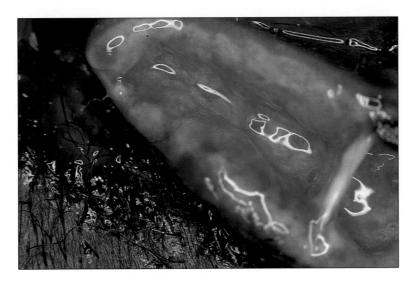

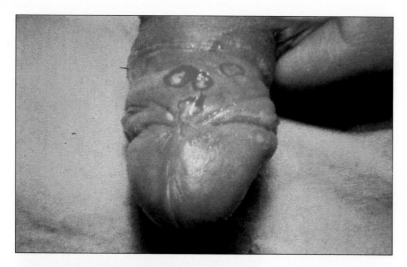

FIGURE 16-13 Four dwarf chancroid lesions on the underside of the penis. These lesions were never vesiculated. Although these small lesions appear initially to be herpetiform, about 10% of chancroid cases present in this way. Many would resolve without treatment over the course of 1 to 3 weeks.

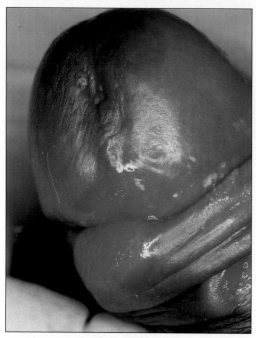

FIGURE 16-14 Chancroid lesion on the glans extending onto the penile shaft. Darkfield examination for spirochetes was positive, as were the rapid plasma reagin screening test and the *Treponema pallidum* hemagglutination assay confirmatory test. In addition, *Haemophilus ducreyi* was grown from the ulcer. In Kenya, about 4% of men who present with genital ulcers have coinfection with both *H. ducreyi* and *T. pallidum*. Another 3% have coinfection with *H. ducreyi* and herpes simplex virus. As a result, etiologic diagnosis is impossible. Because of the inadequacy of clinical diagnosis, all patients should be treated initially with both benzathine penicillin for *T. pallidum* infection and with erythromycin or another effective agent for chancroid. This treatment regimen was used in this patient with an excellent response.

Differential diagnosis of chancroidal lesions

Primary syphilis	Long incubation, usually 2–4 weeks
	Indurated painless ulcer that does not change its shape on squeezing and is usually not purulent
	Adenopathy usually painless
Genital herpes	Vesicles often present with ulcers
	History of recurrent lesions
	Incubation period of 3–7 days
	Usually painful ulcers with painful lymphadenitis
Lymphogranuloma venereum	Primary lesion is transient, painless, and usually not noted
	Groin lesions are chronic, indurated, and often develop sinuses
Donovanosis (granuloma inguinale)	Boggy, indurated, chronic ulcer with beefy red appearance
	Often spreads contiguously from primary lesion onto the groin and continues to intriginous areas of the genital tract

FIGURE 16-15 Differential diagnosis of chancroidal lesions. Syndromic diagnosis is mandatory in most parts of the world. Laboratory information is often not available. *Haemophilus ducreyi* cultures frequently are falsely negative, and there is no reliable serologic test. Darkfield examinations require expertise and technology that often are not available. As a result, all patients should be treated for both syphilis and chancroid. Despite these generalizations, it is still worthwhile to learn the classic features of the various etiologic agents that cause genital ulceration. However, these presenting features must be used carefully because as many as 50% of patients will be diagnosed incorrectly if all ulcerations are expected to be classic. In addition to syphilis, herpes, lymphogranuloma venereum, and donovanosis, other lesions to be considered include neoplasms (particularly squamous cell carcinoma), fungal balanitis, synergistic bacterial infection, traumatic ulcers, and tuberculosis.

Chancroid in Women

Clinical features of chancroid in men and women

	Men	Women
Genital ulcers	Single ulcers common	Multiple ulcers common
	Usually on prepuce or coronal sulcus	Usually vulvar, but anal and cervical ulcers may occur
	Painful ulcers	Painful ulcers on vulva or anus; cervical ulcers asymptomatic
Inguinal lymphadenopathy	30%–50% of cases	Occasionally
	Painful	Painful
	Large nodes suppurate	Suppuration not common
	Usually unilateral	Usually unilateral

FIGURE 16-16 Clinical features of chancroid in men and women. The clinical presentation of chancroid differs in men and women. Men frequently have single ulcers, whereas women typically are noted to have multiple lesions. Lesions in women may be only mildly symptomatic and often go undiagnosed.

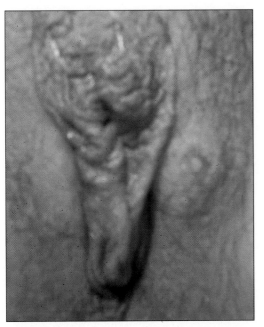

FIGURE 16-17 Small chancroid lesion on the labia majorum. This lesion was only moderately tender, and the patient was brought to medical attention only because she was identified through contact tracing.

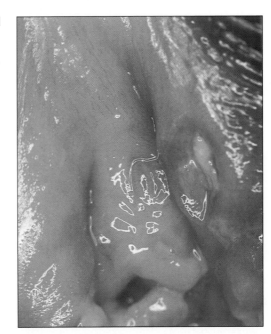

FIGURE 16-18 Chancroid lesion on the inner aspect of the labium majorum. Again, this 6-mm lesion was minimally symptomatic and was not recognized until the patient was examined.

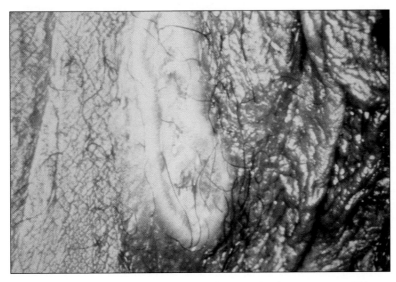

FIGURE 16-19 A longitudinal painful ulcer on the inner aspect of the labia. The common sites of involvement in women are at the entrance to the vagina and include the labia, fourchette, vestibule, and clitoris.

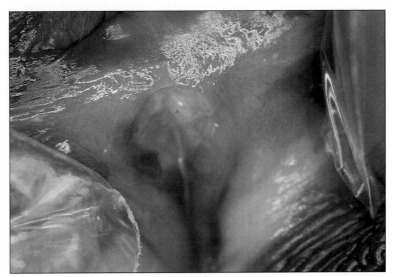

FIGURE 16-20 Periurethral chancroid ulcers. The lesions led the patient to present with complaints of dysuria and frequency. *Haemophilus ducreyi* was cultured from the ulcers.

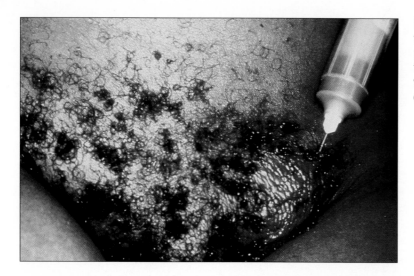

FIGURE 16-21 Aspiration of a left inguinal bubo of 30 mL of pus, which prevents spontaneous rupture and facilitates resolution. The patient had had an ulcer that was treated. However, she continued to have ongoing suppurative lymphadenitis. Cure followed drainage, without the need for additional antibacterial treatment, and the culture of bubo pus was negative for *Haemophilus ducreyi*.

LABORATORY EXAMINATIONS

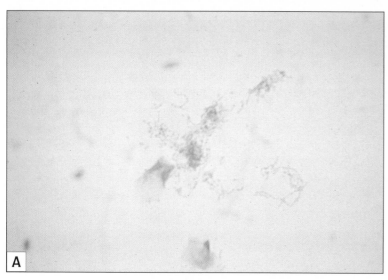

A

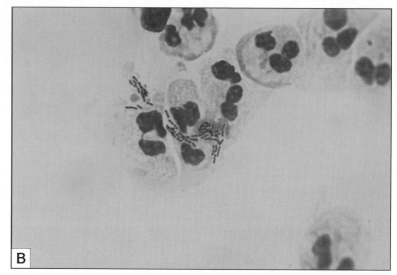

B

FIGURE 16-22 Gram stain of *Haemophilus ducreyi*. **A**, Gram staining of a pure subculture of the organism isolated from a chancroid lesion shows the organisms to be faintly staining, pleomorphic, and arranged haphazardly. **B**, Classically, Gram stains of chancroid lesions are described as showing the organisms in "school-of-fish" patterns. These patterns are seen in only one third to one half of patients, and the finding is not specific for chancroid because other gram-negative rods can have similar arrangements. However, intracellular *H. ducreyi* is usually seen only in patients with chancroid, and Gram stain showing this finding can be a more specific, if insensitive, result from the chancroidal lesion. (Panel 22B *courtesy of* E.J. Bottone, MD.)

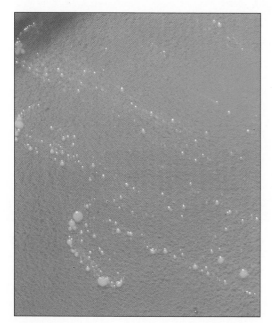

FIGURE 16-23 Culture of *Haemophilus ducreyi*. Culture of *H. ducreyi* is accomplished on gonococcal/chocolate agar supplemented with vitamins and fetal calf serum and made selective with vancomycin (3 mg/L). The organism grows as a pleomorphic yellow-gray colony, which varies widely, from pinpoint to 0.4 mm in diameter. Colonial variants are inconsistent on subculture and do not appear to be cloned genetic characteristics. The colony is very cohesive and can be moved intact with a straight wire. The adherence persists when colonies are suspended in liquid media.

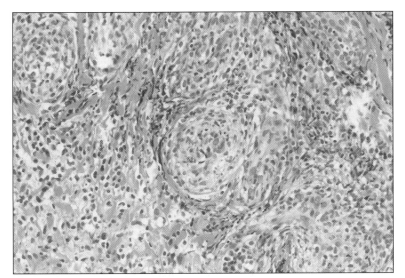

FIGURE 16-24 Histologic examination of the chancroid lesion. An abundance of mononuclear cells can be seen in the ulcer, consisting mostly of CD4- and CD8-bearing lymphocytes as well as macrophages and other tissue histiocytes. In addition, a granulomatous vasculitis is present. (Hematoxylin eosin stain.)

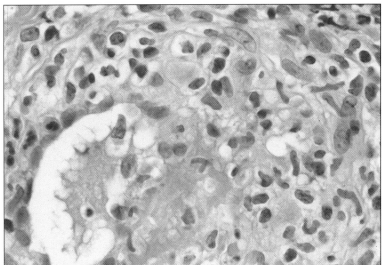

FIGURE 16-25 Biopsy of a chancroid ulcer showing vasculitis with endothelial proliferation and disruption.

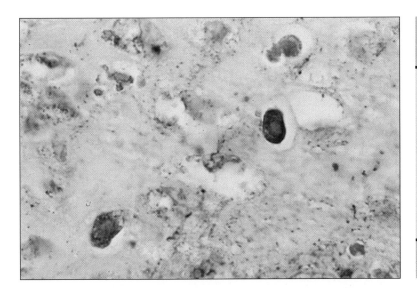

FIGURE 16-26 Monoclonal antibody staining showing coinfection by chancroid and HIV. Monoclonal antibody directed to the gp41 protein of HIV was used to identify HIV-infected mononuclear cells in an ulcer biopsy from an HIV-1–infected patient with chancroid. The cells stained brown with the monoclonal antibody presumably are cells infected with pro-viral HIV DNA. With activation of lymphocytes by cytokines in the chancroid ulcer, a productive HIV infection developed, with viral-laden cells apparent with this special stain. These cells would be very infectious for the sexual partner if intercourse were to occur, supporting the identification of chancroid as a cofactor for HIV infection.

Recommended and alternative treatment regimens for chancroid

Recommended regimens
  Azithromycin 1 g orally × single dose
  Ceftriaxone 250 mg intramuscularly × single dose
  Erythromycin base 500 mg orally 4 times a day × 7 days
Alternative regimens
  Amoxicillin, 500 mg, plus clavulanic acid, 125 mg, orally 3 times a day × 7 days
  Ciprofloxacin 500 mg orally twice a day × 3 days

FIGURE 16-27 Recommended treatment and alternative regimens for chancroid. These five regimens will cure more than 95% of patients with chancroid who are not concurrently infected with HIV. Azithromycin and ceftriaxone offer the advantage of single-dose therapy. Antimicrobial resistance to these regimens has not been well documented. Although two isolates resistant to erythromycin were reported from Asia a decade ago, similar isolates have not been recognized elsewhere. Ciprofloxacin is contraindicated for pregnant and lactating women, children, and adolescents under 17 years of age. (Centers for Disease Control and Prevention: 1993 Sexually transmitted diseases treatment guidelines. *MMWR* 1993, 42(RR-14):21.)

MIC$_{90}$ for recent *Haemophilus ducreyi* isolates	
Sulfonamides	128 µg/mL
Ampicillin	128 µg/mL
Vancomycin	64 µg/mL
Tetracycline	32 µg/mL
Trimethoprim	16 µg/mL
Kanamycin	8 µg/mL
Chloramphenicol	8 µg/mL
Ampicillin/sulbactam	4 µg/mL
Rifampin	0.016 µg/mL
Erythromycin	0.030 µg/mL
Ciprofloxacin	0.007 µg/mL
Ceftriaxone	0.002 µg/mL

MIC$_{90}$—90% minimum inhibitory concentration.

Figure 16-28 Ninety percent minimum inhibitory concentrations (MIC$_{90}$) for recent *Haemophilus ducreyi* isolates. The MIC$_{90}$ expressed here in µg/mL, is that concentration of an antimicrobial agent that will inhibit the growth of 90% of clinical isolates. Ceftriaxone, the quinolones, and erythromycin remained highly effective in almost all geographic areas. Other quinolones in addition to ciprofloxacin are highly active as well. (Ronald AR, Albritton A: Chancroid and *Haemophilus ducreyi*. *In* Holmes D, Mårdh P-A, Sparling PF, *et al.* (eds.): *Sexually Transmitted Diseases*, 2nd ed. New York: McGraw Hill; 1990:263–271.)

Haemophilus ducreyi plasmids coding for antimicrobial resistance	
5.7- or 7.0-MDa plasmid	β-lactamase
3.2-MDa plasmid	β-lactamase (identical to *Neisseria gonorrhoeae* plasmid)
2.6-MDa plasmid	Penicillin resistance
4.9-MDa plasmid	Sulfonamide resistance
Large, conjugative plasmid	Tetracycline resistance
3.0-MDa plasmid	Sulfonamide, kanamycin, and streptomycin resistance
24.4-MDa plasmid	Efficient mobilizing plasmid

Figure 16-29 *Haemophilus ducreyi* plasmids coding for antimicrobial resistance. *H. ducreyi* has acquired a range of plasmids coding for antimicrobial resistance. It is speculated that the 3.2-megadalton (MDa) plasmid was transferred to *Neisseria gonorrhoeae*, resulting in the development of penicillinase-producing *N. gonorrhoeae*.

SELECTED BIBLIOGRAPHY

Centers for Disease Control and Prevention: 1993 Sexually transmitted diseases treatment guidelines. *MMWR* 1993, 42(RR-14):20–22.

Dangor Y, Ballard RC, Exposto FL, *et al.*: Accuracy of a clinical diagnosis of genital ulcer disease. *Sex Transm Dis* 1990, 17:184–189.

Knapp JS, Back AF, Babst AF, *et al.*: *In vitro* susceptibilities of isolates of *Haemophilus ducreyi* from Thailand and the United States to currently recommended and newer agents for treatment of chancroid. *Antimicrob Agents Chemother* 1993, 27:1552–1555.

Martin DH, DiCarlo RP: Recent changes in the epidemiology of genital ulcer disease in the United States: The crack cocaine connection. *Sex Transm Dis* 1994; 21(suppl):S76–S80.

O'Farrell N, Hoosen AA, Coetzee KD, van den Ende J: Genital ulcer disease: Accuracy of a clinical diagnosis and strategies to improve control in Durban, South Africa. *Genitourin Med* 1994, 70:7–11.

CHAPTER 17

Donovanosis (Granuloma Inguinale)

Gavin Hart

EPIDEMIOLOGY

Historical names for donovanosis
Serpiginous ulceration of the groin
Lupoid form of groin ulceration
Chronic venereal sores
Granuloma inguinale
Granuloma contagiosa
Granuloma donovani
Granuloma inguinale tropicum
Granuloma pudendi tropicum
Granuloma venereum
Sclerosing granuloma
Ulcerating granuloma of the pudendum

FIGURE 17-1 Historical names for donovanosis. Donovanosis is a chronic ulcerating disease first described from southeast India in 1882 by Kenneth McLeod, who named the disease serpiginous ulceration of the groin. Since then, many names have been applied to the condition, most being confusing or inappropriate. Granuloma venereum leads to confusion with lymphogranuloma venereum. Until recently, granuloma inguinale was the most widely used name for the disease, but it is particularly inappropriate because the inguinal region is involved in only a minority of cases, and the genitals alone are involved in about 95% of cases (*see* Fig. 17-9). Donovanosis is the most appropriate name because it is short and distinctive and commemorates Charles Donovan who first described the causative organism in 1905. It is the term used in Papua New Guinea and many other areas where the disease is most prevalent. (McLeod K: Précis of operations performed in the wards of the first surgeon, Medical College O Hospital (Rio), during the year 1881. *Indian Med Gaz* 1882, 17:113–123. Donovan C: Ulcerating granuloma of the pudenda. *Indian Med Gaz* 1905, 40:414.)

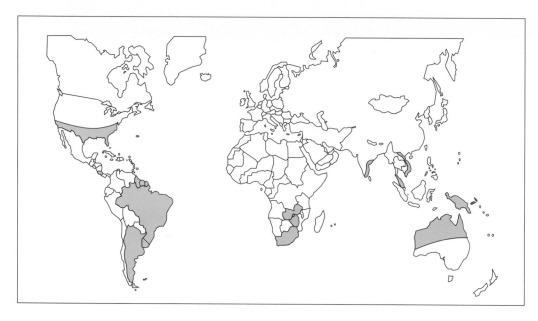

FIGURE 17-2 Worldwide distribution of donovanosis. Donovanosis is now rare in the United States, with fewer than 100 cases reported annually, but outbreaks have occurred. Worldwide, the endemic areas include New Guinea, central Australia, the Caribbean, India (especially the eastern coast), Brazil, Zambia, Zimbabwe, Natal, Vietnam, and Japan. (Rosen T, Tschen JA, Ramsdell W, *et al.*: Granuloma inguinale. *J Am Acad Dermatol* 1984, 11:433–437.) (*Adapted from* Richens J: The diagnosis and treatment of donovanosis (granuloma inguinale). *Genitourin Med* 1991, 67:441–452; with permission.)

ETIOLOGY AND DIAGNOSIS

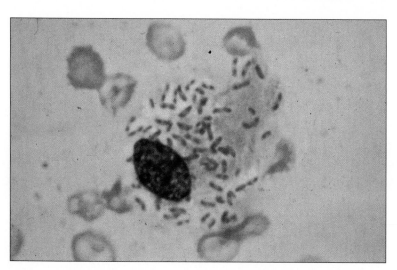

FIGURE 17-3 Donovan bodies. The causative organism of donovanosis is *Calymmatobacterium granulomatis*, formerly called *Donovania granulomatis*, which was first described by Charles Donovan in 1905. The organism is a pleomorphic, gram-negative rod that multiples within host cells. On stained smears, these intracellular organisms are referred to as Donovan bodies. The typical appearance of Donovan bodies is seen in a large mononuclear cell, 20 to 90 µm in diameter. (Giemsa stain; original magnification, × 1000.) The host cell nucleus is usually oval, eccentric, and vesicular or pyknotic. The causative organisms appear as bipolar-staining (closed safety-pin) forms, 1 to 1.5 µm in length and 0.5 to 0.7 µm in diameter, contained in cytoplasmic vacuoles. Smears are best prepared by making an impression from the undersurface of removed tissue (to avoid surface debris and other bacteria) and then air-drying and heat-fixing before staining with Giemsa, Leishman's, or Wright's stain. (Donovan C: Ulcerating granuloma of the pudenda. *Indian Med Gaz* 1905, 40:414.) (*Courtesy of* J. Richens, MD.)

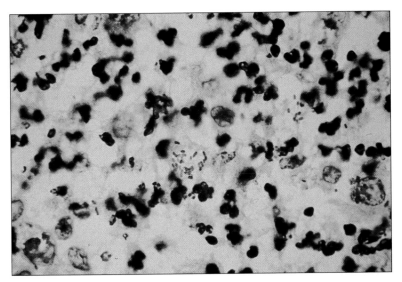

FIGURE 17-4 Black-staining Donovan bodies demonstrated by silver stain. Silver stains are useful, particularly in smears containing few organisms. Typical bipolar-staining organisms are seen in a mononuclear cell in the center of this slide. On the periphery are several cells showing characteristic palisading or clustering of organisms lining the cytoplasmic vacuoles. (Original magnification, × 400.) (Barnes R, Masood S, Lammert N, Young RH: Extragenital granuloma inguinale mimicking a soft-tissue neoplasm: A case report and review of the literature. *Hum Pathol* 1990, 21:559–561.)

Diagnostic techniques in donovanosis

Smear
  Giemsa stain
  Wright stain
  Leishman stain

Histology
  Hematoxylin-eosin stain
  Silver stains
  Thionine azure II basic fuchsin (semithin sections)

Serology
  Indirect immunofluorescence

FIGURE 17-5 Diagnostic techniques in donovanosis. Attempts to consistently grow *Calymmatobacterium granulomatis* in eggs or on artificial media have been unsuccessful. The simplest method of confirming the diagnosis is by demonstration of the characteristic Donovan bodies in smears prepared from active lesions. A small piece of tissue should be removed from a lesion and the underside imprinted on a glass slide (the surface of lesions contains too much debris and other organisms to provide a satisfactory impression). Giemsa, Wright's, and Leishman's stains are all satisfactory for highlighting the Donovan bodies. The general histologic features (dense infiltrate of plasma cells with few polymorphs or lymphocytes; variable epithelial hyperplasia sometimes appearing neoplastic) are insufficiently specific for confirming the diagnosis, but embedded tissue may be used for identifying Donovan bodies. For this purpose, hematoxylin-eosin staining is usually less satisfactory than silver stains, although thionine azure II basic fuchsin also has given good results, particularly when used with semithin sections. Semithin sections are more expensive and time-consuming to prepare but can be useful for difficult cases. A serologic test using an indirect immunofluorescence technique can also be used for difficult cases. (Jain AK, Chandra M, Ganguli DD, Bhargava NC: Utility of semithin sections in the diagnosis of donovanosis. *Indian J Med Res* 1989, 90:270–274. Freinkel AL, *et al.*: A serological test for granuloma inguinale. *Genitourin Med* 1992, 68:269–272.)

Characteristics of Donovan bodies

Donovan bodies	1–2 × 0.5–0.7 µm Bipolar densities result in a closed safety-pin appearance
Mononuclear cell	20–90 µm in diameter Oval, eccentric, vesicular or pyknotic nucleus Vacuolated cytoplasm contains clusters of Donovan bodies, sometimes confined to periphery of phagosomes

FIGURE 17-6 Characteristics of Donovan bodies. The gold standard test for diagnosis of donovanosis is the demonstration of intracellular Donovan bodies in smears or biopsy specimens (*see* Fig. 17-5). The Donovan bodies have bipolar densities that produce a closed-safety-pin appearance and occur in clusters in typical mononuclear cells, 20 to 90 µm in diameter with an oval, eccentric, vesicular, or pyknotic nucleus. The Donovan bodies occur in vacuoles within the cytoplasm and sometimes are confined to the periphery of the phagosomes ("palisading") (*see* Fig. 17-4).

Clinical features of donovanosis

Subcutaneous papule
  Prepuce, coronal sulcus, penile shaft, glans (men)
  Labia minora, fourchette, labia majora (women)
Beefy red protuberant lesion
Direct extension autoinoculation ("kissing" lesions)
Minimal pain
Systemic dissemination (6%)
  Skin, bone, abdominal organs
  Most common in women with cervical lesions

FIGURE 17-7 Clinical features of donovanosis. Donovanosis usually begins as a subcutaneous papule, most commonly involving the prepuce, coronal sulcus, penile shaft, or glans in men and the labia minora, fourchette, or labia majora in women. Ulceration soon occurs to reveal beefy red granulation tissue, which spreads by extension or forms "kissing" lesions by direct contact with adjacent skin. Lesions are generally not painful or indurated unless secondarily infected. Systemic symptoms are absent unless dissemination occurs. Hematogenous dissemination may produce lesions in skin, bone, or intra-abdominal organs. Dissemination is seen most commonly in women with primary lesions on the cervix.

Differential diagnosis of donovanosis

Disease	Distinguishing features
Syphilis	Painless, pale condylomata; subside with penicillin
Carcinoma	Histopathology; nonresponsive to antibiotics
Amebiasis	Histopathology; specific antibiotic response
Lymphogranuloma venereum	Tender lymphadenopathy followed by fibrosis Positive culture for *Chlamydia trachomatis*; positive CFT
Tuberculosis, pyogenic granuloma	Histopathology; bacteriology
Chancroid	Painful (usually multiple) ulceration; tender lymphadenopathy; positive culture for *Haemophilus ducreyi*

CFT—complement fixation test.

FIGURE 17-8 Differential diagnosis of donovanosis. Donovanosis is frequently confused with other diseases. Secondary (and occasionally primary) syphilis may resemble donovanosis, and the two diseases frequently coexist (hence, the serologic test for syphilis is not of significant benefit in clarifying the diagnosis). Condylomata of syphilis are pale, in contrast to the redness of donovanosis lesions; and the latter are unaffected by penicillin therapy, whereas the syphilitic lesions resolve rapidly. Donovanosis is also commonly misdiagnosed as carcinoma, which can be differentiated by histopathologic examination and which does not respond to antibiotics. Amebiasis may be diagnosed by seeing trophozoites on histopathologic specimens and responds to metronidazole therapy but not the antibiotics used for donovanosis. Lymphogranuloma venereum presents predominantly as tender inguinal lymphadenopathy, and culture of *Chlamydia trachomatis* or a high titer (above 1:64) on the complement fixation test confirms the diagnosis. Tuberculosis may be confirmed by histopathologic patterns or detection of acid-fast bacilli. Chancroid usually produces painful ulceration with tender lymphadenopathy and can be confirmed by culture of *Haemophilus ducreyi*.

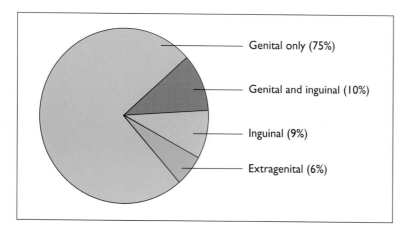

Genital only (75%)

Genital and inguinal (10%)

Inguinal (9%)

Extragenital (6%)

FIGURE 17-9 Anatomic distribution of donovanosis lesions. The actual anatomic distribution of lesions in donovanosis (as well as duration of lesions) varies substantially with patient selection. However, one large study of over 2000 cases found extragenital dissemination in 6% of cases. All studies of any size show that the great majority of cases involve the genitals alone (averaging about 75%), and lesions confined to the inguinal region are relatively infrequent. About 10% of cases present with both genital and inguinal lesions.

Common Morphologic Presentations of Donovanosis

Common morphologic variants of donovanosis

Fleshy, exuberant lesions
Necrotic lesions
Sclerotic or cicatricial lesions

FIGURE 17-10 Common morphologic variants of donovanosis. Donovanosis has diverse patterns of presentations but may be classified into a few general categories. The most common presentation involves fleshy red exuberant lesions that are nontender and tend to bleed on touch. Necrotic lesions are often large and irregular with foul copious exudate. By contrast, sclerotic lesions appear as undermined deep ulcers but have a dry base and do not bleed readily. They are often associated with constriction and distortion of adjacent tissues. Some authors describe an additional "hypertrophic" variant, having a wartlike appearance, but this presentation is less common and may not be clearly distinctive from the other variants.

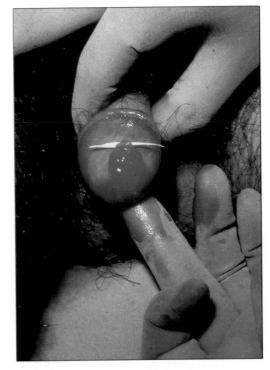

FIGURE 17-11
Fleshy exuberant lesion of donovanosis. Of the common morphologic variants of donovanosis, the most common form is the fleshy exuberant lesion, which is characterized by a red beefy appearance. The genitals are involved in about 90% of infections and are usually the only site of infection. In men, lesions most commonly occur on the prepuce, coronal sulcus, shaft, or glans.

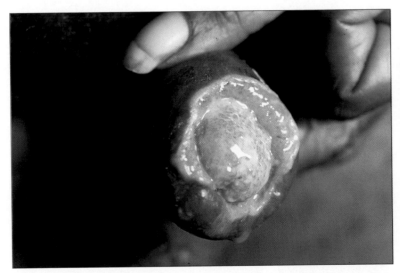

FIGURE 17-12 Necrotic variant of donovanosis. Extensive destruction of the genitals and profuse, foul-smelling exudate are characteristic of necrotic donovanosis. These cases are often diagnosed clinically as carcinoma, and the diagnosis is confirmed only after biopsy prior to amputation. Localized lesions respond rapidly to effective antibiotic therapy (*eg*, trimethoprim/sulfamethoxazole tetracyclines), which produces shrinkage of lesions and disappearance of organisms within 1 week. This lesion healed completely after 3 weeks' treatment with chloramphenicol, 500 mg three times daily.

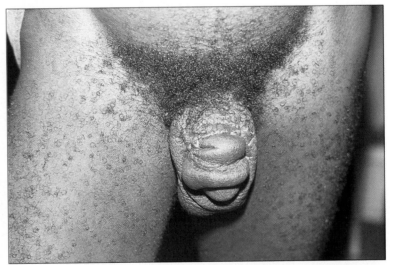

FIGURE 17-13 Cicatricial or sclerotic variant of donovanosis. This variant presents as a dry, bandlike scar around the genitals, frequently associated with lymphedema due to the constrictive nature of the lesion. Biopsy is required to confirm the diagnosis, as direct smears cannot be prepared easily from this type of lesion.

Donovanosis in Men

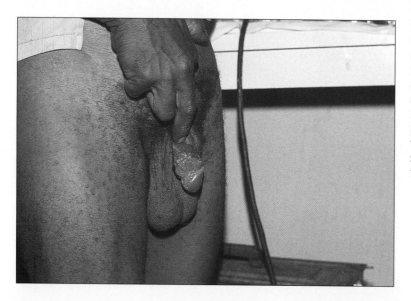

FIGURE 17-14 Typical beefy red lesion of donovanosis on the distal penis. In typical cases, a small papule appears 3 to 40 days after sexual contact, and ulceration through the skin surface soon follows. Lesions are usually painless, unless secondarily infected, and expand slowly by either extension from the periphery or autoinoculation onto adjacent skin. Donovanosis ulcers are not indurated unless secondary infection occurs (in contrast to the primary chancre of syphilis). The extensive destruction of donovanosis results solely from the delay in seeking treatment; in one study, greater than 50% of patients had had lesions for more than 2 months.

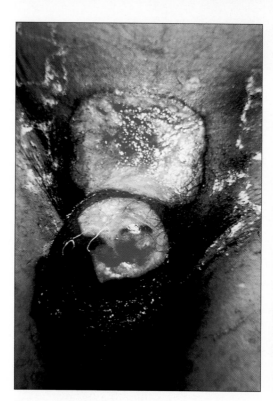

FIGURE 17-15 Complete destruction of the penis by donovanosis. This man aged 30 years had penile donovanosis for 3 months before seeking treatment. The suprapubic lesion was produced by autoinoculation from the penis.

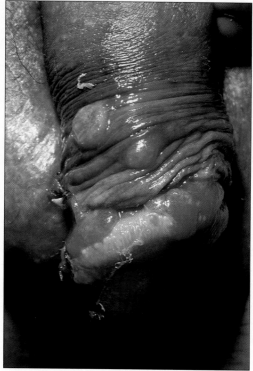

FIGURE 17-16 Multiple nodular lesions of donovanosis, of the fleshy variety, on the penis. The differential diagnosis of donovanosis includes secondary syphilis, ulcerated genital warts, squamous carcinoma, and chancroid. Condylomata lata (of secondary syphilis) are usually pale and flat, in contrast to the beefy red, exuberant lesions of donovanosis. This patient demonstrates lesions with characteristics between those of the classic presentations of the two diseases.

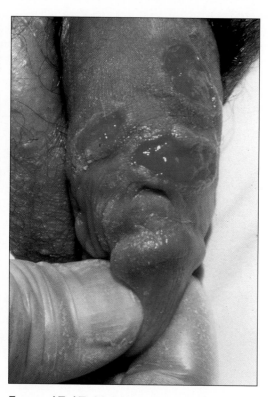

FIGURE 17-17 Multiple granulomatous lesions of the penis. These lesions are ulcerative, rather than displaying the more common protuberant features, but the red granulomatous nature of the ulcer base suggests donovanosis. The lesions could be confused with primary syphilis, although the primary chancre of syphilis is usually solitary. The primary chancre also is usually painless, whereas the lesions of donovanosis may be mildly painful (in contrast to the much more painful lesions of chancroid or herpes).

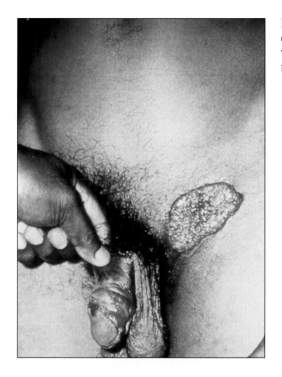

FIGURE 17-18 Inguinal lesion of donovanosis. Inguinal lesions occur in up to 20% of cases, but in more than 50% of these cases lesions also occur on the genitals. In donovanosis, unilateral inguinal lesions are more common than bilateral ones. Typical beefy red penile lesions can also be seen in this patient.

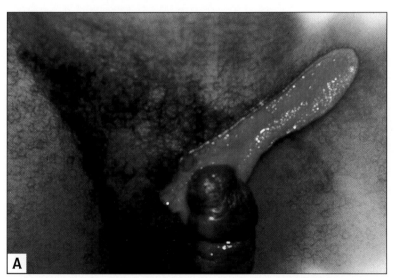

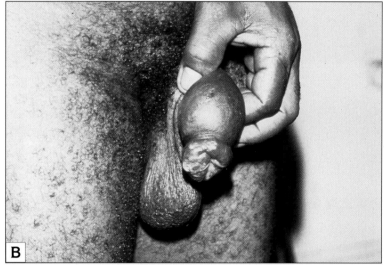

FIGURE 17-19 Inguinal and preputial lesions of donovanosis. Preputial lesions often lead to phimosis, with ballooning of the prepuce and purulent discharge from the constricted preputial opening. This problem is often complicated by concurrent gono- coccal urethritis, which increases the discharge and preputial swelling, while the phimosis hinders diagnosis of the gonococcal infection. **A,** Extensive inguinal and preputial lesions. **B,** Preputial lesions. (Panel 19A *courtesy of* J. Richens, MD.)

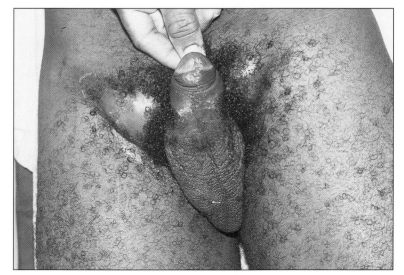

FIGURE 17-20 Donovanosis ulcer of the distal penis with subcutaneous swellings at the base of the penis and bilateral inguinal regions. The swellings are subcutaneous granulomata, which eventually erode through the skin to produce beefy exuberant lesions. Involvement of the lymph nodes is unusual, and suppuration is rare in these swellings (in contrast to the buboes of chancroid and lymphogranuloma venereum, which rapidly suppurate and rupture if not aspirated or treated early in the course of infection).

Donovanosis in Women

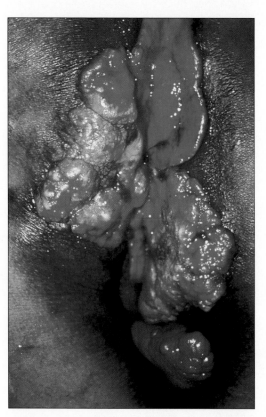

FIGURE 17-21
Beefy red exuberant lesions of donovanosis of the vulva. In women, the most common sites of infection are the labia minora, fourchette, and labia majora. The moist environment facilitates secondary infection of lesions and spread by autoinoculation ("kissing") of adjacent or opposing surfaces. Vulval lesions may extend into the vagina and other pelvic tissues, but lesions in the cervix may occur in the absence of external signs of infection. (*Courtesy of* J. Richens, MD.)

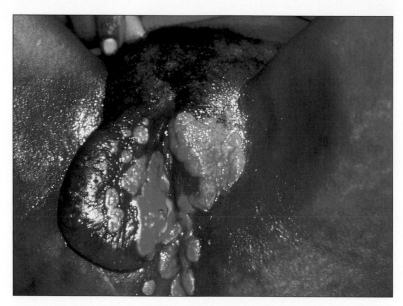

FIGURE 17-22 Vulval donovanosis with labial edema and perianal extension. This common presentation of donovanosis in the woman involves spread of the disease toward the anus and edema of the right labium. In men, severe edema of the scrotum often occurs in association with extensive donovanosis lesions. Edema may persist after successful treatment if the lesions have been longstanding. (*Courtesy of* J. Richens, MD.)

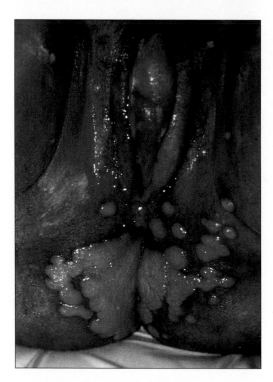

FIGURE 17-23 Extensive vulval and perianal donovanosis. This presentation is difficult to distinguish from condylomata lata of secondary syphilis, particularly because many patients with donovanosis have concurrent positive serologic or clinical findings for syphilis. Donovanosis is suggested by the redness of lesions, in contrast to the paleness of condylomata lata. Condylomata lata rapidly subside after penicillin therapy, whereas donovanosis lesions are not affected by this antibiotic. (*Courtesy of* J. Richens, MD.)

Extragenital Manifestations

Extragenital manifestations of donovanosis
Skin—cheeks, eyelids, nipple
Bones—sternum, ribs, clavicle, vertebrae, skull, joints
Intra-abdominal—colon, liver, uterus, ovary, spleen
Oral cavity
Other—lung, epididymis

FIGURE 17-24 Extragenital manifestations of donovanosis. In over 2000 cases of donovanosis seen by Rajam and coworkers, extragenital lesions occurred in 6% of cases. These lesions can affect virtually any body organ. They are most noticeable on the skin (commonly occurring over the face and thorax) but most commonly affect bones. Intra-abdominal organs may be involved, usually by dissemination from primary cervical lesions. Lesions of the oral cavity, lungs, and epididymis have also been described. (Rajam RV, Rangiah PN, Anguli VC: Systemic donovaniasis. *Br J Vener Dis* 1954, 30:73–80.)

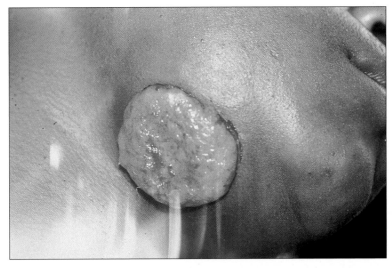

FIGURE 17-25 Donovanosis lesion in the submandibular region. Up to 6% of cases involve extragenital lesions. Skin lesions usually result from autoinoculation of opposing surfaces or spread via clothing or fingers of the patient. However, in some cases, primary extragenital infection occurs (without genital lesions). (Spagnola DV, Coburn PR, Cream JJ, Azadian BS: Extragenital granuloma inguinale (donovanosis) diagnosed in the United Kingdom: A clinical, histological, and electron microscopical study. *J Clin Pathol* 1984, 37:945–949.) (*Courtesy of* J. Richens, MD.)

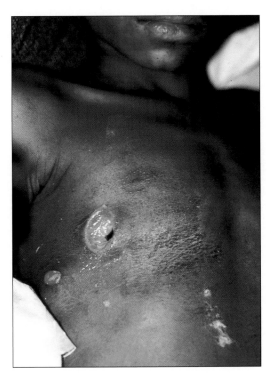

FIGURE 17-26 Granulomatous lesions of the nipple and thoracic wall. This type of lesion frequently occurs by autoinoculation via the patient's hands. (*Courtesy of* J. Richens, MD.)

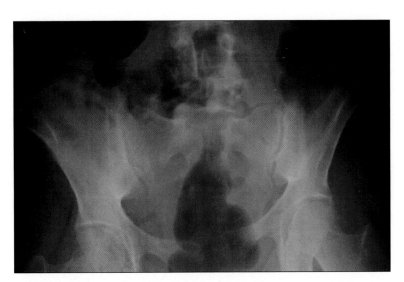

FIGURE 17-27 Erosion and collapse of the lumbar spine from donovanosis. This lesion at L5 was initially diagnosed as tuberculosis, but systemic donovanosis following extensive intrapelvic spread was confirmed at postmortem examination. Systemic hematogenous spread of infection, usually affecting bones, liver, or lungs, is relatively rare. Almost all cases reported have occurred in association with primary cervical lesions. The risk of systemic spread is increased by pregnancy, particularly by delivery or abortion. Systemic donovanosis is associated with severe constitutional disturbance (reflected by high spiking fever, progressive anemia, and weight loss) and a substantial fatality rate. (*Courtesy of* J. Richens, MD.)

Antibiotic therapy for donovanosis	
Tetracycline	500 mg orally 4 times a day
Doxycycline	100 mg orally twice a day
Minocycline	100 mg orally twice a day
Trimethoprim/sulfa-methoxazole	1 double-strength tablet orally twice a day
Erythromycin	500 mg orally 4 times a day
Gentamicin	1 mg/kg intramuscularly twice a day
Streptomycin	1 g intramuscularly twice a day
Chloramphenicol	500 mg orally 3 times a day
Ceftriaxone	1 g intravenously

FIGURE 17-28 Antibiotic therapy for donovanosis. A range of antibiotics is effective against donovanosis. Trimethoprim/sulfamethoxazole is the most widely used drug in India and some other developing countries. Chloramphenicol is the drug of choice in Papua New Guinea. Tetracycline (or doxycycline) is widely used and is probably the most versatile choice in developed countries (being readily available and generally safe). Multiple doses of ceftriaxone or erythromycin can be used for pregnant women. Penicillin is notably ineffective. Of note, treatment should be continued for at least 3 weeks, with some clinicians preferring to extend treatment until the lesions have healed. Response is evident in 7 days, with the lesions decreasing in erythema and friability. Sexual partners should be examined for disease but should not be treated unless lesions are found.

Prevalence of donovanosis in conjugal partners		
Author	Year	Prevalence
Packer, Goldberg	1950	0.4%
Serma	1957	12%
Ramchander, Pankaja	1967	1.6%
Vimla Bai, *et al.*	1969	4%
Lal, Nicholas	1970	52%

FIGURE 17-29 Prevalence of donovanosis in conjugal partners. Although donovanosis is generally considered to be sexually transmitted, some have disputed this view because of disease in the very young or sexually inactive individuals and because of the low infectivity rates in spouses. In fact, widely divergent prevalence rates in spouses have been reported. After an early report from the United States of a prevalence of 0.4%, later reports (all from India) reported rates from 1.6% to 52%. This variation may well be explained by the long variable incubation of the disease (average of 18 days but extending up to 360 days), the extended duration of disease before treatment, and variation in diagnostic capability.

SELECTED BIBLIOGRAPHY

Hart G: Donovanosis: *In* Holmes KK, Mårdh P-A, Sparling PF, *et al.* (eds.): *Sexually Transmitted Diseases*, 2nd ed. New York: McGraw-Hill; 1990:273–277.

Richens J: The diagnosis and treatment of donovanosis (granuloma inguinale). *Genitourin Med* 1991, 67:441–452.

Sehgal VN, Prasad ALS: Donovanosis: Current concepts. *Int J Dermatol* 1986, 25:8–16.

CHAPTER 18

Physical Examination and Diagnostic Techniques

Franklyn N. Judson

EXAMINATION ROOM

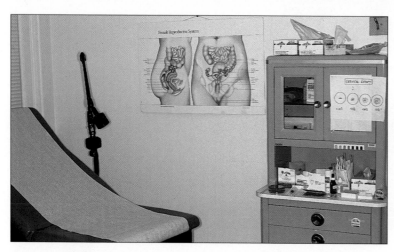

FIGURE 18-1 Examination room. The examination room should be quiet and well illuminated, provide for privacy, and contain all needed supplies and equipment within easy reach.

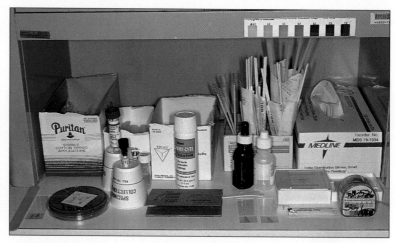

FIGURE 18-2 Supply cabinet. On the cabinet counter, supplies should be arranged so that the physical examination and specimen collection can flow without interruption.

Examination room supplies and equipment

Good examination light
Gloves
Sterile cotton-tipped applicators, calcium alginate urethrogenital swabs on flexible aluminum shafts, and large swabs for cleaning the exocervix
Microscope slides and cover slips
Water-soluble lubricant
10% Potassium hydroxide solution
Physiologic saline solution

Vaginal specula in assorted sizes
Spatula, cytobrush, slide holder, and fixative for Papanicolaou smears
Culture and/or transport media for *Neisseria gonorrhoeae* and *Chlamydia trachomatis*, and herpes simplex virus diagnostic tests
pH paper, 4–7 range
Tissues

FIGURE 18-3 Examination room supplies and equipment. All needed supplies and equipment should be stocked within easy reach in the examination room.

GENERAL PATIENT EXAMINATION

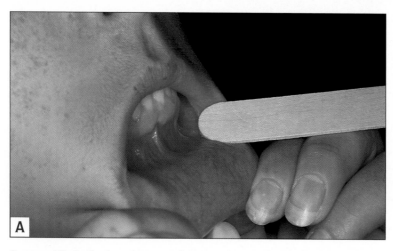

A

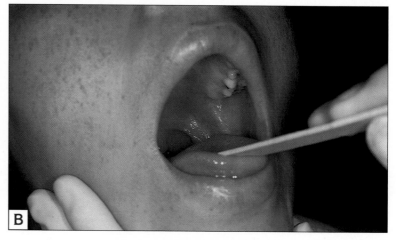

B

FIGURE 18-4 Oral cavity examination. **A** and **B**, Using a sterile wooden tongue depressor, inspect the gums and labial mucosa (*panel 4A*) and then the tongue, buccal surfaces, and oropharynx (*panel 4B*) for enanthema, lesions, and thrush.

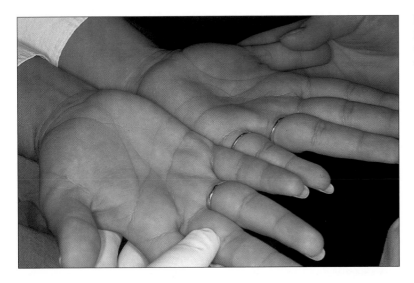

FIGURE 18-5 Inspection of the skin. Looking for rashes and lesions, inspect the face, including the eyes and conjunctivae, trunk, forearms, palms, fingernails, and legs. If a rash consistent with syphilis is present, also inspect the soles of the feet.

GENITAL EXAMINATION OF WOMEN

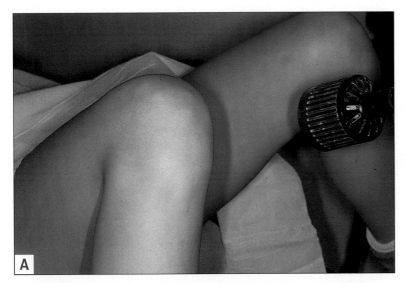

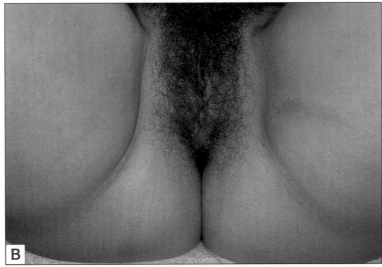

FIGURE 18-6 Patient positioning. **A,** Position the patient on the examination table and cover her with a clean drape that can be extended over the knees. A bright, well-focused, movable examination light should be conveniently placed. Seat yourself comfort- ably at the end of the table, and assist the patient in positioning her legs in the stirrups. **B,** Direct the light so that the external anogenital area can be viewed clearly.

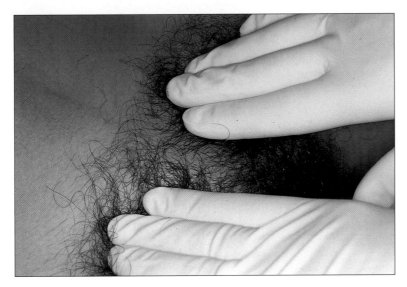

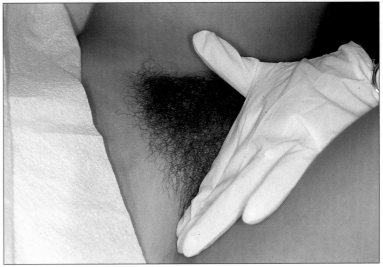

FIGURE 18-7 Examination of skin and pubic hair. Inspect the pubic hair for lice and nits and the underlying skin for rashes and lesions.

FIGURE 18-8 Palpation of lymph nodes. Palpate both inguinal areas, noting any abnormally enlarged lymph nodes or tenderness.

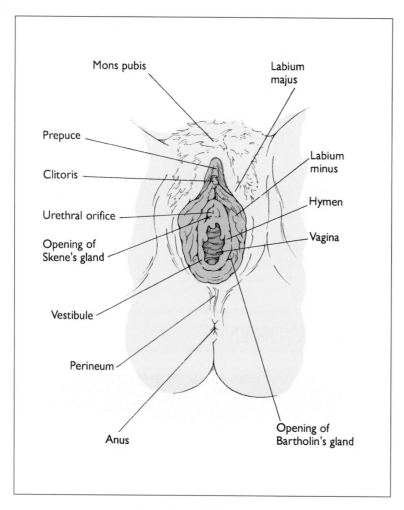

Mons pubis

Labium majus

Prepuce

Clitoris

Labium minus

Urethral orifice

Hymen

Opening of Skene's gland

Vagina

Vestibule

Perineum

Anus

Opening of Bartholin's gland

FIGURE 18-9 Anatomy of the external female genitalia. The external female genitalia, or vulva, include the mons pubis, a hair-covered fat pad overlying the symphysis pubis. The labia majora are rounded folds of adipose tissue; the labia minora, thinner pinkish-red folds that extend anteriorly to form the prepuce, which covers the clitoris. The vestibule refers to the boat-shaped fossa between the labia minora. In its posterior portion lies the vaginal opening, or introitus, which in virgins may be hidden by the hymen. The perineum refers to the tissues between the introitus and anus. (*Adapted from* Bates B: *A Guide to Physical Examination.* Philadelphia: J.B. Lippincott; 1974:188; with permission.)

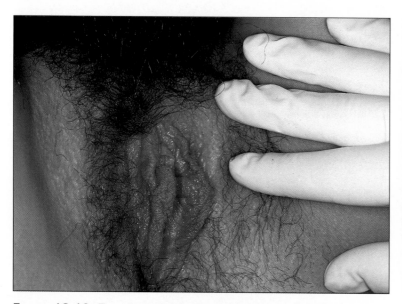

FIGURE 18-10 Examination of external vulvar structures. Examine the mons pubis, labia (*shown*), and perineum.

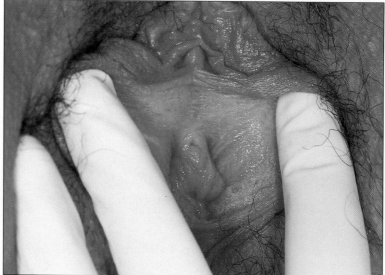

FIGURE 18-11 Examination of vestibular structures. With a gloved hand, separate the labia and inspect the labia minora, clitoris, urethral orifice, and the vaginal opening (introitus). Note any discharge, inflammation, swelling, nodules, tenderness, or masses. If lesions are present, they should be palpated and described.

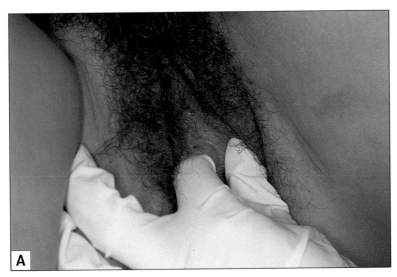

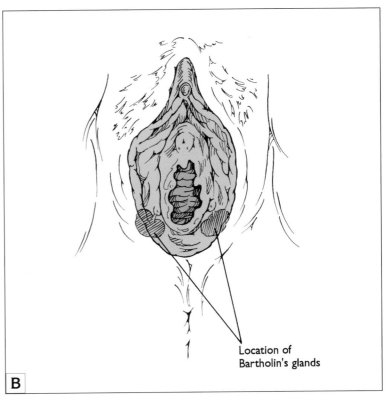

FIGURE 18-12 Palpation of Bartholin's glands. **A,** To palpate the Bartholin's glands, insert the index finger into the vagina near the posterior end of the introitus. Place the thumb outside the posterior part of the labium majorum, and palpate for swelling and/or tenderness. Note any yellow discharge from the gland orifice. **B,** Location of Bartholin's glands. (Panel 12B *adapted from* Bates B: *A Guide to Physical Examination.* Philadelphia: J.B. Lippincott; 1974:189; with permission.)

Location of Bartholin's glands

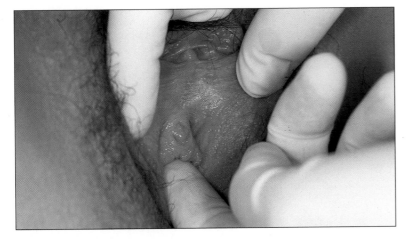

FIGURE 18-13 Examination of the urethra. Insert a gloved finger into the vagina and gently compress the urethra against the symphysis pubis. Milk the urethra from the inside outward, noting any discharge.

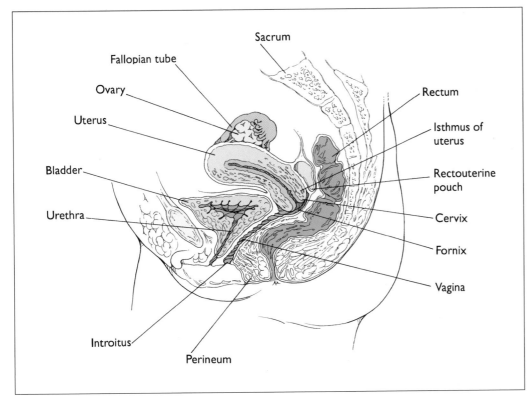

FIGURE 18-14 Anatomy of internal female genitalia. The vagina is a tube extending from between the urethra and rectum upward and back and terminating in the cup-shaped fornix. At almost a right angle to it sits the uterus. Its cervix protrudes into the vagina, dividing the fornix into anterior, posterior, and lateral fornices. A round or slitlike depression, the external os of the cervix, marks the opening into the endocervical canal and uterine cavity. (*Adapted from* Bates B: *A Guide to Physical Examination.* J.B. Lippincott; 1974:189; with permission.)

Labels in Figure 18-14: Sacrum, Fallopian tube, Ovary, Uterus, Bladder, Urethra, Introitus, Perineum, Rectum, Isthmus of uterus, Rectouterine pouch, Cervix, Fornix, Vagina

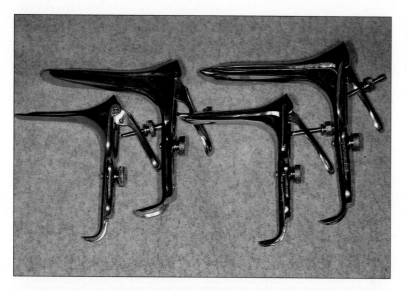

FIGURE 18-15 Vaginal specula. Select a speculum of appropriate size for the patient. Warm water may be used as a lubricant, but do not use other lubricants, as they may interfere with cytologic, cultural, or other diagnostic studies.

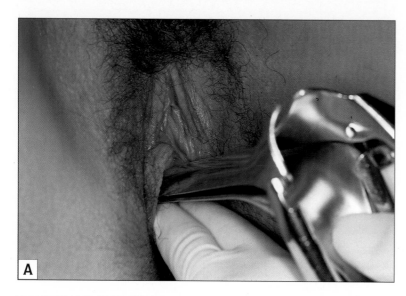

FIGURE 18-16 Insertion of the speculum. **A**, Place two fingers at the introitus and press down on the perineal body. With the other hand, introduce the closed speculum past your fingers in a downward angle. **B**, Slide the speculum along the posterior wall to prevent pressure on the urethra. Avoid pulling on pubic hairs or pinching the labia. (*continued*)

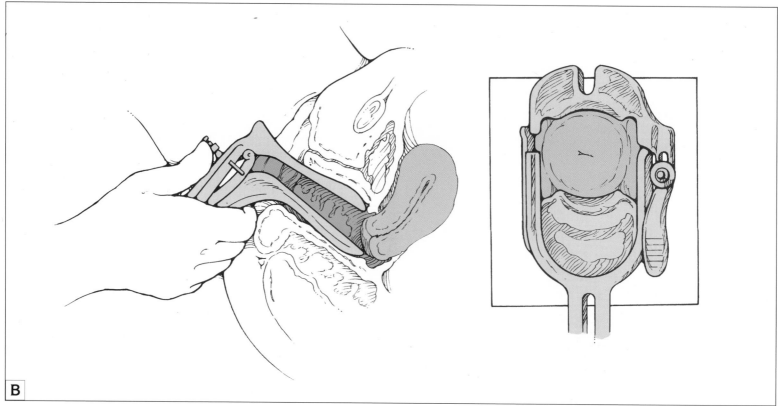

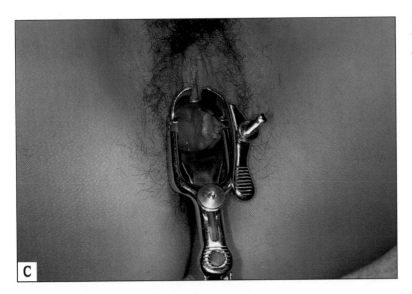

FIGURE 18-16 (*continued*) **C,** After inserting the speculum to its full length, open the valves (cusps) and maneuver them to achieve a clear view of the cervix. Secure the speculum in its open position by tightening the thumbscrew.

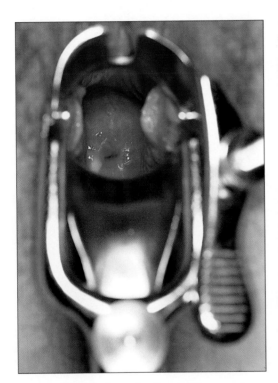

FIGURE 18-17 Examination of the cervix. Inspect the uterine cervix, noting position and color and any nodules, inflammation, ulcerations, ectopy, friability, bleeding, or discharge.

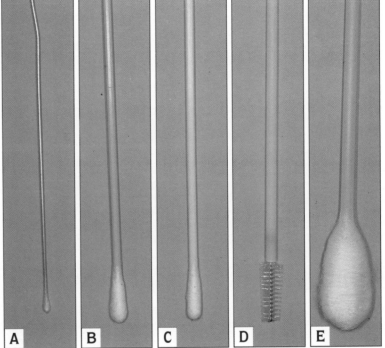

FIGURE 18-18 Swabs and brushes for specimen collection. Swabs and brushes that are commonly used in the collection of specimens to diagnose sexually transmitted infections include **A,** a urethrogenital calcium alginate swab on an aluminum shaft; **B,** a typical cotton-tipped applicator; **C,** a swab specified by its manufacturer for use in a proprietary *Chlamydia* test kit; **D,** a cytobrush; and **E,** a large cotton swab to clean the exocervix.

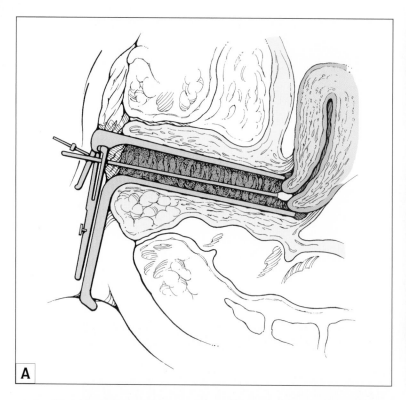

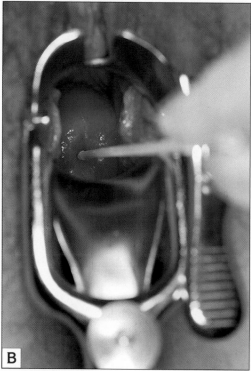

FIGURE 18-19
Specimen collection from the cervix. **A** and **B**, After any vaginal discharge is lightly removed from the exocervix, the cotton tip of a sterile applicator is inserted fully into the cervical canal, rotated for 3 to 4 seconds between the thumb and first two fingers, and removed. Specimens for *Neisseria gonorrhoeae* cultures are obtained first and usually without exocervical precleaning.

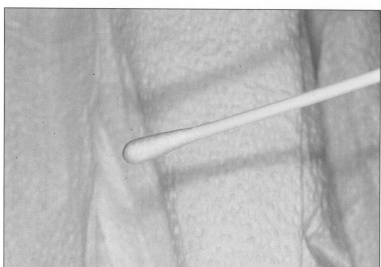

FIGURE 18-20 Visual inspection of endocervical swab. The first endocervical swab specimen should be examined in a bright light, preferably against a white background. Yellow staining indicates pus caused by a cervical infection. The presence of blood may result from cervical friability.

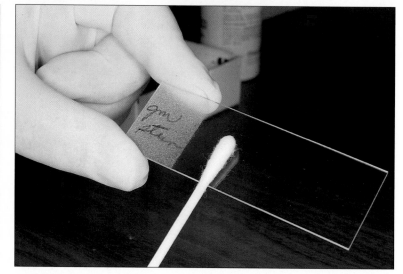

FIGURE 18-21 Cervical Gram staining. The endocervical swab specimen is gently rolled (not rubbed) several times across the middle of a glass microscope slide. The goal is to achieve a thin and evenly spread preparation for staining. Rolling of the swab preserves cellular morphology.

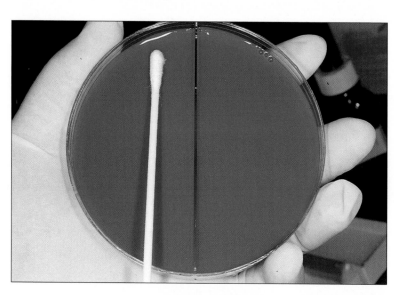

FIGURE 18-22 Cultures for *Neisseria gonorrhoeae*. For best results, a separate swab specimen is immediately transferred to freshly prepared selective medium by gently rotating the cotton tip over approximately one third of the culture plate. The inoculated medium is then sent to the laboratory for cross-streaking and incubation.

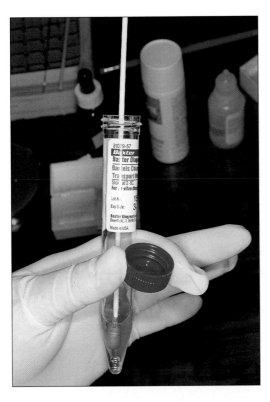

FIGURE 18-23 *Chlamydia* cultures. A separate endocervical specimen is obtained with a cotton-tipped applicator, and then the applicator tip is immersed into a tube of *Chlamydia* transport medium and vigorously swirled. Medium is then expressed from the cotton tip against the inside of the tube. The applicator is discarded, and the specimen tube is immediately refrigerated or placed in an ice bath.

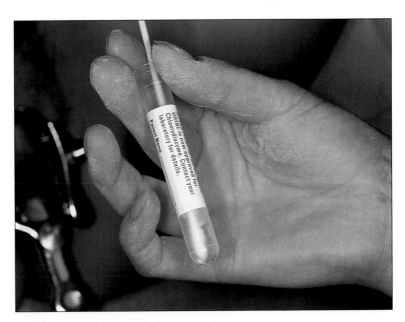

FIGURE 18-24 *Chlamydia* antigen detection. Swabs provided with proprietary test kits are used to obtain endocervical specimens in the manner previously described. Subsequent handling of the swabbed specimen should be according to the manufacturer's specifications.

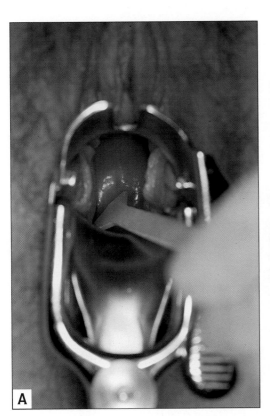

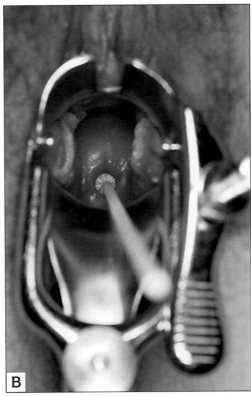

FIGURE 18-25 Papanicolaou smears. Because the epidemiology of cervical cancer is similar to that of many sexually transmitted infections, it is important to offer Papanicolaou smears in the context of clinical services for sexually transmitted diseases. After excess secretions are gently wiped from the surface of the cervix, the following steps are carried out in order and without delay. **A,** To obtain the ectocervical specimen, position an Ayre's spatula as shown and rotate it 360°. It is then set aside. **B,** To obtain endocervical specimen, insert a cytobrush into the cervical canal as shown and rotate it once, one-quarter to one-half turn. (*continued*)

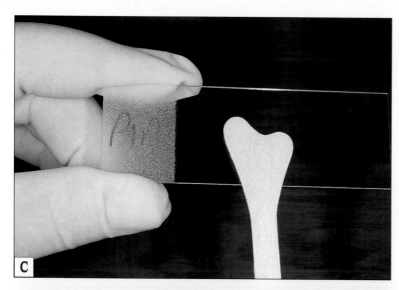

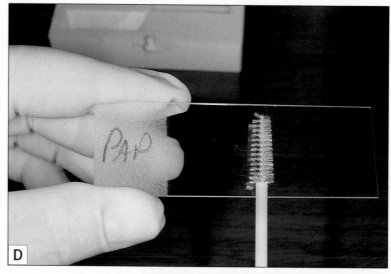

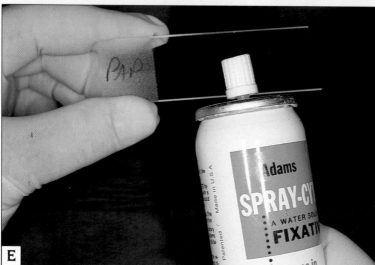

FIGURE 18-25 (*continued*) **C,** With a rotatory motion, apply the material from both sides of the spatula to a glass slide. **D,** With a rolling motion, apply the material from the cytobrush over the portion of the slide containing the ectocervical specimen. **E,** Immediately tilt the slide and spray with fixative until it is dripping wet. Do not touch the slide until it is completely dry.

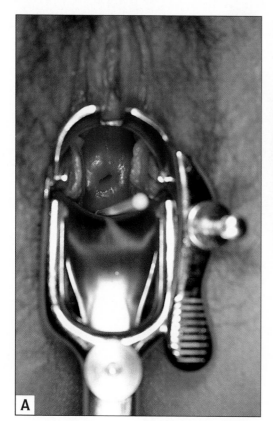

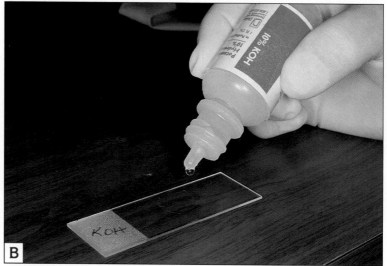

FIGURE 18-26 Wet mount specimens. **A,** Specimens for wet mount microscopy are best obtained with a cotton-tipped applicator from the posterior vaginal "puddle" behind the cervix. **B,** Physiologic saline is used to visualize trichomonads, clue cells, and fungi (usually *Candida* species), and 10% potassium hydroxide solution is used to detect volatile amines associated with bacterial vaginitis ("whiff test") and to better discern fungal elements. Both are available in convenient plastic dropper bottles. One drop of solution is placed in the middle of the glass slide. (*continued*)

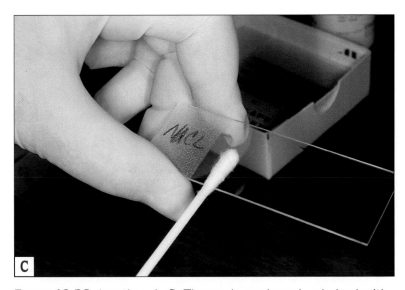

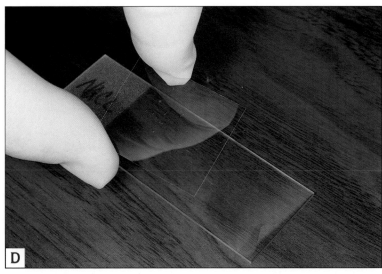

FIGURE 18-26 (*continued*) **C,** The swab specimen is admixed with the drop of solution, and the slide is smelled for the fishy odor of a positive whiff test (10% potassium hydroxide only). **D,** A cover slip is then floated on the slide, and the slide is examined promptly under a microscope.

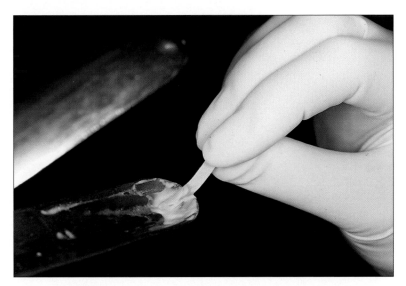

FIGURE 18-27 Vaginal pH. Except during menstruation, the vaginal pH is normally < 4.5 to 5.0. A pH ≥ 5.0 is commonly associated with trichomoniasis and/or bacterial vaginosis and is easily measured with pH test paper (range of 4–7). The test can be performed by rolling a swab specimen on the paper, touching the paper to vaginal fluid in the dependent speculum cusp (*as shown*), or pressing the paper directly against fluid in the posterior vaginal introitus. Also, at this stage of the examination, the vaginal mucosa is best examined as it appears beyond and between the partially opened cusps while the speculum is being withdrawn slowly.

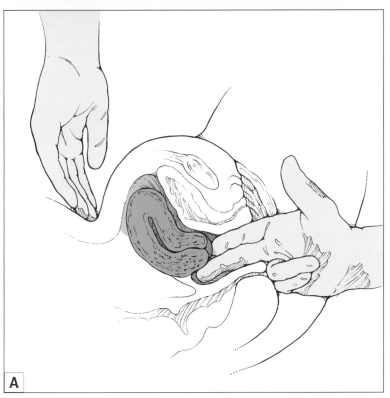

FIGURE 18-28 Bimanual examination. In the examination for sexually transmitted diseases, the primary purpose of the bimanual examination is to detect tenderness and/or masses caused by bacterial infection of the uterine body, tubes, ovaries, and surrounding peritoneum (*ie*, salpingitis or pelvic inflammatory disease). **A** and **B,** After explaining the purpose and nature of the examination to the patient, one inserts lubricated index and middle fingers of one gloved hand into the vagina, bringing them to rest under the cervix. The sign of tenderness on cervical motion, a good indicator of pelvic inflammation, can be evaluated by nudging the cervix with the fingertips. The uterine body, tubes, and ovaries are then palpated in succession by using the fingers of the hand placed on the abdomen to draw these structures firmly down against the underlying intravaginally placed fingers. Normal ovaries are approximately the size of an almond and tender to compression. (*continued*)

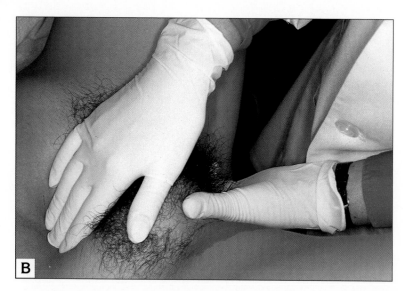

B

FIGURE 18-28 (*continued*)

A. Diagnostic features of common vaginal conditions: Symptoms

	Physiologic	Bacterial vaginosis	Trichomoniasis	Candidiasis
Vulvar irritation	0	0 to +	0 to +++	0 to +++
Dysuria	0	0	0 to +; internal or external	0 to ++; external
Odor	0	0 to +++	0 to ++	0
Discharge	0 to +	0 to ++	0 to +++	0 to +

B. Diagnostic features of common vaginal conditions: Signs

	Physiologic	Bacterial vaginosis	Trichomoniasis	Candidiasis
Labial erythema	0	0	0 to +++	0 to +++
Vaginal tenderness	0	0	0 to ++	0 to ++
Discharge				
Consistency	Floccular	Homogeneous with bubbles	Homogeneous with bubbles	Thin to curdy
Color	White	Gray-white	Yellow-green in 25%; frothy in 25%	White
Adherence	0	0 to +++	0	0 to +++
pH	≤ 4.5	> 4.5	> 4.5	≤ 4.5
Whiff test	0	+++	0 to ++	0

FIGURE 18-29 Diagnostic features of common vaginal conditions. Clinical features that may be diagnostically useful in differentiating the infectious vaginitides are summarized. The scale of 0 to +++ suggests both the frequency and severity of the finding. There is considerable variation from patient to patient. **A.** Symptoms. **B.** Signs. (*continued*)

C. Diagnostic features of common vaginal conditions: Microscopic examination

	Physiologic	Bacterial vaginosis	Trichomoniasis	Candidiasis
Epithelial cells	Normal	Clue cells (90%)	Normal	Normal
PMN/epithelial cells	≤ 1	≤ 1	> 1	Variable
Flora	Rods	+++ coccobacilli; + motile curved rods	Rods	Rods
Pathogens	—	—	Trichomonads (≈ 50%–70%)	Yeasts and pseudohyphae (≈ 50%)

PMN—polymorphonuclear neutrophil.

FIGURE 18-29 (*continued*) **C,** Microscopic examination. Most patients can differentiate external from internal dysuria, the former associated with vulvovaginitis and the latter with urethritis or cystitis. Motile curved rods are observed in small numbers in many patients with bacterial vaginosis. These rods probably belong to the genus *Mobiluncus.* One polymorphonuclear neutrophil (PMN) per epithelial cell may be considered normal in vaginal discharge. Excess PMNs may indicate an inflammatory vaginitis (including purulent or desquamative vaginitis) or may result from a coincident cervicitis that is dumping PMNs into the vaginal pool. Note that the sensitivity of microscopic examination for trichomonads or yeasts is considerably less than 100%. (Sobel JD: Desquamative inflammatory vaginitis: A new subgroup of purulent vaginitis responsive to topical 2% clindamycin therapy. *Am J Obstet Gynecol* 1994, 171:1215–1220.) (*Courtesy of* M.F. Rein, MD.)

GENITAL EXAMINATION OF MEN

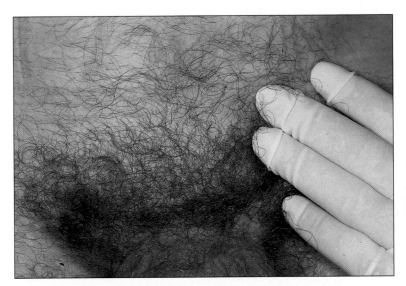

FIGURE 18-30 Inspection of skin and pubic hair. A genital examination begins with good illumination and full exposure of the area from the umbilicus to the knees. Before one attends to any obvious disease, it is important to proceed through all the routine steps of the examination. This will avoid oversight of other potentially important findings. First, briefly inspect the skin of the upper legs and abdomen. Then, inspect the pubic hair for lice and nits and the underlying skin for rashes and lesions (*as shown*). The skin of the crural areas and scrotum should also be inspected for rashes and lesions.

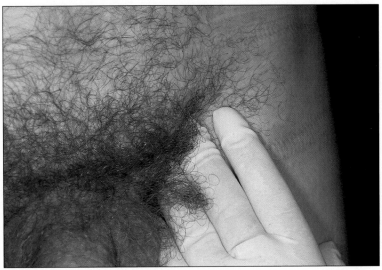

FIGURE 18-31 Palpation of lymph nodes. Palpate both inguinal areas, noting any abnormally enlarged lymph nodes or tenderness.

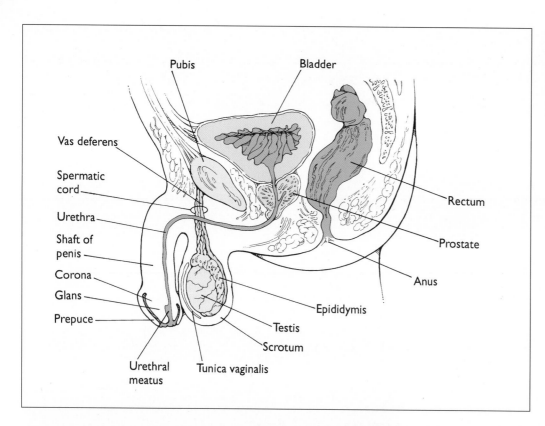

FIGURE 18-32 Anatomy of male genitalia. At the end of the penis is the cone-shaped glans with its expanded base, or corona, and the urethral meatus at its tip. The urethra is located ventrally in the shaft of the penis. (*Adapted from* Bates B: *A Guide to Physical Examination.* Philadelphia: J.B. Lippincott; 1974:79; with permission.)

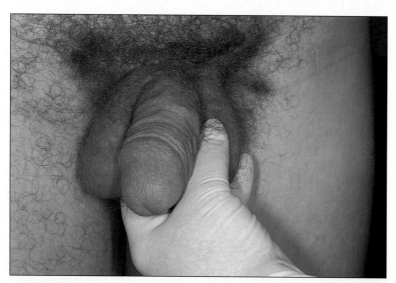

FIGURE 18-33 Scrotal examination. To detect any abnormal scrotal tenderness, masses, nodules, or testicular anatomy, gently palpate each testis and epididymis between the thumb and first two fingers.

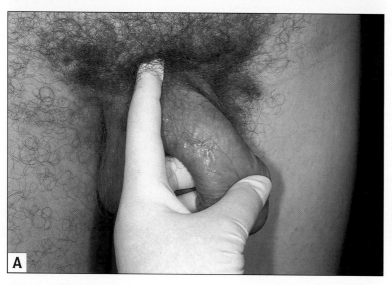

A

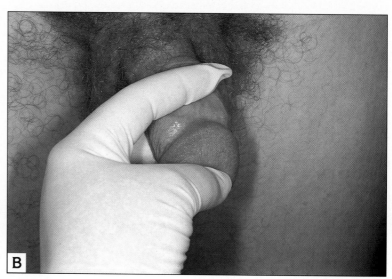

B

FIGURE 18-34 Penile examination. **A,** Inspect the shaft of the penis with one gloved hand. **B,** Retract the foreskin, and inspect the glans and coronal sulcus for rashes and lesions.

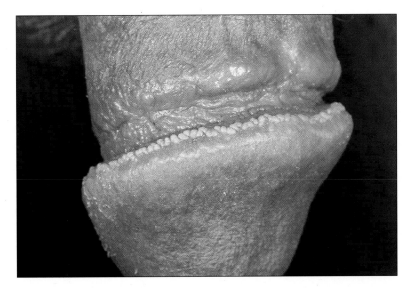

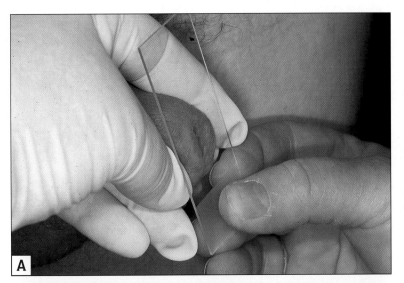

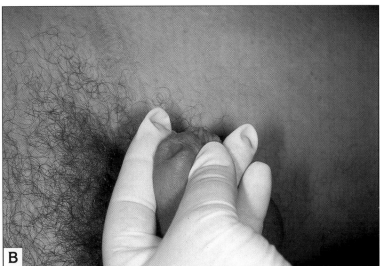

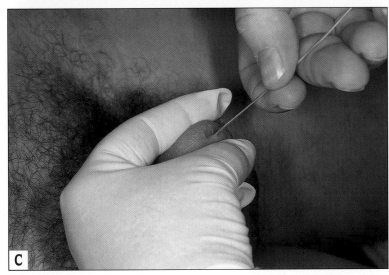

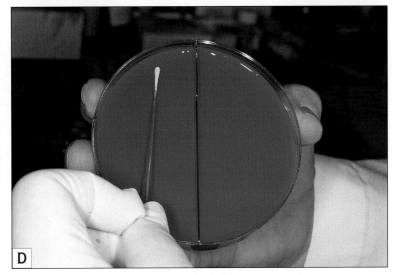

FIGURE 18-35 Pearly penile papules. These hypertrophic papillae appear in perfectly symmetrical, parallel rows on the corona and are a variant of normal anatomy. They should not be confused with genital warts caused by human papillomavirus.

FIGURE 18-36 Examination of the urethral meatus and specimen collection. The urethral meatus should be examined for discharge and lesions. **A**, If an obvious discharge is present it should be described in terms of quantity (scant, moderate, or profuse) and quality (clear or mucoid, white or cloudy, or yellow or purulent) and smeared directly on a slide by drawing the smooth surface across the meatus at an angle that delivers a thin, uniform preparation. If there is no overt discharge, the distal urethra should be stripped and the meatus reexamined. **B**, In men, urethral specimens for gonorrhea or chlamydial cultures or *Chlamydia* antigen detection tests are usually obtained with a urethrogenital calcium alginate swab on a flexible aluminum shaft. If there is no discharge, it is best to compress the meatus with gloved thumb and forefinger until it opens. **C**, Then, the swab is carefully inserted 2 to 3 cm into the urethra with a rotary motion. **D**, For gonorrhea culture, the specimen should be immediately transferred to freshly prepared selective medium by gently rotating the swab over approximately one third of the culture plate. The inoculated medium is then sent to the laboratory for cross-streaking and incubation.

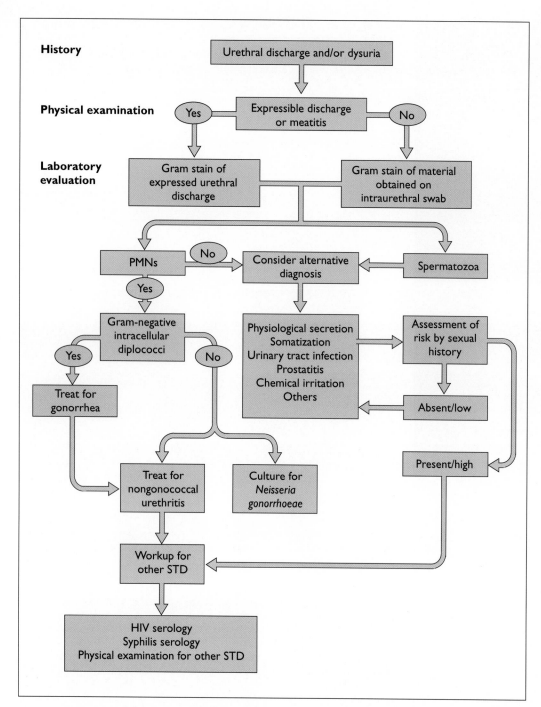

FIGURE 18-37 Approach to the patient with urethral symptoms. Some clinicians believe that the presence of expressible urethral discharge indicates infection, even in the absence of polymorphonuclear neutrophils (PMNs) on Gram stain. Vigorous self-examination can elicit a benign urethral discharge that usually contains no PMNs. Spermatozoa are gram-positive ovoids that pale toward the acrosomal cap. Their presence suggests that the perceived discharge is in part ejaculum. Even small numbers of PMNs on Gram stain suggest urethritis. In symptomatic men, the sensitivity of the Gram stain for *Neisseria gonorrhoeae* approximates 95%. Nongonococcal urethritis cannot be diagnosed by Gram stain in the presence of gonorrhea, and because some 20% of heterosexual men with gonorrhea also carry *Chlamydia trachomatis*, treatment for gonorrhea should include a regimen capable of eradicating chlamydial infection as well. (STD—sexually transmitted disease.) (*Courtesy of* M.F. Rein, MD.)

ANORECTAL EXAMINATION

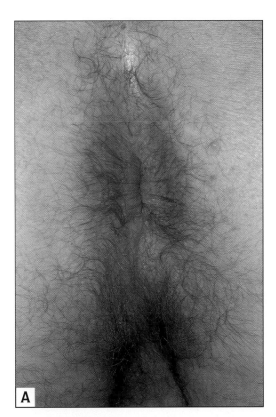

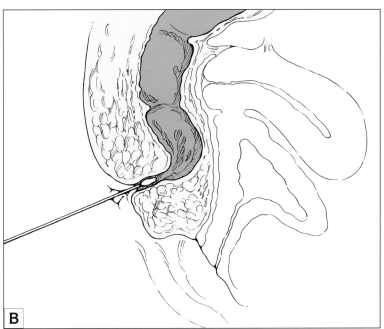

FIGURE 18-38 In homosexual men who report recent receptive anal intercourse or who have symptoms referable to the anorectum, anoscopy may be included as part of a clinical examination for sexually transmitted diseases. The patient is asked to bend over the end of an examination table and rest his upper body on his arms. **A,** The perianal area and perineum are inspected for rashes and lesions. **B,** If indicated, blind anal canal and/or rectal culture specimens are collected before application of the lubricant. A sterile cotton-tipped swab is inserted approximately 1 inch into the anal canal. If the swab is inadvertently pushed into feces, another swab should be used to obtain the specimen.

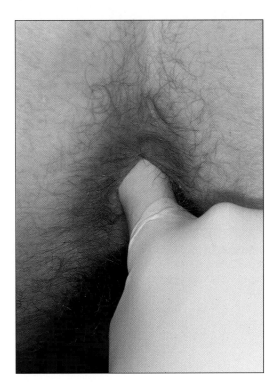

FIGURE 18-39 Digital rectal examination. A standard digital rectal examination is performed with a well-lubricated, gloved index finger.

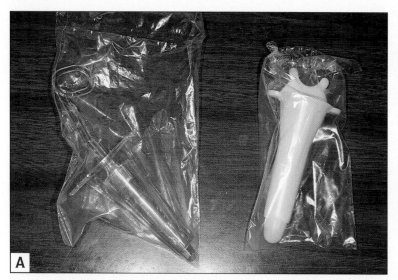

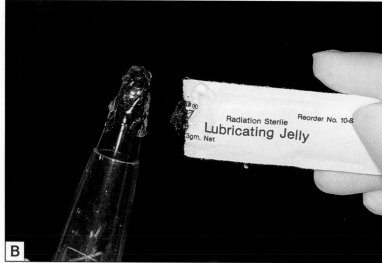

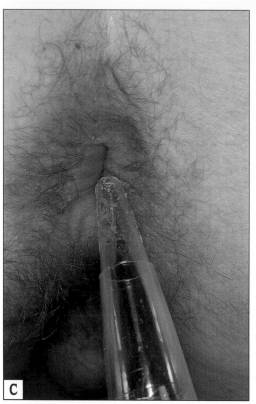

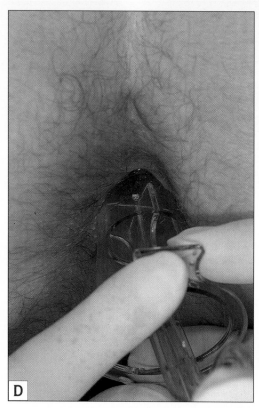

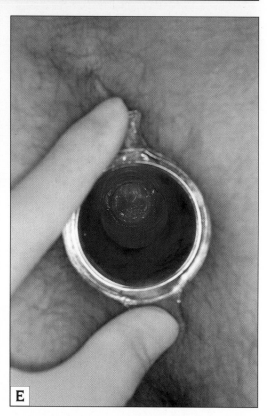

FIGURE 18-40 Anoscope examination. **A**, Two sterile, packaged anoscope models are pictured. **B**, The obturator is lubricated. **C** and **D**, The anoscope is inserted and secured in viewing position. **E**, The anal canal and distal rectal mucosa are inspected. Pus, mucopus, lesions, or mucosal friability should be noted. Additional cultures and/or biopsy specimens can be taken through the anoscope.

SELECTED BIBLIOGRAPHY

Judson FN: Clinical facilities for sexually transmitted disease control. *In* Holmes KK, Mårdh P-A, Sparling PF, *et al.* (eds.): *Sexually Transmitted Diseases*, 2nd ed. New York: McGraw Hill; 1990.

Judson FN (ed.): Sexually Transmitted Diseases. *Clin Lab Med* 1989, 9(3):369–593.

Wentworth BB, Judson FN, Gilchrist MJR (eds.): *Laboratory Methods for Diagnosis of Sexually Transmitted Diseases*, 2nd ed. Washington, DC: American Public Health Association; 1991.

INDEX